COVID-19 in South, West, and Southeast Asia

Aslam and Gunaratna bring together a broad analysis of the responses of states in Asia to the threats presented by the COVID-19 pandemic in its early phase.

While the impact of the pandemic has undoubtedly been disastrous, it has also taught many lessons about social, political, economic, and security norms in modern civilization. The contributors to this book look at how these lessons have been learned—often the hard way—by a range of states including India, Pakistan, Sri Lanka, Singapore, Indonesia, Thailand, Brunei Darussalam, and Jordan, as well as by international organizations including ASEAN. They look at a range of issues, going beyond the most apparent healthcare concerns to also look at challenges such as the gig economy, terrorism, extremism, religious identity, and cybersecurity. Using these country-based case studies, this book establishes a framework for understanding these challenges and establishing best practice and scalable solutions for addressing them.

A valuable resource for scholars and practitioners trying to understand how the world will and won't be changed by the impact of COVID-19, especially in the realms of security, society, and economy.

Mohd Mizan Aslam is a former professor in Security Studies at the Naif Arab University for Security Sciences in Riyadh, Saudi Arabia and a senior fellow at the Global Peace Institute London.

Rohan Gunaratna is the professor of Security Studies at the S. Rajaratnam School of International Studies, Nanyang Technological University, Singapore.

COVID-19 in Asia

COVID-19 in South, West, and Southeast Asia

Risk and Response in the Early Phase

Edited by Mohd Mizan Aslam and Rohan Gunaratna

Routledge
Taylor & Francis Group

LONDON AND NEW YORK

First published 2023
by Routledge
4 Park Square, Milton Park, Abingdon, Oxon OX14 4RN

and by Routledge
605 Third Avenue, New York, NY 10158

Routledge is an imprint of the Taylor & Francis Group, an informa business

© 2023 selection and editorial matter, Mohd Mizan Aslam and Rohan Gunaratna; individual chapters, the contributors

British Library Cataloguing in Publication Data
A catalogue record for this book is available from the British Library

Library of Congress Cataloging in Publication Data
A catalog record for this book has been requested

ISBN: 978-1-032-27223-8 (hbk)
ISBN: 978-1-032-27224-5 (pbk)
ISBN: 978-1-003-29190-9 (ebk)

DOI: 10.4324/9781003291909

Typeset in Galliard
by Deanta Global Publishing Services, Chennai, India

Contents

Figures

Tables

Contributors

Mamdouh Abdelhameed Abdelmottlep (SJD) is a professor of Police Administration and Law Enforcement at Naïf Arab University for Security Science (NAUSS) and an executive chairman at the International Police Science Association (IPSA), Prof. Mamdouh is interested in the research and studies related to the fields of police science, law enforcement, and criminal justice administration. He has numbers of studies, research and published literatures in policing. He has extensive experience in police training, security education, and international academic cooperation. In addition to Founding the International Police Science Association (IPSA), he innovated the World Internal Security and Police Index (WISPI) which measures the capacity and efficiency of police and security service providers to address the internal security issues worldwide. His efforts contributed to the development of the police in several countries. He has won and received many international awards, most notably the 2014 CRIMINOLOGIA.IT, awarded by the United Nations, and the 2016 Distinction Medal, awarded by the United Arab Emirates for developing Arab Police Science and Security Education.

Ainuddin Iskandar Lee Abdullah was born in 1974 in Johor Bharu, the capital of the southern-most state of Malaysia. He enrolled at SRJK (C) Chung Hwa, Ipoh and continued his secondary school at Sekolah Tuanku Muhammad, Kuala Pilah Negeri Sembilan. Ainuddin received BA and MA in History and Sociology from the National University of Malaysia (UKM) in 1998 and 2000. He was conferred a Philosophy Doctorate (PhD) from the Northern University of Malaysia (UUM) in 2000. Ainuddin started his career as a tutor at UUM and is currently a senior lecturer at the School of International Studies (SOIS). Ainuddin's forte are on the constitution, politics, administration, economics, and comparative politics of Malaysia. He has actively been involved in research and leadership roles since his campus life, when he was an Exco Member of the student association—Persatu, UUM. He was also appointed as a research fellow at the Institute of Tun Dr. Mahathir's Thoughts (IPDM) and the Northern Corridor Research Centre (NCRC) UUM. He was also appointed to the evaluation panel for the Ministry of Higher Education research grant committee. He then went on an attachment to the Malaysian

Journal of Society and Space (GMJSS), UKM as an editorial board member. In 2000, he was appointed to a Malaysian Qualification Agency (MQA) expert panel to evaluate academic programs at all higher education institutions in Malaysia.

Mohammed Hussain Ahmad is currently the deputy rector of Sultan Sharif Ali Islamic University (UNISSA), Brunei Darussalam. Prior to this appointment, he taught at both UNISSA and the University of Brunei Darussalam (UBD). His research interests include the study of Hadith and its sciences, the network of Malay and Arab scholars, the traditional Malay religio-intellectual culture, Arabic manuscripts, Malay-Jawi manuscripts, and Malay scholars. He has published several articles, book chapters, and a book entitled *Islam in the Malay World: Al-Falimbani's Scholarship.*

Saud Al-Sharafat is a Brigadier-General (Ret), Jordanian General Intelligence Directorate (GID). He is a member in the National Policy Council (NPC), Jordan, 2012-2015, adviser on National Security and Strategic Studies at European Centre for Counterterrorism and Intelligence Studies, and expert at Wikistrat Crowdsourced Consulting, USA. He is the author of two books: Globalization and Terrorism: Flat World or Deep Valleys? 2011. Global Terrorism and Extremism: Phenomena struggle and Paradigm Conflict in the Era of Globalization, 2016. Al-Sharafat is a member of Jordanian Writers Association. His areas of expertise focus on globalization, terrorism, intelligence gathering and analysis (OSINT), counter-terrorism intelligence, online radicalization, political islam, middle east politics, and Jordanian affairs. Al-Sharafat writes analytical studies and articles commenting on the worldwide impact of the global terrorism and globalization for: Mominoun without Borders institute for studies and research- Morocco, The Washington Institute for Near East Policy, The Geopolitics (TGP), European Centre for Counterterrorism and Intelligence Studies, and Hafryat magazine- Egypt. Al-Sharafat received the Medal of Long-Term Sincere Service Badge in General Intelligence Directorate, June 8, 2004, and The Order of Independence 3rd Degree, awarded in presence of the late King Hussein, June 10, 1998.

Muhammad Amir Rana is the director of Pakistan Institute for Peace Studies (PIPS). He was a founder member of PIPS when it was launched in January 2006 and had previously worked as a journalist with various Urdu and English daily newspapers from 1996 until 2004. He has also given lectures at several universities and security institutes in Pakistan and abroad. He has worked extensively on issues related to counter-terrorism, counter-extremism, and internal and regional security and politics. He has published widely in national and international journals, professional publications, and magazines. He writes regularly for *Dawn*, Pakistan's leading English newspaper. He is also the editor of Pakistan Annual Security Report, PIPS' English research journal "Conflict and Peace Studies," and Urdu monthly magazine "Tajziat."

Mohd Mizan Aslam is a senior academician at the Universiti Malaysia Perlis (UniMAP), and the founder and first director of the Malaysian Research Institute of Strategic Studies (MyRISS). Mizan was conferred Honorary Major by the Malaysian Armed Forces in 2016 due to his contribution in security and CVE initiatives. He is also a national expert panel in rehabilitation programs to terrorist inmates nationwide. He is a writer for numerous books, conference papers, journals, proceedings, newspapers, magazines, keynote speakers, and TV and news columnist. Mizan is actively involved in fellowships abroad as Executive Council of Benevolent Fund for Outstanding Students (BFOS), Hadramowt, Government of Yemen and Executive Advisor QATAR Guest Centre, Doha Qatar. Mizan held position as an adjunct professor at the School of Arts and Humanities, Universitas Ubudiyah Indonesia (UUI), Acheh, Indonesia. Mizan was also appointed as visiting professor at the Centre for Civilization and Peace Study, Ibnu Haldun University, Besheksehir, Istanbul, Turkey in 2017. Mizan was involved in developing a National Action Plan on CVE with the Home Ministry of Malaysia and was also appointed as senior fellow at the Islamic and Strategic Studies Institute (ISSI-CONCAVE).

Ruetaitip Chansrakaeo is a lecturer in Public Administration Programme at Valaya Alongkorn Rajabhat University under the Royal Patronage, Thailand. She obtained a bachelor of Laws from Thammasat University and a master of Arts in Political Science from the Institute of International Studies, Ramkhamhaeng University, Thailand. Now she has completed her doctorate degree in Criminology, Justice and Social Administration at Mahidol University, Thailand. She started her teaching career at Bangkokthonburi University where she was the head of the public administration program and taught related courses with public policy, development and administration and civil society and people's politics. Her ongoing current research is titled "European Union's Policy on Foreign Terrorist Fighters: Lesson Learned for ASEAN," funded by Chulalongkorn University.

Vajira H. W. Dissanayake is the dean of the Faculty of Medicine, University of Colombo. He is also the chair and senior professor of Anatomy; the director of the Human Genetics Unit; and the chair of the Specialty Board in Biomedical Informatics at the University. He was the president of the Sri Lanka Medical Association in 2012 and the president of the Commonwealth Medical Association from 2016 to 2019. He was elected a fellow of the National Academy of Sciences of Sri Lanka in 2013 in recognition of his outstanding contribution to the field of medicine. He was awarded the national titular honor of Vidya Jyothi by his excellency the President for outstanding scientific and technological achievement in 2019.

Rohan Gunaratna is a professor of Security Studies at the S. Rajaratnam School of International Studies, Nanyang Technology University, and the founder of the International Centre for Political Violence and Terrorism Research, Singapore. He received his masters from the University of Notre Dame in the

US where he was a Hesburgh Scholar and his doctorate from the University of St Andrews in the UK where he was a British Chevening Scholar. A former senior fellow at the Combating Terrorism Centre at the United States Military Academy at West Point and the Fletcher School of Law and Diplomacy, Gunaratna was a visiting fellow at the Washington Institute for Near East Policy. The author of "Inside al Qaeda: Global Network of Terror" (University of Columbia Press), Gunaratna edited the Insurgency and Terrorism Series of the Imperial College Press, London. A trainer for national security agencies, law enforcement authorities, and military counter-terrorism units, he interviewed terrorists and insurgents in Afghanistan, Pakistan, Iraq, Yemen, Libya, Saudi Arabia, and other conflict zones. For advancing international security cooperation, Gunaratna received the Major General Ralph H. Van Deman Award.

Khuram Iqbal is an associate professor and the head of the International Relations Department at the National Defense University, Pakistan. He obtained his doctorate in Policing, Intelligence, and Counter-terrorism from Macquarie University, Australia and masters in Strategic Studies from Nanyang Technological University (NTU), Singapore. Prior to joining NDU, Dr. Iqbal was attached with the Centre for Transnational Crimes Prevention, Australia and the International Centre for Political Violence and Terrorism Research, Singapore, where his research focused on South Asian security. Dr. Iqbal has also held fellowships at prestigious Chinese institutes including the China Institute of International Studies (CIIS) and the National Defense University of People's Liberation Army of China, where he worked on the global implications of the Belt and Road Initiative. Huram's research interests include Political Violence and State Response, Radicalization and Violent Extremism, Guerilla Warfare and Insurgency, Suicide Terrorism, Chinese Security and Foreign Policy, Rise of Asia, and China Pakistan Economic Corridor

Kapila Jayaratne is a consultant community physician currently working as the National Programme Manager for Maternal and Child Morbidity and Mortality Surveillance at the Family Health Bureau—Ministry of Health, Sri Lanka. Dr. Jayaratne graduated from Faculty of Medicine, University of Colombo and obtained masters and doctorate in Community Medicine from the Postgraduate Institute of Medicine of University of Colombo. He had his post-doctoral training at the University of Melbourne, Australia. He is the national focal point for surveillance of maternal deaths, maternal suicides, maternal near misses, infant deaths, birth defects, and injury-related child deaths. Dr. Jayaratne has carried out numerous studies in maternal and child health. He has contributed to reshaping maternal and child health service delivery by translating lessons learnt out of maternal and feto-infant deaths into practice in the country. During the COVID-19 pandemic, Dr. Jayaratne coordinated at central level maintaining maternal and child health services, care for the suspected COVID-19 pregnant mothers, and review of maternal and perinatal mortality during the lockdown period. He was the lead in formulating an exit strategy from the College of Community Physicians of Sri Lanka (CCPSL) for the country and the capital city. Dr. Jayaratne is the CCPSL media coordinator on COVID-19 pandemic and published an article showcasing the success story of Sri Lanka. He is a member of the Presidential Task Force to Prevent Transmission of Covid19 Virus within Military Establishments of Sri Lanka. He was a past president of Perinatal Society of Sri Lanka and served as the Honorary Secretary of the Sri Lanka Medical Association.

Palitha Karunapema is the director of Health Promotion and publicity at the Health Promotion Bureau of the Ministry of Health, Sri Lanka—the national risk communication focal point for the current COVID-19 response. Dr Karunapema obtained his MBBS from the Faculty of Medicine, University of Colombo, and obtained masters and doctorate in Community Medicine from the Postgraduate Institute of Medicine of the same university. He is a constant community physician with over 20 years of experience in the field of public health. He worked as a program manager at the Non-Communicable Disease directorate, director of the National Rehabilitation Hospital, and director of Quarantine. Palitha was the national focal point for International Health Regulation (IHR) from 2015 to 2019. He contributed immensely to improving health security preparedness in Sri Lanka being a lead advocate. He was the point of contact for coordinating the Joint External Evaluation mission and was instrumental in developing National Action Planning for Health Security for Sri Lanka. Dr. Karunapema was also responsible for developing public health contingency plans for point of entries and standard operating procedures for ports and airports' public health activities in Sri Lanka. He has represented Sri Lanka in many international forums on health security. Palitha is also a long-standing member of the National Advisory Committee on Communicable Diseases, National Biosafety and Biosecurity committee, National Influenza Committee, and National IHR Steering Committee in Sri Lanka. He is currently a representative of the Presidential Taskforce for COVID-19 prevention in Sri Lanka and also serves as an advisor to WHO IHR COVID-19 emergency committee.

Rachel Kumendong serves as the admission and administration staff for International Teachers College (ITC), Universitas Pelita Harapan. She earned a bachelor's degree in International Relations, majoring in ASEAN studies, from Universitas Pelita Harapan, Karawaci, Indonesia with a scholarship program. She has been exposed to the international community by joining several Model United Nations (MUN) Conferences, National Assembly of International Relations Students, and having experience of conducting on-job-training abroad at the Indonesian Embassy in Manila, Philippines. Her area of interest is related to international politics and security, the study of terrorism and counter-terrorism, and international development. Recently, she just published her first article entitled "The Reasoning Behind The Philippines' Strategy to Combat Global Terrorism Under the Administration of President Rodrigo Duterte (2016–2018)."

Adil Rasheed is a research fellow at the Manohar Parrikar Institute of Defence Studies and Analyses (MP-IDSA) in New Delhi since August 2016. He has been a researcher and political commentator in various international think tanks and media organizations for over 17 years. He was a senior research fellow at the United Services Institution of India (USI) for two years from 2014 to 2016, where he still holds the honorary title of Distinguished Fellow. He was a researcher at the UAE's premier think tank The Emirates Center for Strategic Studies and Research (ECSSR) for eight years (2006–2014), where, in addition to research and publishing several papers and articles, he interviewed many distinguished international leaders such as former US Secretary of State Leon Panetta, former Prime Minister of Malaysia Tun Mahathir Mohamed, Nobel laureate Muhammad Yunus, the first Executive Chairman of UNMOVIC in Iraq Hans Blix, former NATO Chief Jaap de Hoop Scheffer, etc. He has initiated the Counter-Radicalization Task Force at the MP-IDSA. He is also currently writing a book on "Counter-Narratives and Strategic Communication against Jihadist Radicalization."

Joshua Snider is a faculty member at UAE National Defense College in Abu Dhabi. His research focuses on sectarian political violence and terrorism, with a particular focus on Southeast and South Asia. He is particularly interested in violent religiosity in Middle East and South-Southeast Asia and how states make and execute P/CVE policy. Prior to arriving in UAE, Joshua spent 8 years in Malaysia where he was a faculty member in the School of Politics, History and International Relations at the University of Nottingham's Malaysia Campus in Kuala Lumpur. In addition, Joshua has consulted for national governments and international organizations on matters related to CVE program development. Before embarking on an academic career, Joshua worked for the Canadian government and in the public affairs consulting industry. He earned his PhD in politics in 2015 from the University of Newcastle, Australia.

Tulus Suryanto is a professor in accounting; the head of Master Sharia Economy Program, Postgraduate Raden Intan State Islamic University (UIN), Lampung, Indonesia; and an adjunct professor at the School of Management (SOM) in the Asia e University. Tulus is the chairman of the Indonesian Lecturer Forum and President of the Islamic Development Studies Network (IDSN). He is the founder and chief editor in International Business and Accounting Research Journal, Ikonomika: Journal of Islamic Economics and Business, and Finance, Accounting and Business Analysis Journal (FABA). He is the reviewer of the international journal Scopus index. He has written a lot of research and published in reputable journals, including Beyond Muamalah Principles in Digital Payment Education and its Impacts on Corruption Prevention in Indonesian Public Sectors. Journal of Social Studies Education Research Vol. 11 No. 3 (2020), 46-64 and The Influence of Liberalization on Innovation, Performance, and Competition Level of Insurance Industry in Indonesia. Sustainability, Vol. 12 No. 24 (2020), 10620.

Edwin Tambunan is an associate professor at the Department of International Relations, Universitas Pelita Harapan. He obtained a bachelor's degree in International Relations from Padjadjaran University. Then he continued his postgraduate studies in the Political Science Program, Concentration in International Politics, at Gadjah Mada University. Edwin completed his doctoral program in International Relations from the School of History and International Relations, Flinders University, Adelaide. His primary interests are security, conflict, and peace. Recently, he initiated Youth and Peace Program to educate students sensitive to conflict and acquire peace skills. He is also active in the Academic Forum for Peaceful Papua (Forum Akademisi Papua Damai-FAPD).

Kenneth Yeo Yaoren is a research analyst at the International Centre for Political Violence and Terrorism Research (ICPVTR), a specialist center of the S. Rajaratnam School of International Studies (RSIS) based in Singapore. His primary research focuses on terrorism in Southeast Asia and specializes in Islamist terrorism in the Philippines. Kenneth has written for *The Diplomat*, RSIS Commentary, Channel News Asia, the Defense Post, East Asia Forum, and the Counter-Terrorism Trends and Analyses (CTTA). Topics Kenneth has written about suicide terrorism in the Philippines, foreign fighters in Mindanao, kidnap for ransom tactics, developments in terrorist fundraising, developments in extremist charities, and general developments of Islamist terrorism in the Philippines. Privately, Kenneth volunteers as a case manager for the Meet-the-People Session in Singapore. Through this, he has a deep appreciation for the government's policy and helps youths and residents to understand the complex policy decisions made by the government in Singapore.

Ahmad F. Yousif is currently a lecturer at the Faculty of Usuluddin, Sultan Sharif Ali Islamic University, Brunei Darussalam. Dr. Yousif previously taught at the International Institute of Islamic Thought and Civilization (ISTAC), the University of Winnipeg in Canada, and the University of Brunei Darussalam. He has written a number of books and published over a dozen articles in the fields of Islamic Studies and Social Sciences.

Acknowledgments

This work would not have been possible without the strong support of the Universiti Malaysia Perlis (UniMAP) and the International Centre for Political Violence and Terrorism Research (ICPVTR), Nanyang Technological University (NTU), Singapore who helped make this book a reality.

I and Professor Rohan would like to thank our colleagues and friends, especially to Malaysian Research for Strategic Studies (MyRISS) and S. Rajaratnam School of International Studies (RSIS), NTU for the stimulating discussions, working together for deadlines, and for all the productive time we have had in last few months along this journey.

I and Prof. Rohan would like to thank Mr. Clifford Gere and Ms. Siavalee Wijayawardhana in Singapore and USA who helped us in copy-editing this book. A special thanks are due to both, who gave their time to read and edit our manuscript. I would like to thank Prof James Veitch in New Zealand, and The Honourable Yemeni Ambassador in Kuala Lumpur, Dr. Adel Bahamid for the support and critical comments toward this book. I also would like to express my gratitude thanking the Vice Chancellor of UniMAP, Prof. Dr. Zaliman Sauli, the Dean Prof. Dr. Salleh Rashid, and HoD Dr. Sharmini Abdullah for their support for research. My special thanks to Lieutenant General Datuk Hasagawa Abdullah and Prof. Datuk Dr. Ahmad Mujahid Ahmad Zaidi from National Defence University Malaysia (UPNM) for their visionary leadership in the formative years of these initiatives.

We are grateful to Prime Minister of Malaysia, Dato' Sri Ismail Sabri bin Yaakob, for contributing the foreword to our book. We also thank Mr. Prime Minister for his personal interest and care, as well as an advanced endorsement of our book. Your honesty, recommendation and advice helped us refine our ideas throughout the productive process.

We are eternally grateful to Mr. Simon Bates, Mr. Subhayan Chakrabarti, and the team at Routledge, Taylor and Francis Group for taking a chance on us and welcoming us again into the Routledge Area Studies, Politics and International Relations. We acknowledge and thank Routledge's publishing team for making this book a reality.

Last but not the least; we would like to thank our family for supporting us spiritually, endless love, prayers, and encouragement through this exciting journey.

Mizan & Rohan.

Introduction

Mohd Mizan Aslam & Rohan Gunaratna

This book comprises a collection of COVID-19 responses in Asia in the early phase. It provides a rich selection of perceptions and field studies on the world's most critical issue of the time as scholars, analysts, and practitioners from all over Asia express their opinions through various distinctive perspectives in the formative phase. A critical analysis of explicit threats and responses posed by COVID-19 to Asian society is presented in this book. It presents a thorough and significant analysis of nationwide studies concerning the responses and challenges with regard to COVID-19, indicating more stable and distinct methods in managing the pandemic from the very early stage. Contributors consist of prominent scholars in various areas such as security, economics, public health, ICT, bioterrorism, politics, and religion. These cross-country specialists consist of distinguished Asian analysts, in addition to highly deemed ex-military officers, journalists, economists, academics, medical practitioners, and overall outstanding commentators.

The COVID-19 pandemic is broadly discussed in this book as more than just a disaster, whilst recognizing that it has taught and carries on to teach many lessons about social, political, economic, and security norms in modern civilization. It explores the countries' responses to the pandemic. The majority of scholars are of the opinion that the post-pandemic era will not be a continuation of the pre-pandemic trajectory. The situation is referred to as "extraordinary" since the "new normal" in the post-pandemic era may never be achieved, for better or worse, under typical conditions. The advantageous and cost-effective tenants of a system adapted to fight the novel Coronavirus pandemic will be sustained, as well as work-from-home incentives, online economization and communication, and even some leisure activities and gig economic activities.

This book deliberately meets the principal agenda of putting together a collection of initiatives engaged by countries in Asia to create and implement a functional environment across regions post COVID-19 at the very early stage. It also describes the basic steps involved in forming an efficacious response, which will be illustrated by case studies from different countries. The aim of this book is to provide a practical framework backed by case studies. Therefore, it includes an illustration of country-based case studies on COVID-19 responses and real-life experiences for employing such a right approach in numerous settings. This

DOI: 10.4324/9781003291909-1

book aims to assist in reinforcing the established framework and to give a clear understanding of the challenges faced in translating theory into practice by the authorities. Inherently, it intends to imply that the best notions should be taken into perspective when constructing a COVID-19 early response.

Complexity is the most vital issue in outlining the best solution to COVID-19. Nonetheless, this is the perfect time for us to establish specific platforms to re-examine needs and wants. Therefore, this task has emerged as a major policy concern and has challenged states in their COVID-19 formative responses. The contents of this book portray that progressive initiatives have utilized a milieu of soft and hard response strategies that involve understanding, containing, fighting, and preventing COVID-19. The idea of a framework for fighting COVID-19 is not the least bit straightforward. It is complicated and entails a thorough study of a variety of factors that will be optimistically responded to by the overall system. The outcome of the book looks at the understanding of the impact and threat COVID-19 poses to the Asian communities and intends to assist governments and policymakers to review the entire pandemic-related policy, in order to prevent their countries from declining into chaos as a result of the COVID-19 pandemic.

Mizan Aslam, in Chapter 1, examines terrorism-related activities in Malaysia and its neighboring countries amidst the COVID-19 pandemic. Malaysia's strong links to terrorist groups and cells in the region are well documented and undeniable. Jemaah Islamiyyah (JI) and ISIS made a significant impact on terrorism-related activities in Malaysia and its wider networking. In the year 2020, during the COVID-19 pandemic and following the arrest of Ustad Arif, Indonesian security sources indicated that he had sleeper cell links to Malaysia, but have not been profiled. Inspector-General of Royal Malaysia Police (RMP) Datuk Seri Abdul Hamid Bador also confirmed the existence of sleeper cells in 2019. The sleeper cell is trained and sent out by an organization to infiltrate the targeted society or organization and then remains dormant, sometimes for a long time until being activated, possibly by a pre-arranged signal or a particular series of events. The release of Abu Bakar Baa'syir from Jakarta Prison has made a significant alert to regional security communities. Potential terrorists are being effectively monitored in Malaysia, with the widespread use of VPN and other secure messaging apps such as Telegram, Signal, BiP as well as platforms on the dark web. Even though physical contact could not take place, the radical ideology can be continuously scattered using online platforms. The indoctrination of radical ideologies across Southeast Asia is well connected with the availability of access to the internet, which mainly happened because of incentives given in stimulus packages by pandemic-affected countries that, at the same time, created more space for online radicalization.

A medical doctor from Sri Lanka discusses the COVID-19 response by the medical department of Sri Lanka in Chapter 2. Dr. Kapila Jayaratne, Dr. Vajira Dissanayake, and Dr. Palitha Karunapema talk on the progression of COVID-19 in the country. Their writing is aimed at documenting some of the essential elements of Sri Lanka's response to the COVID-19 pandemic. It is safe to say that Sri

Lanka has come out strongly through its response to the COVID-19 pandemic during the past few months baring for the economic fallout. Sri Lanka's success so far lies in the reliance on the suppression of the pandemic curve by implementing multi-faceted, multi-stakeholder, and society-oriented strategies with leadership from health and law enforcement authorities, backed by the highest level of political commitment. Sri Lanka has also shown that basic public health measures and technology are both vital when facing a situation such as this. The country has reaped the benefits of its long-standing investment and reliance on a strong system of public health, coupled with the appropriate use of modern technology in its response to the COVID-19 pandemic. Strong high-level political will, top-down approach, and judicious interventions contributed to controlling the virus on the island. The authors also talked about the challenges faced by the Sri Lankan government. The main challenges encountered were: initial difficulties in logistics supply for real-time PCR testing; communities with irresponsible behavior not complying with guidelines; conflicting messages on wearing face masks; food supply chain management in the early days of the lockdown due to sudden imposition of the curfews; financial difficulties faced by the daily-waged labor force; compromised care for the non–COVID-19 patients; controversy over disposal of dead bodies due to cultural sensitivities of different ethnic groups; unexpected clusters originating from a navy camp and a rehabilitation center with exponential increase of cases; and the continuous influx of imported cases. Being located next to India, which is currently reporting the second largest outbreak in the world, Sri Lanka should not underestimate its very high vulnerability to frequent waves of COVID-19.

Khuram Iqbal's chapter focuses on Pakistan's response to COVID-19. In the face of ongoing global recession, Pakistan is also set to face severe economic issues during the COVID-19 pandemic. Pakistan's GDP growth is expected to fall to –2% in 2020 according to IMF estimates. Pakistan's economy is largely reliant on the exports and services sectors. Foreign remittances also make up an important part of Pakistan's economy standing at USD $21 billion in 2018–2019, almost equivalent to Pakistan's exports. In such a scenario, any significant impact to national economy can raise the threat to security level. The coming part looks into how the economic situation has developed so far for Pakistan and what Pakistan is doing to contain it. Professor Khuram looks into Pakistan's security strategy by incorporating both traditional and non-traditional aspects in its national security policy after the COVID-19 pandemic due to the threats it poses to both traditional and non-traditional security areas. In order to achieve this, Pakistan needs to incorporate disease control and counter-epidemic exercises in military strategy, as well as improve civil-military cooperation for disease control. In this regard, Pakistan can also learn from China's military-civilian cooperative emergency response to disease prevention and control, which incorporates various laws mandating military-civilian cooperation, information sharing, and joint operations to prevent and control infectious diseases. The Chinese cooperation framework also mandates China's People's Liberation Army (PLA) to initiate the emergency research mechanism in case of any health emergency or infection outbreak. In view of the Indian strategic posturing during the pandemic, it is unlikely that Pakistan may witness any paradigm shift in its security agenda. National security calculation will continue to be dominated by the traditional threat of Indian hegemonic design, perceived or real. Given a weak economy, Islamabad can ill-afford a "tit-for-tat" response to New Delhi's growing defense expenditure. Rather, cooperation in dealing with non-traditional security threats such as COVID-19 will offer a rare window of opportunity to partner in a noble mission to protect billions of South Asians against the modern plague.

Amir Rana in Chapter 4 explores terrorism activities in Pakistan during COVID-19. Basically, Pakistan lifted the COVID-19-related lockdown on August 10, 2020 after having employed strict to smart lockdown strategies for about five months. During these months, the security landscape of Pakistan did not witness any major shift. However, the frequency and intensity of terrorist attacks slightly increased from May to July, particularly in North Waziristan district of Khyber Pakhtunkhwa and the restive southwestern province of Balochistan. Meanwhile, violent Sindhi nationalist groups launched a number of attacks against the security forces in Sindh. Similarly, in June, Balochistan Liberation Army (BLA) militants attacked the Pakistan Stock Exchange (PSX) building in Karachi, where law enforcement personnel were alert enough to kill all four attackers; however, three security guards and one police officer also lost their lives before the attack was successfully foiled. Hizbul Ahrar, a breakaway faction of militant group Jamaatul Ahrar, has perpetrated two attacks in 2020 at Rawalpindi district of Punjab. However, linking this relative increase in terrorist attacks with the pandemic is difficult. But it certainly indicates that the terrorist groups continue to demonstrate the capacity to plan and conduct attacks from the tribal belt to Karachi, despite the government's claims of counter-terrorism successes. Terrorists could be eyeing the opportunities created by the pandemic, but they are, apparently, waiting to take any major action in that regard. To fully reactivate their operational networks, they would have to reconnect to their support bases in the country, besides increasing recruitment and fund-raising efforts. Amir Rana also talks on Pakistan's complicated internal security landscape due to both internal and external threats. The internal security dimension not only includes threats from hard-core radical and sectarian terrorist groups but also from groups that promote religious extremism and intolerance. The latter pose a different sort of critical challenge because such groups can mobilize their support bases to cause more damage to the economy, the social cohesion of society, and the global image of the country. COVID-19 has created space for sectarian and radical groups, who tend to spread hate, including in cyberspace. In the beginning of the pandemic, while Sunni extremists and activists blamed the Shia pilgrims returning from Iran for the spread of the COVID-19 infection in Pakistan, the Shia activists accused the Tablighi Jamaat tours and gatherings for the spread of the virus. Posts and messages rife with sectarian hate speeches also went viral on social media platforms.

Adil Rasheed in Chapter 5 discusses about COVID-19 and the threat and early response in India. Dr Rasheed explains that India's response to the COVID-19 crisis has been like the three-dimensional chess game played in the television series "Star Trek" with "health," "economy," "social," and "political" fronts panning out at separate levels and yet inter-connected to a grand strategy. In order to score a decisive victory, the Indian central and state governments have had to not only consider the pros and cons of their coordinated actions, but have had to keep tabs on an unknown and unpredictable adversary, the elusive coronavirus. Again, as in the game of chess, some of the best-laid plans have tended to go awry and have not necessarily delivered the intended results. The challenge and the costs involved for India in fighting this pandemic, both in humanitarian as well as in economic terms, have been enormous. For a nation with 1.3 billion people of which 275 million (22 percent) live below the poverty line, the big question was whether the overstretched administrative machinery and weak public healthcare system could prevent a pandemic from causing a major humanitarian crisis. Rasheed also explains, by mid-June 2020, India became the *fourth country worst hit by the coronavirus* after the US, Brazil, and Russia. Whereas the disease was on the decline in other parts of the world, the pace of coronavirus transmission in the country started picking up dramatically after the lockdown. Authorities in the states of Maharashtra, Tamil Nadu, Delhi, Gujarat, and Uttar Pradesh feared an acute shortage of intensive care units and ventilators in the coming months. The Harvard Global Health Institute director Ashish K. Jha feared that India might become "the global epicenter" of the coronavirus pandemic and believed India had 50,000 unreported pandemics a day already, which might rise to 200,000 cases a day by August 2020. Many experts believed the disease had already entered the stage of community transmission in the country and averred that because of the migrant workers' mass exodus, the focal point of the pandemic will soon "shift from urban centers like Delhi, Mumbai, Ahmedabad to second- and third-tier cities and even district towns." The grim prospect of doctors, nurses, and paramedics falling sick of the disease in large numbers was highly worrisome. It seemed unlikely for the government to re-enforce lockdowns given the precarious state of the economy and it had very few options other than going for aggressive testing and sequestering, as well as enforcing the wearing of masks. However, there was a silver lining amidst dark clouds hovering on the horizon. The country was also ardently hoping that a vaccine would also be produced at least by early 2021 so that the threat of a major humanitarian crisis is averted.

In Chapter 6, Kenneth Yeo Yaoren focusses on Singapore's response to COVID-19. Singapore has experienced three waves of outbreaks, and possibly a fourth. The first wave of infection was introduced by tourists and employees coming from the Chinese Wuhan province. The second wave was induced by Singaporeans repatriated from Europe and North America. The third wave of infection exploded at the migrant worker's dormitories which led to the exponential increase of infected cases in Singapore. The government then imposed a lockdown from April 2020 which was expected to terminate in early June 2020. However, fears of a potential fourth wave loomed as Singapore adopted a "three steps forward, two steps back" approach. In this chapter, Kenneth details the government's priorities and responses in each phase of the crisis. The core strategy of the Singapore government was to "save lives and livelihoods." However, means to achieve the objective changed significantly due to the dynamic situation. The government of Singapore maintained a gold standard in the management of the pandemic for an extended period of time as discussed by Kenneth. This was attributed to the ingenuity and prudence of the incumbent government as they contained the virus effectively by redirecting resources and manpower to critical sectors. Nonetheless, oversight from the authorities resulted in the explosion of cases in migrant dormitories; exposing the untold story of Singapore's success. Despite its initial shock, authorities did not flinch and enacted a litany of policies to address the escalation of threat. This included the implementation of a circuit breaker to interdict community transmission while mobilizing the whole government and nation to aid the migrant worker's community. Within the span of two months, authorities recovered from the migrant worker crisis and prepared to lift the circuit breaker. Authorities remained watchful about the situation and adopted a cautious approach in lifting the circuit breaker measures. They acknowledged that policies could only minimize the transmission of the COVID-19 virus and governments depended on scientists to develop a vaccine. Conclusively, Singapore's COVID-19 story is one of resilience and fortitude. The government of Singapore mobilized the whole of society to combat COVID-19 promptly and efficiently despite some oversights. This could only be achieved by amassing political goodwill and trust between government and society over the years, one which is unique to Singapore.

Ruetaitip Chansrakaeo discusses on responses, health preparedness, and policy direction amidst the deadly COVID-19 attack in Thailand in Chapter 7. COVID-19 has been declared a dangerous transmissible disease since March 1, 2020 under the 2015 Communicable Diseases Act. If anyone finds a suspected case or persons that meet the COVID-19 criteria, reporting to disease control officers within 3 hours was mandatory. Under Section 5, The Minister of public health is responsible for and oversees the implementation of this Act and is also authorized to appoint officers for communicable disease control, issue Ministerial Regulations for additional acts and issue Rules or Notifications for the implementation of this Act. Under Section 6, the Minister shall be empowered in the notifications by and with the advice of the Committee to prescribe for the purposes of preventing and regulating communicable diseases: (1) names and symptoms of dangerous communicable diseases and communicable diseases under surveillance, (2) classification of any ports of entry in the Kingdom as foreign transmissible disease control checkpoints and cancellation of international communicable disease control checkpoints; and (3) immunization. Ruetaitip recommends strategic considerations regarding Thailand's national security preparedness to these new emerging infectious threats by emphasizing on preparedness system capacity development and health security system as follows: (a) Preparedness system capacity development; 1. The continuing development of the national readiness system, in the same way, should be given priority by the central, provincial, local, and related sectors. 2. Regional and local agencies should prepare state staff information, resources and accounts, and volunteers who are consistent with the types of mutual benefit disasters that take place in the area. 3. The development of guidelines for the integration of databases and information security networks for national preparedness and the national disaster data warehouse so that they can be used to support the management and coordination of disaster management and to exchange information for use among agencies for collaboration. 4. Courses and manuals for government agencies should be created with private and public sectors to be ready to face all forms of threats especially in risky areas. 5. The Ministry of provincial administration organization should arrange training and practice within and between departments to prepare to handle all forms of threats through participation of the private and public sectors. (b) Health security system: 1. Governments should commit themselves to taking action to address health safety risks while leaders should coordinate and monitor national health security investments in order to coordinate them with improvements to routine public health and healthcare systems. 2. The capacity in health security should be transparent and regularly measured. The results of these external assessments and self-assessments should be published at least once every two years. 3. New funding mechanisms to address epidemic and pandemic preparedness gaps are needed and should be set up urgently. 4. Thailand should at least annually test its health security capabilities and publish post-action reviews. Therefore, the government must commit to a functioning system by holding annual simulation exercises. It should be recognized that these recommendations will not succeed if the relevant factors are not met.

In Chapter 8, Rachel Kumendong and Edwin Tambunan discuss about the global security crisis, COVID-19 threat, and response in Indonesia. From the initial cases in March 2020, this pandemic has caused the country to undergo double crises: public health crisis and economic crisis. It hit all sectors of life such as economic, social, political, and security of the country. However, the rising threat brought by COVID-19 virus was not proportionally responded to by the government of Indonesia and this was proved by the sluggish and uncoordinated policy. Both authors also discuss Indonesia's past experiences in dealing with outbreaks which do not serve as a solid foundation to deal with the current pandemic. COVID-19 is the first human-to-human transmission that ever happened in the country. The complex interests in domestic politics also contributed to an uncertainty of how the country would deal with the virus. The pandemic has also resulted in multidimensional threats to the country. Due to the pandemic, Indonesia experienced an economic blowback due to the decline in tourism sector, loss of many MSME business, and millions of workers being laid off. The informal sectors and low-income workers were the most affected by this pandemic. In politics and security, the unpreparedness of the government caused major uncoordinated policies which could be an opportunity to delegitimize the government. The responses of the government toward the COVID-19 pandemic can be understood from three periodical categories: defensive responses, initial responses, and mixed responses. In the early time of the pandemic, the government seemed to downplay the threat of COVID-19 and prioritized its policy on how to save the country's economy. Furthermore, the government became more alert when Indonesia announced its first cases on March 2, 2020, followed by more responsive policies such as the formation of COVID-19 Task Force, improved public health infrastructure, and economic stimulus to ensure the survival of the country. Entering the second month of the crisis, the government appeared to issue more agile and compelling policies such as the implementation of large-scale social restrictions (PSBB) and the country's preparation to enter the "new normal." Indeed, the magnitude of the COVID-19 pandemic crisis accentuated the need for strong and relevant policies during the time of crisis to ensure the survival of the country and importantly its people. In regard to policy formulation, the government should not only focus on using an economic approach, but also involve multi-disciplinary advice from public health researchers, social scientists, and related parties to create a more comprehensive policy. Further, it should be taken into account the importance of effective crisis communication to support the policy formulation process. This pandemic has shown how poor Indonesia's public health infrastructure is.

In Chapter 9, Ahmad F. Yousif and Mohammed Hussain Ahmad precisely explain about the sociological observation of the religious identity in Brunei Darussalam during COVID-19. During the COVID-19 era in Brunei Darussalam, the government along with the private sector took serious steps and formulated specific policies to treat and control the virus. Among the measures taken after the partial "lockdown" was announced were total closure of religious worship places, closure of educational institutions and change in the learning system to distance online method, closure of health clinics with exception to emergencies, shutdown of sports and recreational facilities and related activities, forbiddance of social gatherings such as public weddings and postponement of all national celebrations, and others. In addition, the Brunei government closed all national borders and suspended flights in and outside the country, except for special chartered flights related to medical supplies and/or to bring Bruneian citizens home, particularly overseas students. It also barred international visitors from entering the country, including transiting at the international airport. While the government took drastic measures to control the virus, people in Brunei welcomed the new policies and tried to work together to follow the international standard required by WHO and Brunei's specific regulations. The Diplomat (international current affairs magazine for the Asia-Pacific region) stated that Brunei "has earned a much more honourable distinction this time around (for) winning the war on the coronavirus." The authors also discuss two main questions that need to be addressed in the context of Brunei's era of COVID-19. Firstly, does the high level of religious commitment correlate positively with COVID-19, on individual, family, community, societal, and international perspectives? Secondly, how do the policies and regulations proposed by the Brunei government during the pandemic period lead to reinforcing an individual's religiosity and reshaping Islamic commitments? Responses to the above and other questions are demonstrated nicely through discussion in their chapter.

In Chapter 10, Tulus Suryanto and Mizan Aslam explore the economic impact of COVID-19 in ASEAN region. Based on literature studies that have been carried out on five ASEAN countries (Indonesia, Malaysia, Brunei Darussalam,

Thailand, and Singapore), there has been a large increase in the revival of the Islamic economy financial sector and halal products. The resilience of Islamic finance is allegedly related to applying justice and transparency, which minimizes social inequality. The extraordinary resilience shown by the Islamic finance industry is facing a current economic turmoil. The market share strategy by utilizing digital technology, restructuring, and mergers has strengthened Islamic finance and become a driving force for the economy in the midst of "new normal" conditions. Still, this research did not find any big implications of COVID-19 for six other Islamic economy sectors, namely Muslim-Friendly Travel, halal food, modest fashion, halal pharmaceuticals, halal cosmetics, and halal media and recreation. It is essential to focus on Islamic finance. But it does not rule out the possibility of pursuing the right policies for the sustainability of other sectors of the Islamic economy.

Ainuddin Lee in Chapter 11 discussed COVID-19 as a serious global pandemic. As of April 28, 2020, infected patients were present in 185 countries and there were more than 3,000,000 cases reported worldwide, with more than 210,000 fatalities. The outbreak began in China, but the number of cases outside of China exceeded those in China by March 15, 2020, and rose at an exponential rate (Kevin J. Clerkin, 2020). The study human mobility (in parentheses) is one of the main factors that contribute to the worldwide dissemination of microorganisms. The spread of coronavirus disease 2019 (COVID-19) was reported to transmit to neighboring countries with relocation diffusion. With most of the studies focusing on China, Western Europe, and the USA, little is known about its evolution and genome variability in Southeast Asian (SEA) countries. SEA is home to more than half a billion or 9% of the world's population. As the region grapples with a surge in infection cases since March 2020, it is important to investigate purported mutations and the role of geographical proximity in shaping the genetic structure of the SARS-CoV-2 in SEA countries. On March 4, 2020, the World Health Organization (WHO) outlined that only nine of the eleven countries have the capacity to test for COVID-19, suggesting that the lack of testing facilities could hinder the preparedness and response planning of these countries toward COVID-19. Among the SEA countries, Malaysia, Thailand, and Singapore employ a large number of migrant workers, with Malaysia being the top importer with approximately 2.23 million people.

In Chapter 12, Saud Al-Sharafat focuses on the securitization of COVID-19 crisis in Jordan. With all measures taken by the Jordanian government to deal with the coronavirus, it is clear now that the virus has changed the "behavior" of the state and society in a broad and profound way. The securitization process was one of the most important manifestations of this change in the conduct of the state, especially in the short term. It also became clear that Jordan, through securitization, avoided a "Pyrrhic victory" over the virus, with many losses of life and property. Dr Saud also explains why the Jordanian government passed twelve defense orders, during the period (March 2 to May 3, 2020) to deal with the virus, all of which are subject to the application of the armed forces and security agencies. In all these "defense orders," the government has dealt with institutions in the public and private sectors and citizens of all walks of life, such as soldiers in war with the virus. Securitization deepened in Jordan as a result of "functional actors" like: media, academia, non-governmental agencies and think tanks, and Jordanian individuals themselves, since they help frame storylines about the existentially threatening nature of the virus" add to the failure of relevant ministries such as: industry and trade, labor, social development, and transportation to deal with the virus crisis (i.e. failure to distribute bread to homes in Jordan), so the armed forces and security agencies intervened clearly and explicitly to fill the vacuum and perform the task instead. The coronavirus in Jordan has gone beyond identifying the disease as a "critical public health crisis" due to concerns that a medical emergency would not provide the speed and agility necessary for dealing with the virus and to prevent its spread. Jordan's "securitization model" has in many ways proven itself as an effective, quick, and strict way to mobilize all needed resources available in the face of the pandemic, in order to preserve lives and properties before the disease is able to infect a large proportion of the population. Dr Saud also recommended Jordan to ensure that the political process continues with the implementation of appropriate safety standards. Both the withdrawal of the military and removal of all aspects of securitization in public life and elections will further confirm that Jordan's securitization strategy is applied only when necessary and will not permanently hinder the country's societal freedoms in the long term.

In Chapter 13, Joshua Snider talks on the Indo-Pacific region which has been particularly hard-hit by the COVID-19 pandemic. The Philippines, in particular, has been disproportionately impacted by the pandemic conditions. In addition to already grinding levels of economic inequality, the pandemic brought new and unwelcome challenges to an already fragile state. The country faced economic vulnerability at the best of times, born from a mix of over-reliance on OFW and remittances, elite captures of the economy, subsistence employment, corruption, and frequent natural disasters. These factors and more make the Philippines uniquely vulnerable and generally lacking in society-level resilience mechanisms to cope with long-term pandemic conditions. Beyond the country's general economic precariousness, the impact of the pandemic on the simmering ethno-religious conflict in the south of the country remains a point of concern. Despite a peace agreement with the mainstream insurgent elements, in recent years the conflict has been driven by recalcitrant violent extremist movements that challenge the state and pose a threat to communities. The Philippines' VEO space has undergone a transformation in recent years. While legacy movements such as Abu Sayyaf have always maintained linkages with regional and international Jihadist movements, post-Arab spring conflicts have further radicalized and internationalized the local VEO space. In 2017, two new ISIL-linked VEOs—Bangosmoro Islamic Freedom Front and the Maute Group (BIFF) —occupied the Marawi region and waged against the armed forces of the Philippines in a brutal months-long confrontation. The synergistic effects of the ferocity of this iteration of violent extremism and the state's response to it have diminished prospects for either a swift military victory or a negotiated settlement. Moreover, there is concern that the state is over-reaching and in particular that the Duterte government's new suite of anti-terror laws could further alienate Muslim Malays in the South without addressing any of the root causes.

In Chapter 14, Mamdouh Abdelmottlep concludes this volume with the analysis on the security threats and challenges of the coronavirus outbreak. Mamdouh discusses medical emergencies that require coordination and rapid response from public health officials in the country and supportive bodies of public emergency states. Security, police, and law enforcement agencies' roles may include enforcing public health orders (such as quarantine or travel restrictions), securing surrounding areas where the epidemic outbreaks, securing healthcare units, controlling the crowded people, investigating suspected biological terrorism scenes, or protecting national vaccines or other drug stocks. In cases of epidemic outbreaks on a wide scale, such as Corona, the security, police, and law enforcement officials will resort to balance their resources and efforts among these new responsibilities and daily service requirements on the security of the community and safety of its individuals. This policy declares the main issues assigned to security, police, and law enforcement officials to be solved following the health emergency states and preparing for emergency health conditions in the future, including epidemics and biological terrorism incidents. It is hoped that security, police, and law enforcement officials carefully consider the issues that require a solution in the planning operation for all dangers in their departments. Public safety and responded issues discussed here may be considered relatively new in this era of security work. Therefore, it requires more coordination and cooperation between various police and security agencies on the one hand and between the other bodies concerned in law enforcement on the other hand. This policy tackles the security challenges, which relate directly to security, police, public security, state security, Ministry of Interior, and its parallel agencies.

Rohan Gunaratna in the final chapter speaks on planetary health that concerns itself with a need for serious governance, posing a threat to the sustainability of our human civilization, environment, and the planet. Specifically, it seeks to confront three areas of challenges: "imagination challenges," such as failing to account for long-term human or environmental consequences of human progress; "research and information challenges," such as underfunding and lack of scope in research; and "governance challenges," such as delayed environmental action by governing bodies determined by unwillingness, uncertainty, or non-cooperation. Likewise, nutrition and diet are important contributors to and indicators of planetary health. Scientists speculate that human population growth threatens the carrying capacity of the planet. Diets, agriculture, and technology must adjust to sustain population projections upward of 9 billion while reducing harmful consequences on the environment through food waste and carbon-intensive diets. A focus of planetary health research will be nutritional solutions that are sustainable for the human species and the environment, and the generation of scientific research and political will to create and implement desired solutions. In January 2019, an international commission created the planetary health diet.

Conclusion

This book relates the best response to COVID-19 in Asia in the early phase. Other than transforming the future of Asia on the whole, the pandemic also altered human lifestyles from how it was previously; new policy, rules, and regulations were constructed in high-level meetings attended by a special task force, every one of them closely confirmed by the government's strict instruction to the nation. The disparity between the rich and poor aggravated when millions of people became unemployed, especially fresh graduates. Asia required a cohesive response to the COVID-19 pandemic. The arrival of the pandemic allows the opportunity for the creation of early-fast-active response adjacent to the nation's priorities, as well as to re-evaluate the dissemination of resources accordingly, particularly in an Asian context. Forthcoming priorities should correspondingly be dealing with new norms, elevating developing nations from poverty, and undertaking the future economy, social, health, and food and health crises as issues pertaining to the pandemic response.

We believe this book can be used as recommended reading for a course in an academic institute or a policy-oriented class. The edited volume could be assigned as core reading material for undergraduate and post-graduate courses and modules. In addition, it can be used as a reference for academic studies and research. The country case studies within the book intend to provide a guide for policymakers, ministries, and law enforcement agencies in developing the best functional post–COVID-19 response. This book is also relevant for online and offline conference proceedings; it can be used as a guide for policymakers and governments who are looking to understand best practices from all around the world in response to the pandemic.

1 Extremism in Southeast Asia amidst Pandemic COVID-19

Mohd Mizan Aslam

Introduction

Southeast Asia's (SEA) strong links to terrorist groups and cells in the region is well documented and undeniable. Abu Sayyaf Group (ASG), Jemaah Islamiyyah (JI) and Islamic State (IS) made a significant contribution in terrorism-related activities in the region and its wider global networking. ASEAN countries at the 3rd Sub-Regional Meeting on Counter-Terrorism and Transnational Security in December 2020 discussed the issue of COVID-19 being used as a means for terrorists to spread COVID-19 as an improvised tactic of a biological attack. This is relevant because The Mujahidin of Eastern Indonesia (MIT) leader Ali Kalora has claimed that the virus was a divine retribution against China for its treatment of the Uighurs, and against other major economies that battled ISIS.

The U.N. counter-terrorism chief Vladimir Voronkov warned that terrorists are exploiting the COVID-19 pandemic and appealing to new "racially, ethnically, and politically motivated violent extremist groups" that the IS, which lost its self-declared caliphate in Iraq and Syria in March 2019, is still carrying out attacks in the two countries and seeking to reconstitute an external operations capability. Assistant U.N. Secretary-General Michele Coninsx reiterated that IS affiliates have emerged in many places, including Southeast Asia, while Britain's Foreign Office minister of state, James Cleverly, urged greater attention to terrorist misuse of social media and other new technologies and the longer-term impact of COVID-19 on "the terrorism dynamic."[1]

In April 2020, amidst pandemic COVID-19 and following the arrest of Ustad Arif, Indonesian security sources indicated that he has sleeper cell links to Malaysia, but has not been profiled. Former Inspector General (IGP) of Royal Malaysia Police (PDRM) Datuk Seri Abdul Hamid Bador also confirmed the existence of sleeper cells in 2019.[2] This is something that should be taken seriously as research shows that a sleeper is trained and dispatched by an organization to infiltrate the targeted society or organization and then remains dormant, sometimes for a long time until being activated, perhaps by a prearranged signal or a certain chain of events. The pandemic slowed down terrorism-related activities but the threat is intact.

DOI: 10.4324/9781003291909-2

The release of Abu Bakar Ba'asyir from Jakarta Prison has made a significant alert to the regional security community. Ba'asyir, eighty-two years old, is the former head of JI, an Al-Qaeda proxy group operated in SEA. JI is the most dangerous militant group established in SEA which is based in Maahad Ittibaussunnah Kuala Pilah Negeri Sembilan, Malaysia. JI was established in 1993 and the main factor behind the deadliest "Bali Bombing" that killed 202 people; mostly Australians and Britons. Ba'asyir has mentioned that he will continue his radical preaching till the end of his life. Moreover, JI also created other factions such as Jamaah Anshorut Tauhid (JAT) and Jamaah Anshorut Daulah (JAD), which are actively involved in a series of attacks in Indonesia and the Philippines.

In relation to the release of Ba'asyir from Gubung Sindur Correction Centre in West Jakarta, the Head of E8, Special Branch Counter Terrorism Unit, Normah Ishak, made a statement that Abu Bakar Ba'asyir's release in Indonesia had no influence in Malaysia or that he is only followed by a small group of people who warrants examination. The concern is how potential terrorists are being effectively monitored in Malaysia, with the widespread use of VPN and other secure messaging apps such as Telegram, Signal, BiP as well as dark web. Physical contact could not happen during the pandemic and because of the Movement Control Order (MCO), but radical indoctrination continued to flourish using online platforms.

Normah also claimed the pandemic prevention measures had minimized such threats while adding that previous JI members had been rehabilitated and their offspring have no interest in what their parents have gone through with the group.[3] She also added that Ba'asyir has no influence in Malaysia as he is only followed by a small group of people who were already being watched by the Indonesian authorities. She did acknowledge that there were JI members in Malaysia but were constantly monitored by police and that Putrajaya's deradicalization program has been a success. While these statements must come as a relief to Malaysians, they do present some curious points of discussion.

Meanwhile, Indonesia's National Counter-Terrorism Agency's (BNPT) director for enforcement, Eddy Hartono has acknowledged that although there have been no major terrorist attacks during the pandemic, terrorism cells in Indonesia "are not sitting back and relaxing." He stated that terror cells are actively recruiting, spreading their ideology, raising funds, and conducting training and that the only thing that has slowed down during the pandemic is the sending of militants to join the ranks of the Islamic State in Iraq, Syria, and Afghanistan.[4]

Southern Philippines has similar patterns of terrorist activities, with Mindanao now been described as a center of transnational terrorism in Southeast Asia and has become a boot camp co-opting regional "jihadists" to join their cause. The goal is to establish an Islamic nation turning to the caliphates in countries including Indonesia, Malaysia, Brunei, Southern Thailand, and Mindanao.[5] Militants travel between Malaysia's eastern state of Sabah, Indonesia's shared island of Sebatik and the adjacent Sulu archipelago in the Philippines, the home territory of the IS-aligned Abu Sayyaf Group (ASG). To underscore matters, a 2018 Merdeka Centre survey showed that Muslims in Malaysia are more likely to support global terror groups, including the IS and JI, than their counterparts in other South-East Asian nations. Based on the above discussion, it can be reasonably said that the threat of terrorism still exists in Malaysia amidst the pandemic COVID-19.

The coronavirus pandemic forced countries to impose lockdowns and close their borders, leading to a drop in public events and gatherings, as well as a sharp slowdown in travel. These meant that, for the most part, extremist terrorism has dropped off the headlines and seen a dip in impact. But the threat still exists, as incidents like the beheading of a schoolteacher in France and the discovery of new training sites in Indonesia show. The following are some of the trends which could be expected:

Jemaah Islamiyyah and Regional Threat

It may be too early to get a full picture of the impact of COVID-19 on terror recruitment and radicalization; however, it may have potentially multiplied its reach. Some extremists have begun promoting COVID-19 conspiracy theories to win a following, claiming the virus is a hoax by governments and that the vaccine causes serious illnesses and is genetically controlled. Britain's Head of Counter-Terrorism Police Neil Basu warned recently that these conspiracy theories could radicalize a small minority to violence and hatred. The main concern is that online radicalization has allowed all these theories, and various forms of terrorism, to now thrive 24 hours a day, seven days a week, internationally.

The Mujahidin of Eastern Indonesia (MIT) leader Ali Kalora believed the virus was a divine retribution against China for its treatment of the Uighurs, and against other major economies that battled ISIS, which MIT had sworn allegiance to. This confidence spurred a series of attacks on policemen and police informants in Sulawesi, seen in a footage which was uploaded on social media groups in a bid to win new recruits.

While Malaysia has destroyed JI's networks in the country following the 2002 Bali bombings, a number of its leaders and bomb makers remain on the run. The recent arrests in Indonesia of two key bomb makers involved in the 2002 Bali blasts, Taufik Bulaga and Aris Sumarsono,[6] coupled with Malaysia's confirmation of sleeper cells within the country, should be of concern. The recent and upcoming release of detained militants, including JI spiritual leader Abu Bakar Ba'asyir is a concern, as some may be set on returning to their old ways. This underscores why security agencies in Malaysia must continue to be on high alert.

Following the recent arrest of a little-known cleric named Ustad Arif who turned out to be the leader of JI, Indonesian security sources indicated that he had sleeper cell links to Malaysia, but have not been profiled. After the 2002 Bali bombings, JI had split into two factions. One faction believed in violent jihad and supported Al-Qaeda and later the Islamic State, while another focused on "jihad proselytization." Arif has allegedly revealed that JI has been regenerating and is estimated to have recruited 6,000 people into its ranks. Security sources also stated that JI has no plans for terror attacks in the immediate to short-term time span due to the disruption in JI leadership and due to the involvement of the US and its allies in the Middle East, positioning it at the top of its strike list. Ustad Arif, 54, from Klaten, Central Java, with his supposedly deep knowledge of Islam, is a highly respected member of the group. Arif led JI for only eight months before being arrested. He was the second JI leader to be arrested within the last two years. Arif's predecessor, Para Wijayanto, was arrested in July 2019 and sentenced by a court to seven years' imprisonment this year on terrorism charges as well as for sending JI members to Syria to fight alongside opposition rebels there. Following Wijayanto's arrest, police discovered he had restructured and rebuilt JI into an organization that had moved away from donations and robberies as its main source of income into an organization with business interests in palm oil plantations and other commercial sectors.

At least 96 young militants underwent training there, with many going to Syria to fight alongside terror group Al-Nusra Front. JI members are also running businesses, including oil palm plantations and cleaning service contractors, to finance terror activities while of *pesantren* or religious boarding schools have remained active in propagating hardline teachings where many of its militants were nurtured in recent decades.

Also arrested was JI's expert bomb maker, Upik Lawanga (aka 'Professor'), in January 2021. He had been on the country's most-wanted list for fourteen years and allegedly assembled many of the bombs that were set off in Poso, Central Sulawesi, from 2005 to 2007. Among the terror attacks linked to Upik were the two 2005 blasts at Tentena market in Central Sulawesi, which killed twenty-two people. He was a Malaysian student, Dr. Azahari Hussein. Azahari made the bombs for the 2002 Bali attacks that killed 202 people, including 111 Australians. He was killed in a shoot-out with police in East Java in 2005 and was known as one of the deadliest and most lethal bomb-makers in the region, and police have long worried that he had passed on his skills to his students. Azahari was known to be extremely meticulous, surveying a target and its location before setting out to assemble bombs and ensure they could inflict "massive destruction." Terrorism analysts from Malaysia and Singapore have however opined that there was no indication of JI's reactivation in Malaysia at this time and close monitoring by the authorities continued. The leader of JI has been arrested in Indonesia along with one of the group's expert bomb makers according to sources (reported December 10, 2020). JI was behind all the deadliest terror attacks in Indonesia from 1998 to 2010 before it was weakened by the Indonesian counterterrorism police (Detachment 88). There are indications that the network has been on the rise again lately, accumulating business interests in palm oil plantations as well as the mining industry to fuel its activities.

Malaysia has destroyed its networks, and further arrests in Indonesia following the 2002 Bali bombings have reduced much of its leadership. Furthermore, its links with Al-Qaeda were also disrupted whereby a number of its leaders and bomb makers remain on the run even after the group was banned in 2008. It is clear that they have not shifted from its aim of establishing an Islamic state in the region.

The recent arrests of JI's key players have helped neutralize the threat but they have also highlighted that the group has evolved and expanded its reach as it maintains its militant leanings and tries to gain a greater foothold in the public sphere to win support for its eventual aim. As was reported in March 2021, a two-story house in Central Java was used by JI to train recruits in handling weapons and assembling bombs.

Malaysia: Terrorism amidst Pandemic COVID-19

After 20 years' imprisonment, for the first time two Malaysians and one Indonesian with Malaysian Permanent Residence status were charged in the martial court of the US. Riduan Isamuddin aka Hambali, a key man for Osama bin Laden's Al-Qaeda network in South-East Asia, and his two Malaysian lieutenants Mohammed Farik Amin (Selangor) and Mohammed Nazir Lep (Johor) will be formally charged for their terror acts. Farik and Nazir will become the first Malaysians to be charged with terrorist activities in a US court. All three were implicated in the Bali bombings in 2002, in which 202 people were killed, and the 2003 bomb attack at the JW Marriott Hotel in Jakarta which killed 12 people.

Farik and Nazir have also been implicated in a planned Al-Qaeda plot to crash a hijacked plane into the seventy-three-story Library Tower/US Bank Tower in Los Angeles. Intelligence sources reported that the two were arrested in a joint operation involving the CIA and Thai police in Bangkok in 2003. Hambali, their mentor, was arrested a few days later. They were subsequently held in Camp Delta in Guantanamo Bay, Cuba, by the US. The Malaysians had also received arms training in Afghanistan.[7]

In responding to the developments, Inspector-General Police Tan Sri Abdul Hamid Bador had stated that such a decision was a long time coming as justice must be served and that thwarting the threat of terrorism in the country remained a priority for Royal Malaysian Police (RMP). Datuk Ayob Khan Mydin Pitchay, the former RMP Counter-Terrorism Division (E8) head, was previously quoted as saying that the Malaysian duo was high-ranking members with a great deal of influence. "There is a high possibility that they might return to their militant ways and join other groups, especially the Islamic State group if they are released."

Hambali has strong ties with Malaysia as his wife, Noralwiza Lee Abdullah, a Malaysian from Sandakan, Sabah was also detained under the Internal Security Act in 2003 but was released in 2007. Relevant sources have tried to locate Noralwiza at present but have been unsuccessful. There are indications that she may have moved to Cianjur, West Java in Indonesia, to be with Hambali's family, including his siblings.

Malaysian Yazid Sufaat, a US-trained biochemist, was also recruited by Hambali directly, as stated in court testimonies.[8] He was detained under the then Internal Security Act (ISA) in December 2001, for his alleged involvement with Osama bin Laden's Al-Qaeda. He was released in 2008, but re-arrested five years later and again in 2017 after a brief release. Yazid was then rearrested in 2013 under the Security Offences (Special Measures) Act (SOSMA) and sentenced to four years for recruiting new members into the Islamic State terror group. Following that release, Yazid was again detained in December 2017 after authorities discovered that he had been recruiting fellow inmates into Al-Qaeda while in detention.

In 2019, he was released after the Prevention of Terrorism Board[9] considered all aspects of Yazid's condition while he served his sentence, including his behavior and whether he had fully repented. This is despite being described previously by other sources as "unrepentant." Whether the early release of such hardened terrorists is wise and whether they can be truly rehabilitated and allowed to mingle with society is left to be seen. Recidivism is still under control and not many cases are reported; however, the possibility for ex-detainees to regroup and end up in jihad battlefields such as Rafi Udin and Ustaz Lotfi cannot be ignored. As long as the opportunity is there, recidivism also has a potential.

Terrorism-Crime Nexus

Malaysia currently has seventy-two known and active criminal gangs that could overrun the country with criminal activities, if left unchecked. The link to terrorism should not be overlooked as many hardened criminals end up incarcerated. The concern about prisons contributing to the spread of extremism and the nexus between convictions and terrorism have been mentioned repeatedly by academics and practitioners. Looking at the stages of radicalization from pre-radicalization to action, it is clear that selected individuals are targeted by recruiters. According to RMP Criminal Investigation Department deputy director Datuk Dev Kumar, Malaysia currently has seventy-two known and active criminal gangs that could overrun the country with criminal activities if left unchecked. Among the 72 gangs identified, 49 were confirmed to have been established in 2013, while 23 others were established in 2015 with a total number of 9,042 active members.[10]

While this presents worrying data from a traditional security perspective, the link to terrorism should not be overlooked as many hardened criminals end up incarcerated. It has been researched in other countries that prisons have been a hotbed for terrorist recruitment for both the skill sets they possess (weapons handling for example) and their susceptibility to violence or even for redemption at any cost (where recruits believe their past wrongs can be erased by carrying out jihadist agendas). The concern about prisons contributing to the spread of extremism and the nexus between convictions and terrorism has been mentioned repeatedly by academics and practitioners. Looking at the stages of radicalization from pre-radicalization to action, it is clear that selected individuals are targeted by recruiters.[11]

In his speech in conjunction with the Asia/Pacific Group (APG) Annual Typologies Workshop Bank Negara Malaysia (BNM), deputy governor Marzunisham Omar stated there have been growing concerns that terrorist groups are using the COVID-19 pandemic to advance their propaganda and fundraising efforts. Although the risk seems muted at the moment due to strengthened border enforcement, online activities and financial transactions related to terrorism could easily go under the radar of authorities. Bank Negara, as a regulator, should strive to facilitate this transformation while being cognizant and vigilant of the risks that it can pose to the stability and integrity of the financial system, including ML/TF.

This statement echoes the statement of Dian Triansyah Djani (Indonesia), Chair of the 1267 Committee (UN Security Council) November 2020 has recorded that terrorist groups are using the outbreak of the COVID-19 pandemic to advance their propaganda and fundraising efforts. A further major concern is the increase in terrorist acts committed by lone actors and by individuals and groups embracing what is referred to by several Member States as "extreme right-wing" terrorism or "racially and ethnically motivated terrorism." These various groups and individuals have demonstrated their ability to adapt to the current unprecedented situation resulting from the COVID-19 pandemic by continuing to exploit new technologies for radicalization, recruitment, and fundraising purposes, among other things.[12]

Fintech and the Risk of Terrorism

Bank Negara Malaysia (BNM) has issued five Digital Banking licenses in 2022 and had issued the anticipated digital banking framework recently, which followed a six-month public consultation period. BNM stated that the licensing framework was created to "enable innovative application of technology to uplift the financial well-being of individuals and businesses and foster sustainable growth" which includes expanding "meaningful access" and "promoting responsible usage of suitable financial solutions to unserved and underserved segments."

Digital banks will be required to comply with the requirements under the Financial Services Act 2013 (FSA) or Islamic Financial Services Act 2013 (IFSA), including standards on prudential, Shariah, business conduct and consumer protection, as well as on anti-money laundering and terrorism financing. This is important as while the fintech revolution brings significant benefits to countries, it also raises concerns when certain entities, in particular terrorist networks, use new technologies to augment their power and resources.

A 2018 study commissioned by the European Parliament's Policy Department for Citizens' Rights and Constitutional Affairs had detailed the terrorist financing risks associated to the adoption of virtual currencies (VCs). According to the report, even while conventional methods of fundraising still present concerns, VCs could represent a new frontier for lone actors and small terrorist cells, especially for young people who are fluent in the use of the internet and digital technologies. The fertile fintech environment, which is destined to grow, could potentially pose significant risks that should be monitored closely.

Money Laundering

It was reported that the Indian intelligence agencies are believed to have intercepted financial transactions suggesting that a Malaysian-based Rohingya outfit, trained in Myanmar, may be in an advanced stage of orchestrating a terror strike in that country by a group led by a woman. The woman leading the alleged terror attack plan was sent from Malaysia to Myanmar for training and had planned to infiltrate India through Bangladesh or Nepal. The likely targets mentioned were Ayodhya, Bodhgaya, Srinagar, and Punjab.

Indian authorities were also investigating whether these suspicious India-centric transactions (some USD $200,000) allegedly routed from Kuala Lumpur to fund the operation, had links with controversial preacher Zakir Naik, who is currently a Malaysian permanent resident. The RMP have however stated that they have not received any official report on Zakir Naik's alleged terrorist involvement from Delhi.

Malaysia is arguably more polarized now in terms of race and religion than at any point in her history. Politicians and leaders discharging subjective and narrow views in mainstream and closed groups for ulterior objectives, often being lauded, is now the norm. The effect of such sentiments could adversely influence a fragile mind. Malaysia needs to be cognizant of this and remain vigilant.

Indonesia: Terrorism amidst Pandemic COVID-19

According to reports,[13] scores of Rohingya women missing from a refugee camp in Indonesia have been trafficked into Malaysia to reunite with their husbands. Just over 100 refugees remain at the camp in Lhokseumawe on Indonesia's northern coast, well down from the almost 400 who arrived in separate boat landings between June and September 2019. Neither local authorities nor the UN could account for the whereabouts of the women, who are feared to have enlisted traffickers to help them cross the Malacca Straits into Malaysia. This underscores the gaps in monitoring and security.

In Malaysia, more than 100,000 Rohingya live on the margins of society in Malaysia, registered as refugees but not allowed to work, forcing the men into illegal construction and other low-paid jobs. This is a relevant concern from a counter-terrorism and prevention of violent-extremism perspective.

Research indicates that radicalization does, in fact, happen in refugee camps. Also, the treatment of refugees in those camps makes a massive difference. Extremely poor camp conditions, including lack of sanitation/hygiene, isolation, hostility from host countries, lack of regular access to food/water/other supplies, lack of education and/or work opportunities, overcrowding, failure or lack of mental health and other medical services, and extreme restriction of movement are all tied to increased risks of radicalization. Some, such as a lack of education, have been tied to an increased risk even if it is the only factor present, but all combinations of any of these factors pose definite risks.

Studies also show that in refugee camps where these factors have been deliberately avoided or rectified such as in Jordan, where refugees (who otherwise share the same traits, origins, etc. as refugees in surrounding areas) were made citizens and granted work permits, the risk of radicalization is significantly lower than in regions with worse conditions for refugees. In other words, petty policies towards refugees and refugee camps are directly associated with a higher risk of radicalization.[14]

Most Southeast Asian extremist groups have already been linked to the latest Rohingya crisis in some way. For example, there have been media reports of hundreds of jihadists from regional countries training for terrorist operations in Myanmar, or being put on standby to go to Bangladesh.[15] It is not clear if any of these reports are accurate, but the possibility of increased terrorist activity in Malaysia on behalf of the Rohingyas needs to be taken seriously especially when refugees slip through the "net" for whatever motive, and cannot be accounted for. This is critical because in 2019, four Rohingyas were arrested in Malaysia for an extortion racket to fund the Arakan Rohingya Salvation Army (ARSA) including one who was believed to have links to a pro-Isis terror cell.[16]

The Indonesian police's anti-terror squad has arrested 228 suspects in terrorism cases this year according to sources. Some of the terrorism cases which became the spotlight were the arrests of twenty-three terrorist suspects from the outlawed Jemaah Islamiyah (JI) group between November and December 2020. JI seeks to establish an Islamic state in the region including Malaysia. Among the arrests was Upik Lawanga (also known as Taufik Bulaga) who had been on the run for fourteen years as he was involved in bombings in Central Sulawesi province between 2004 and 2006 and Zulkarnain (also known as Aris Sumarsono) is believed to be involved in the Bali bombings of 2002.

He was also thought to have led the squad involved in the suicide bombing at Jakarta's JW Marriott Hotel that killed twelve people in 2003. He was a fugitive for nineteen years and was capable of assembling high-explosive bombs and firearms. No escalation of threat levels to Malaysia has been reported although police are aware of sleeper cells and are being vigilant based on intelligence gathered following the arrests.

The Philippines: Terrorism amidst Pandemic COVID-19

The threat of terrorism and violent extremism in the Philippines, especially in Mindanao, the country's second-largest island, is severe and persistent. The current COVID-19 pandemic has also provided some new challenges to countering violent extremism (CVE). The following briefly outlines the background of extremist groups in the Philippines and highlights how the pandemic has influenced such activities. The roster and alignment of groups operating within the Philippines have fluctuated, but terrorists and rebels have been consistently motivated by two overarching ideologies: *Islamist extremism* and *Communism*.

During the last two decades, a diverse mix of Islamist extremist groups has operated throughout the Philippines. These groups are unstable: their splinter frequently converge in tactical alliances and fluctuate between committing criminal acts, mounting insurgency against the government, and carrying out terrorism as their primary pursuits. The overarching political goal of these groups is to expel the Christian majority from Mindanao and establish an autonomous or independent Islamic state there for Filipino Muslims, who are commonly referred to as the Moro or Bangsamoro people.

As the MILF[17] began to adopt a more favorable stance toward autonomy, as opposed to complete independence, more-radical factions split from the group. One such faction is the *Bangsamoro Islamic Freedom Fighters* (BIFF), which split from the MILF in 2010 and declared its allegiance to *the Islamic State of Iraq and Syria* (ISIS) in July 2014. In 2013, the BIFF's leader, *Mohammad Ali Tambako*, left to form a new group, the *Justice for Islamic Movement* (JIM), allegedly in reaction to disagreements within the BIFF over his decision to attack civilian communities. The BIFF and JIM have since reconciled and allied against the Philippine government. The MILF produced another splinter group at about the same time that the BIFF emerged. This second new group was known as the Maute Group or the Islamic State in Lanao.

Arguably, the most notorious extremist group in the Philippines is the *Abu Sayyaf Group* (ASG), which parted ways with the MNLF in 1991 to form the smallest but most radical of the MNLF's splinter groups. The ASG was the first Filipino Islamist extremist organization to be named to the U.S. Department of State's list of foreign terrorist organizations, having been designated in 1997. The ASG joined the BIFF in pledging allegiance to ISIS through videos posted on social media in July 2014, straining its relationship with Al-Qaeda.

Despite its origin as part of the MNLF and its connections to Al-Qaeda and ISIS, for much of its existence, the ASG has engaged primarily in violent criminal behaviors with no clear political or ideological agenda other than material gain. As such, it has never been included in peace negotiations with the government.

Other Islamist extremist groups targeting the Philippines include *Ansar al-Khilafah* (AKP), which emerged in 2014 through a video pledging allegiance to ISIS, and the Indonesian, Al-Qaeda-affiliated terrorist network *Jemaah Islamiyah* (JI), which occasionally collaborates with selected Filipino terrorist groups. In addition to influencing and supporting other jihadist groups in the region, ISIS has established its own branch in the Philippines[18] (ISIS-Philippines), earning its own designation on the U.S. Department of State's foreign terrorist organizations list in February 2018.

The group's terror tactics rely heavily on suicide bombings against the Philippines government and civilian targets (particularly Catholic establishments) and U.S. affiliated targets (namely the U.S. embassy). According to one analysis, the Philippines' landscape of Islamic extremist actors, combined with its vulnerable populations alienated from the government, has made the country "ISIS" the greatest hope for a revival of its caliphate.

Communist Terrorist and Violent Extremist Groups

Although the Philippines government's efforts to counter and contain the Islamist extremist separatist movement have taken center stage in recent years, the government's longest-running campaign has been against the Communist coalition formed by the *Communist People's Party* (CPP); its armed wing, called the *New People's Army* (NPA), and its political wing, called the National Democratic Front (NDF). The CPP-NPA has members throughout the Philippines, including in Manila, and, as of 2009, it had just shy of 5,000 members, down from its strength of 25,200 in its 1987 heyday. The CPP-NPA has launched more terrorist attacks than any other group in the Philippines, and it has a wider geographic reach within the Philippines than its Islamist extremist counterparts.[19]

The 1980s saw the emergence of two CPP-NPA splinter groups: The *Alex Boncayao Brigade* (ABB) and the *Revolutionary Proletarian Army* (RPA). In 1997, the ABB and RPA converged to form a political arm called the *Rebolusyonaryong Partidong Manggagawàng Pilipinas* (RPM-P). The RPM-P entered into a peace agreement with the Philippines government in 2000, and it has even engaged in legitimate politics by entering candidates in elections. The ABB and RPA continue to act as the RPM-P's armed wing, but they have not perpetrated any major attacks in recent years.

The Philippines faces a very high level of threat from terrorist and extremist activity, ranking in tenth place on the Global Terrorism Index's 2020 list of countries most affected by terrorism and continues to face grave security challenges on multiple fronts. Despite a slight reduction in terrorist activity (from 2019), the Philippines remains the only Southeast Asian country to be ranked in the ten countries most impacted by terrorism.

Terrorism Trend in Philippines During the Pandemic

Drivers of radicalization in the Philippines consist primarily of push factors that steer an individual down the path of violent extremism such as socioeconomic pressures and pull factors that attract an individual to the idea of joining a terrorist or violent extremist group. For example, an individual living in extreme poverty (a push factor), if left to his or her own devices, might not join a terrorist group to make a living unless the terrorist group was offering financial incentives (a pull factor).

Groups will seek to gain legitimacy, expand their support base and boost recruitment during COVID-19. Scholars of counterterrorism highlight the importance of economic conditions which act as fuel for terrorism and the value of economic and social policies as countermeasures. An essential tenet in fighting terrorism lies in promoting economic growth and combating inequality. The pandemic-induced economic slump across vulnerable areas in the Philippines may further cement the support and presence of these organizations in various affected communities.

Inadequate state relief during the COVID-19 pandemic will be an opportunity for terrorist networks to raise and move funds. If these groups remain outside the purview of the state authorities responsible for countering terrorism financing, they will be able to finance their activities with relative ease. When resources are funneled towards more immediate COVID-19 needs, more cracks will appear in social services and welfare systems to the benefit of terrorist financing and recruitment. Terrorist groups and their front organizations will exploit these weaknesses to gain legitimacy and boost recruitment.

Terror-linked charities that provide public goods and social services must be watched closely. Al-Qaeda affiliates have used charities to exploit crises to gain legitimacy and recruit militants. In Southeast Asia, JI has a history of recruiting through the provision of social services. They provided long-term relief for victims of the 2004 Aceh tsunami and 2006 Yogyakarta earthquake. JI charities provided family support, health care, and welfare for victims affected by these crises. Aid provided by terror-linked charities helps terror groups gain legitimacy, not only among their immediate beneficiaries but also among the broader population. With the travel-restricting COVID-19 pandemic, forcing many into unemployment, many could soon become more vulnerable than ever to extremist groups.

Adding to this, following the unhappiness caused by mosque closures to curb the spread of COVID-19, a BIFF leader, *Sheik Muhiddin Animbang*, alias *Commander Kagi Karialan*, urged fighters to launch attacks against government assets because they were "destroying Islam" by disallowing congregation in mosques. This appears to be a strong pull factor in the current climate. BIFF militants are mainly located in the densely forested and mountainous regions of Maguindanao and Cotabato. There, loose firearms and explosive materials are not difficult to acquire. Hence, an armed assault at a police or military outpost south of Mount Piapayungan of Maguindanao and Cotabato cannot be ruled out.

Mindanao has also been described as "a mecca of transnational terrorism in Southeast Asia and has become a boot camp co-opting locals to join their cause." The goal is to establish a fundamentalist Caliphate in countries that include Indonesia, Malaysia, Brunei, the southern province of Thailand and Mindanao. Militants traveling between Malaysia's eastern state of Sabah and the adjacent Sulu archipelago in the Philippines, the home territory of the IS-aligned Abu Sayyaf Group (ASG) have been well documented.

These sorts of pull factors are especially potent as the Christian majority has long perceived Muslims as being "troublemakers and violent," and many, if false, associate Muslims with terrorism, particularly because of the high level of terrorist activity in Muslim areas of Mindanao. Indeed, attacks by Islamist extremist groups have exacerbated tensions between the Muslim and Christian communities, with both sides feeling persecuted either by the attacks themselves or by the government's often heavy-handed militant response, which has grown even harsher under the leadership of Duterte (push factor).

There is no consensus on which push/pull factor is the most important. However, CVE scholars and practitioners agree that the main drivers of radicalization are poverty and economic hardship, ethnic and religious marginalization and disenfranchisement, and frustration with the government.

Singapore: Terrorism amidst Pandemic COVID-19

It has been reported that a thirty-three-year-old radicalized Malaysian working as a cleaner in Singapore has been deported to Malaysia.[20] Mohd Firdaus Kamal

Intdzam was arrested under the Internal Security Act (ISA) in July 2020 for planning to travel to Syria with his Singaporean wife to take up armed violence for the terrorist group Islamic State in Iraq and Syria (ISIS). After investigations were completed, Firdaus had his work pass canceled and he was handed over to the Malaysian Special Branch in August 2019. In addition to traveling to Syria to take up arms, Firdaus was also apparently willing to carry out attacks against countries which he deemed to be oppressing Muslims, or which he saw as being hypocritical for aligning themselves with the West.

Prosecutors are expected to request that the case be transferred to the Kuala Lumpur High Court. According to the Internal Security Department (ISD), the man's thirty-four-year-old wife, a religious teacher who was radicalized by him and wanted to go with him, has been placed on a restriction order (RO) for two years with her teaching accreditation suspended. Investigations revealed that Firdaus started being radicalized in 2016 when he went online to deepen his religious knowledge and was exposed to pro-ISIS content. Firdaus was convinced by early 2018 that ISIS was fighting for Islam and that its use of violence to create an Islamic caliphate was justified.

He also actively posted materials promoting ISIS and armed jihad on his social media accounts and even created an ISIS flag which he hung at home to show his loyalty to the group. He believed armed jihad, or struggle in the name of Islam, was compulsory for all able-bodied Muslim men.

Singapore Lone-Wolves of Terrorist

A sixteen-year-old Singaporean student has been detained under the Internal Security Act (ISA) for planning to attack two mosques and kill worshippers in Singapore on March 15, 2020 marks the second anniversary of the Christchurch terror attacks. A Protestant Christian of Indian ethnicity is the first detainee to be influenced by far-right extremist ideology and the youngest person detained under the ISA for terrorism-related activities to date, according to the Internal Security Department (ISD).[21] The student was found to have made detailed plans and preparations to conduct terrorist attacks using a machete against Muslims at two mosques. He had also watched Islamic State in Iraq and Syria (ISIS) propaganda videos and concluded that ISIS represented Islam and that Islam called on its followers to kill non-believers.

His original plan was to use a rifle similar to that used by Tarrant but gave up the idea only when he realized that it would be difficult to get his hands on one, given Singapore's strict gun-control laws. Similar to Tarrant, he had prepared two documents which he intended to disseminate before his attacks—one as a message to the people of France to stand against Muslims, and the second as an unfinished manifesto detailing his hatred for Islam.

The ISD said its investigation to date indicated that the youth had acted alone and that there was also no indication that he had tried to influence anyone with his extreme outlook or involve others in his attack plans. It was also reported that his immediate family and others in his social circles were not aware of his attack plans and the depth of his hatred for Islam. While it may be convenient to note that this teenager acted in isolation without being "noticed," it is more likely that the warning signs went unnoticed.

Similar to Tarrant, current society in this region is likely geared towards Islamic radicalization and a certain "profile" of a terrorist. The greater system (educators, family members, etc.) may have been ill-prepared to notice the cues, although social media, including the gaming community, could have contributed to reinforcing the detainee's indoctrination. Based on existing lone-wolf terrorist profiling research, the following needs to be considered:

1. Lone-wolves tend to create their own ideologies that combine personal vendettas with broader political or religious grievances. When did this process begin? Brenton Tarrant's process began at age twelve.[22]
2. Traditional terrorists do not suffer from any identifiable mental illness but lone-wolves are likely to suffer from some form of psychological disturbance. Was he suffering from any observable anxiety: abuse at home, bullying at school, etc.?
3. Was the detainee a loner? If so, when did it start?
4. As already been determined in this case, even though lone-wolves are by definition unaffiliated with a terrorist organization, they may identify or sympathize with extremists.
5. In terms of prevention, lone-wolf terrorism does not take place in a social vacuum. While lone-wolves may physically isolate themselves from society, at the same time they communicate with others through spoken and written statements (manifestos, for example).

   It is commonly assumed that lone-wolves have a critical advantage in avoiding detection before and after their attacks because most of them do not communicate with others regarding their intentions. On the contrary, it appears that they are doing precisely that but the "system" is slow in tracking these cues.

The case in Singapore demonstrates yet again that extreme ideas can find resonance and radicalize, regardless of race, gender, age, or religion.

Way Forward

Malaysia, Indonesia, the Philippines, Singapore, and ASEAN countries demonstrated their commitment to combat terrorism at the 3rd Sub-Regional Meeting on Counter-Terrorism and Transnational Security on December 1, 2020. The meeting explored two main issues: "The Impact of COVID-19 on the Counter-Terrorism and Transnational Security Environment" and "Foreign Terrorist Fighters (FTFs) Regional Preparedness." This is crucial as a June 2020 paper by the United Nations (UN) Counter-Terrorism Committee Executive Directorate assessed that restrictions on international travel due to COVID-19 could affect the movement of FTFs.

The paper also forewarned of the potential long-term impact of COVID-19 on national counter-terrorism budgets and international cooperation. These issues could create opportunities for FTFs who may be forced to adapt their travel methods. In Southeast Asia, FTFs could resort to more illicit travel by exploiting the seas. The archipelagic geography and high maritime traffic in Southeast Asia make border security a constant challenge. This challenge provides a conducive environment for the clandestine movement of people and goods. Illicit maritime activities are a longstanding problem in the region and might worsen over time. COVID-19 could affect maritime security measures such as coastal surveillance as states re-direct national resources to fight the pandemic.

The economic impact of COVID-19 could drive more disenfranchised people in coastal communities to resort to piracy to supplement their incomes. The risk of people becoming radicalized is also higher as they spend more time online due to movement restrictions. The Tri-Border Area[23] has also been in the spotlight for terrorist activities. INTERPOL led an operation codenamed "Maharlika III" from February to March 2020 based on intelligence on common routes that criminals and terrorists use to travel in the area. Apart from the Tri-Border area, the Straits of Malacca and Singapore is also another crucial sea line of communication, especially for cargo vessels.

The use of cargo vessels is one way that FTFs could adapt their travel methods. For example, in March 2020, the US Justice Department reported that Islamic State (ISIS) supporter Muhammad Masood attempted to travel to ISIS territory in Syria in part via a cargo vessel. Research indicates smuggling activities have been endemic in this waterway since as far back as the 1800s. In 2020, the Singapore Strait recorded a sharp increase in such incidents from 2019 to 2020, according to a recent report by the Regional Cooperation Agreement on Combating Piracy and Armed Robbery against Ships in Asia (ReCAAP). The rise in piracy incidents might be indicative of other illicit maritime activities, which could facilitate illicit travel.

The possibility of the COVID-19 virus slipping through border control measures is also a cause for concern as it is feared that illicit travel could be one of the means for terrorists to spread COVID-19 as an improvised tactic of a biological attack.

Notes

1 Retrieved   from   https://apnews.com/article/race-and-ethnicity-coronavirus -pandemic-united-nations-terrorism-united-states-71fe8fc4b22317609d8d9c1 31c297582
2 https://www.thesundaily.my/local/message-pertaining-terror-cell-members-in -sibu-bintulu-not-true-GJ874558
3 Malaysia detained four men in 2013 in its first Isis-linked arrest, a figure that increased to 82 in 2015 and peaked at 119 a year later. There were 106 people arrested in 2017 and 85 in 2018. Only 7 were detained in 2020.
4 https://www.channelnewsasia.com/news/asia/indonesia-terrorism-attack -recruitment-plot-COVID-19-bnpt-13959304
5 https://manilastandard.net/mobile/article/344618

6 Altogether, the Indonesian police in 2020 have arrested more than thirty militants linked to JI.
7 Retrieved from https://www.thestar.com.my/news/nation/2021/01/24/finally-in-the-dock-after-18-years
8 Retrieved from https://www.malaysiakini.com/news/314941
9 Retrieved from https://www.todayonline.com/world/msian-911-militant-yazid-sufaat-who-targeted-spore-released-johor-detention-centre
10 Retrieved from https://www.malaymail.com/news/malaysia/2021/02/17/malaysia-on-path-to-becoming-gangsters-paradise-senior-police-official-warn/1950414
11 Retrieved from https://journals.sagepub.com/doi/pdf/10.1177/1477370819828946
12 Retrieved from https://www.un.org/press/en/2020/sc14363.doc.htm
13 Retrieved from https://www.freemalaysiatoday.com/category/world/2021/02/02/missing-rohingya-trafficked-into-malaysia-from-indonesian-camp/
14 Retrieved from https://www.um.edu.mt/library/oar/bitstream/123456789/51831/4/19MCRMS007.pdf
15 Retrieved from https://www.lowyinstitute.org/the-interpreter/rohingyas-new-terrorist-threat
16 Retrieved from https://www.scmp.com/week-asia/geopolitics/article/3019396/militant-rohingya-group-raises-funds-malaysia-extorting-money
17 The Moro National Liberation Front (MNLF) is the oldest Islamic extremist group in the Philippines. It was established in 1971 to fight for an independent Muslim Mindanao. The Moro Islamic Liberation Front (MILF) which split from the MNLF in 1978 to pursue a more Islam-focused agenda in conjunction with the quest for Moro independence supplanted the MNLF as the primary organization conducting negotiations with the Philippine government for a Muslim autonomous region.
18 ISIS-Philippines was instrumental in orchestrating the siege of Marawi in 2017, and ISIS-affiliated militants managed to capture the city at the outset of the battle. Despite its eventual defeat in Marawi at the hands of the Philippine military, ISIS spun its initial victory to its advantage, featuring the battle heavily in its recruitment propaganda.
19 The NPA was the most active terrorist organization in the Philippines and was responsible for over 35 percent of deaths and 38 percent of terror-related incidents in 2019, at 98 and 132, respectively.
20 Retrieved from https://www.straitstimes.com/singapore/radicalised-malaysian-cleaner-held-and-deported
21 Retrieved from https://www.straitstimes.com/singapore/16-year-old-detained-under-isa-for-planning-terrorist-attacks-at-two-mosques-in-singapore
22 Retrieved from https://www.rnz.co.nz/news/national/432610/christchurch-gunman-s-racist-views-traced-to-when-he-was-12-report
23 Comprising the Sulu/Celebes seas between Indonesia, Malia, and the Philippines.

Bibliography

Abu Bakar Djalloh. (2020). Increased Terror Attacks in Africa Amid Coronavirus Pandemic. Retrieved on the 10th of April 2020 from: https://www.dw.com/en/increased-terror-attacks-in-africa-amid-coronavirus-pandemic/a-53066398
Adriana Rodriguez. (2020). These Countries Have No Reports on Coronavirus Cases. But Can They be Trusted? Retrieved on the 07th of May 2020 from: https://www

.usatoday.com/story/news/world/2020/05/06/COVID-19-which-countries -have-no-coronavirus-cases/3076741001/

Ali, K. A. M. (2008). Aspek Kualiti, Keselamatan Dan Kesihatan di Kalangan PKS Makanan: Satu Sorotan Kajian. *Jurnal Teknologi* 49(1).

Aslam, M. M. (2005). Asian and Globalization: An Analysis from Tun Mahathir's Perspectives. Paper presented at the International Conference of Asian Scholars. Shanghai.

Aslam, M. M. (2008). Operational and Ideological Challenges in Islamic Militancy in Malaysia: The Case of Kumpulan Militan Malaysia (KMM). In Md Yatim Othman (Ed.), *Malaysia in Various Issues: A Collection of Essays.* New Zealand: Victoria University of Wellington.

Aslam, M. M. (2009). A Critical Study of Kumpulan Militan Malaysia, its Wider Connections in the Region and the Mplications of Radical Islam for the Stability of South East Asia. (Ph.D Thesis), Victoria University of Wellington, New Zealand.

Aslam, M. M. (2016). Drugs and Cross Border Terrorism. Keynote Paper Presented at the 1st International Joint Conference on Drugs, Social Sciences and Technology (DRUGSTECH), 30–31st October 2016. Universitas Ubudiah Indonesia, Banda Acheh, Indonesia.

Aslam, M. M. (2019a). *Cross Border Terrorism in Terrorist Rehabilitation and Community Engagement di Malaysia and Southeast Asia.* London: Routledge.

Aslam, M. M. (2019b). *Artificial Intelligence (AI) Belum Cukup Bagus. Special Column in Harian Metro, 13th June 2019.* Kuala Lumpur: Media Prima.

Aslam, M. M. (2020). Pemahaman Agama Ketika Wabak. Terbitan Malaysiakini pada 11 April 2020. Dilayari pada 11 April 2020 di laman sesawang. https://www .malaysiakini.com/columns/520063

BBC News. (2019). Venezuela Crisis: Maduro Warns of Civil War. Retrieved on the 03rd of May 2020 from: https://www.bbc.com/news/world-latin-america -47112284

Chu, K. Y., & Gupta, S. (1998). *Social Safety Nets: Issues and Recent Experiences.* Washington, DC: IMF.

Damin, Z. A. B. (2016). Dasar Kerajaan dan Isu Makanan di Malaysia. Tesis PhD. Perpustakaan UUM.

Daniel De Simone. (2020). Sudesh Amman: Who Was the Streatham Attacker. Retrieved on the 03rd of March 2020 from: https://www.bbc.com/news/uk -51351885

Daud, S. et.al. (2020). *Pelan Tindakan Majlis Tindakan Kos Sara Hidup Negara, 2019–2022.* Putrajaya: KPDNHEP.

Daud, S. (2020). *Dasar Pembangunan dan Populisme di Malaysia.* Bangi: Penerbit UKM.

Dharvi, V. (2020). COVID-19 Crisis Prolongs Kashmir Lockdown. Retrieved on the 13th of April 2020 from: https://www.dw.com/en/COVID-19-crisis-prolongs -kashmir-lockdown/a-53088317

DW. (2020). IS Takes Advantage of Coronavirus to Ramp Up Attacks in Iraq & Syria. Retrieved on the 06th of May 2020 from: https://www.dw.com/en/is -takes-advantage-of-coronavirus-to-ramp-up-attacks-in-iraq-syria/a-53321781

Ghebreyesus, T. A. (2020, 13 April). WHO Director-General's Opening Remark at the Media Briefing of COVID-19 – 13 April 2020. Diakses daripada laman web World Health Organization: https://www.who.int/dg/speeches/detail/who

-director-general-s-opening-remarks-at-the-media-briefing-on-COVID-19--13 -april-2020 pada 3 Mei 2020.

Global Humanitarian Response Plan, April–December 2020. United Nation Coordinated Appeal April–December 2020.

Gunaratna, G., Jerard. J., & Rubin, L. (2011). *Terrorist Rehabilitation and Counter-Radicalisation.* London: Routledge.

Gunaratna, R. (2015). Global Threat Assessment: A New Threat on the Horizon? Counter Terrorist Trend and Analysis. *A Journal of International Centre for Political Violence and Terrorism Research*, S. Rajaratnam School of International Studies, 7(1), January/February 2015, 5.

Gunaratna, R. (2018). Counterterrorism: ASEAN Militaries' Growing Role – Analysis. *RSIS Commentaries.* March 14. Retrieved on the 01st of June 2018 from https://www.rsis.edu.sg/wp-content/uploads/2018/03/CO18042.pdf.

Gunaratna, R., & Ali, M. (2014). *Terrorist Rehabilitation: A New Frontier In Counter-terrorism.* London: Imperial College Press.

Hechter, M. (1992). The Dynamics of Seccession. *Acta: Socioogica*, 35: 267–83.

Idris Okuducu. (2020). DAESH/ISIS Increases Attacks in Iraq Amid Virus. Retrieved on the 11th of May 2020 from https://www.aa.com.tr/en/middle-east/daesh-isis-increases-attacks-in-iraq-amid-virus/1832517

Interview with Perlis Special Branch Director, Royal Malaysia Police. Dated: 06th of May 2020.

Interview with Yemen's Ambassador. Dated: 13th of April 2020.

Interview with Yemen's Ambassador. Dated: 28th of August 2018.

Kalbana, P., & Chan, D. (2020, 2 Mei). A Longer Wait Could Have Resulted in More Losses in Revenue. New Straits Times. Retrieved on the 03rd of May 2020 from: https://www.nst.com.my/news/nation/2020/05/589227/longer-wait-could-have-resulted-more-losses-revenue pada 2 Mei 2020

Katjuscia, M. (2012). *Inter Internal colonialism in Western Europe: The Case of Sardinia.* Barcelona: University of Barcelona Press.

Kementerian Kesihatan Malaysia. (2020). Malaysia Memulakan Kajiselidik Solidariti Global. Retrieved on the 15th of April 2020 from: http://www.moh.gov.my/index.php/database_stores/store_view_page/21/1425

Kementerian Kewangan. (2020). Laporan Laksana Ketiga: Pelaksanaan Pakej Prihatin Rakyat. Dilayari pada 25 April 2020 dari laman sesawang: https://www.treasury .gov.my/pdf/Teks-Ucapan-Laporan-LAKSANA-PRIHATIN-Ketiga.pdf

Kementerian Pertahanan. (2020). Kekang PATI, Keselamatan Negara Terus Diperketat, Kawal Pendatang. Dilayari pada 27 April 2020 dari laman sesawang: http://www.mod.gov.my/ms/mediamenu/berita/701-kekang-pati-kawalan-sempadan-negara-terus-diperketat-diperhebat

Kementerian Pertanian. (2020). Bekalan Makanan Negara Mencukupi. Dilayari pada 13 Aril 2020 dari laman sesawang: https://www.moa.gov.my/documents /20182/197571/Bekalan+Makanan+Negara+Konsisten+dan+Mencukupi.pdf /78833140-e787-4751-8b21-586cfef7f5e8

Koya, Z. (2020, 2 Mei). Be Prepared to Live with COVID-19 for the Next Two Years, Says Dr Jemilah. Diakses daripada laman web The Star: https://thestar .com.my/news/nation/2020/05/02/be-prepared-to-live-with-COVID-19-for -the-next-two-years-says-dr-jemilah pada 2 Mei 2020.

Kruglanski, A., Belanger, J., & Gunaratna, R. (2019). *Three Pillars of Radicalization: Needs, Narratives & Networks.* Oxford: Oxford University Press.

Mat, B., Othman, Z., & Omar, M. K. (2018). Anjakan Paradigma dalam Kajian Keselamatan Insan di Asia Tenggara. *Akademika* 88(1): 193–207.

McCarthy, N. (2020). COVID-19 Death Toll Surpasses Vietnam War. Retrieved on the 01st of May 2020 from: https://www.statista.com/chart/21545/deaths-from-the-coronavirus-and-vietnam-war/

Ross, P. (2020). Why Do New Disease Outbreak Always Seems to Starts in China? Retrieved on the 12th of April 2020 from: https://www.realclearscience.com/blog/2020/02/18/why_do_new_disease_outbreaks_always_seem_to_start_in_china.html

Samad, J. (2020). COVID-19: The New National Security Threat. Retrieved on the 01st of April 2020 from: https://www.freemalaysiatoday.com/category/opinion/2020/03/31/COVID-19-the-new-national-security-threat/

Shafie, N. S. M. (2014). Kajian tahap penilaian amalan keselamatan makanan di premis makanan sekitar alam mesra Kota Kinabalu. Universiti Malaysia Sabah. http://eprints.ums.edu.my/14674/(Unpublished).

Shamsudin, M. N. (2016). Urban Agriculture: A Way Forward to Food and Nutrition Security in Malaysia. *Procedia - Social and Behavioral Sciences*, 216·January.

Stanislaus, R., Amy, Y. S., & Benny, J. M. (2020). Collaborative Governance in Terrorist Rehabilitation Program in Indonesia. Concept Paper for book proposal by Aslam, M.M. & Gunaratna, R.

Suhor, S., Yusoff, S. S., Ismail, R., Aziz, A. A., Razman, M. R., & Talib, K. A. (2014). Kesihatan dan Keselamatan Makanan: Kesedaran Pengguna dan Peruntukan Perundangan Kanun. Disember.

Tamburino, L., Bravo, G., Clough, Y., & Nicholas, K. A. (2020). From Population to Production: 50 Years of Scientific Literature on How to Feed the World. Elsevier Sciencedirect. March. https://www.sciencedirect.com/science/article/pii/S2211912419301798.

United Nation. (2020). Update on the Secretary General's Appeal for Global Ceasefire. Retrieved on the 10th of April 2020 from: file:///Users/mariyani/Downloads/Update%20on%20SG%20Appeal%20for%20Ceasefire,%20April%2020 20%20(2).pdf

Veena, B. (2020, 2 Mei). Do it in Stages, Say Health Expert. Diakses daripada laman web New Straits Times. https://www.nst.com.my/news/nation/2020/05/589215/do-it-stages-say-health-expert pada 2 Mei 2020.

Waxman, O., & Wilson, C. (2020). How the Coronavirus Death Toll Compares to Other Deadly Events From American History. Retrieved on the 30th of April 2020 from: https://time.com/5815367/coronavirus-deaths-comparison/

William, C. D. (2006). *Lone Star Rising*. Texas: A&M University Press.

Yassin, M. M. (2020, 1 Mei). Teks Perutusan Khas YAB Tan Sri Dato' Haji Muhyiddin bin Haji Mohd Yassin, Perdana Menteri Malaysia sempena Hari Pekerja. Putrajaya: Pejabat Perdana Menteri.

2 COVID-19

Threat and Response in Sri Lanka

Kapila Jayaratne, Vajira Dissanayake, and Palitha Karunapema

Introduction

Sri Lanka is a middle-income island country located at the southern tip of the Indian subcontinent with a population of 21.4 million (Figure 2.1). The country boasts a high human development index. It also claims impressive health indices with low maternal mortality (32 per 100,000 live births) and infant mortality (8.2 per 1000 live births) (Central Bank of Sri Lanka 2019). Sri Lanka has a well-organized public health system covering each household of the country. A hierarchy of public health personnel originating at the grassroot level and extending up to the higher administrative level operates, providing essential public health services including disease prevention and control. A western-qualified medical doctor is reachable within a 5 kilometer radius of any household. Similarly, a network of eighty-seven tertiary care hospitals manned by different clinical specialists and equipped with intensive care facilities are located throughout the island (Fernando 2000, Ministry of Health 2018).

Progression of COVID-19 in the Country

The first local case of COVID-19 was identified in Sri Lanka on March 11, 2020. The patient was a foreign tour guide. Figure 2.2 illustrates the progression of the epidemic in the country since then.

The epigraph of COVID-19 cases shows three peaks; a community cluster in April 2020, an outbreak in a navy camp in May, and a much larger outbreak in a drug addicts rehabilitation center in July.

As of August 31, 2020, there were 3,012 real-time PCR confirmed cases—both asymptomatic and symptomatic, 2,868 recovered patients, and 132 active cases with 12 deaths. All cases encountered at the time were imported cases (returnees from other countries) (Figure 2.3). The last local case was detected on August 3, 2020. At present, the country has more or less successfully flattened the curve with only reporting of sporadic imported cases.

The Response

With the reporting of the first local case in early March 2020, realizing the need for urgent and aggressive action, the health and non-health authorities executed

DOI: 10.4324/9781003291909-3

Population	: 21.8 Million
Total Area	: 65610 Sq Km
GDP	: 4079 USD
Poverty Head Count Index	: 8.9%
Literacy	: 92.5%
Education enrolment	: 96.3%
Human Development Index	: 0.780
Life Expectancy	: 75.5 years
Access to safe water	: 91.9%
Persons per doctor	: 1203

Figure 2.1 Country Profile—Sri Lanka. Source: Author, collected from various sources.

a cascade of measures. Figure 2.4 depicts some of the initial key interventions implemented in relation to the reported cumulative number of cases over time.

The three main response strategies that could be adopted at country level in a pandemic of this nature include—totally containing the outbreak at a very early stage, flattening the curve, and raising health system capacity (WHO 2020). Sri Lanka's strategy was to "flatten the curve." Every effort was made to prevent the progression of the disease to community transmission, since it would be very

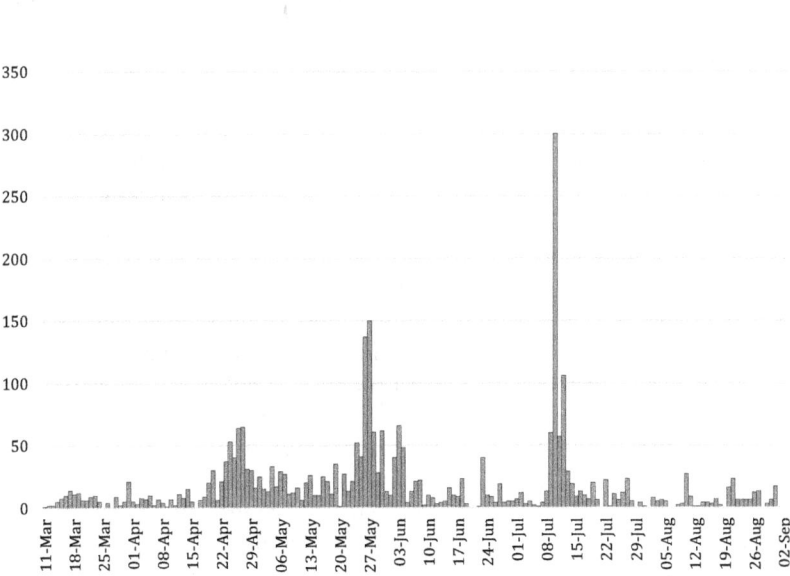

Figure 2.2 Epigraph of COVID-19 Cases in Sri Lanka. Source: Author, collected from various sources.

```
Imported Cases (Returnees from other countries)
Foreigners      - 40
Sri Lankans     - 1079

Local Cases
Navy Camp cluster & their close contacts        - 950
Kandakadu cluster & their close contacts        - 630
Others                              - 313
Total Number Confirmed              - 3012
Total Number Recovered                      - 2868
Total Number of Deaths                      - 12
Active cases                        - 132
```

Figure 2.3 Sri Lanka COVID-19 Situation Report—August 31, 2020. Source: Author, collected from various sources.

difficult to stop the exponential increase of cases once community transmission occurs (Jayaratne et al 2020a).

Sri Lanka strategically implemented many key interventions far ahead of other countries. The key pillar, country-level coordination, planning, and monitoring, was at its maximum. A unified and effective command system was put in place by setting up a National COVID-19 Task Force even before a single death was reported. This was done with strong political leadership provided by the President, the Prime Minister, and the Minister of Health. The National COVID-19 Task Force included the Minister of Health, the Director General of Health Services, and the Army Commander who gave strategic operational leadership and other key health and non-health stakeholders. The effort was facilitated by the strict enforcement of the quarantine act backed by development and implementation of local health guidelines to cover all aspects of the response ranging from social distancing and other public health measures, to early detection, early reporting, contract tracing, self-isolation, quarantine, case definition, real-time PCR testing, case management, disposal of dead bodies, health education, and social mobilization. The health response was backed by the law enforcement agencies, including the state intelligence services, that enabled rapid identification and quarantining of contacts. Sri Lanka was one of the few countries that successfully utilized technical support from the National Intelligence Services to assist in identifying second and third contacts of confirmed COVID-19 cases (Maddumage 2020). When a COVID-19 positive case was found, the health and law enforcement authorities worked in coordination to control cluster formation and prevent community transmission.

Epidemiological surveillance played a critical role in the country's effective pandemic response. The Epidemiology Unit of the Ministry of Health is the national focal point for communicable disease control and prevention in the country. National-level surveillance capacity was intensified by mobilizing the entire

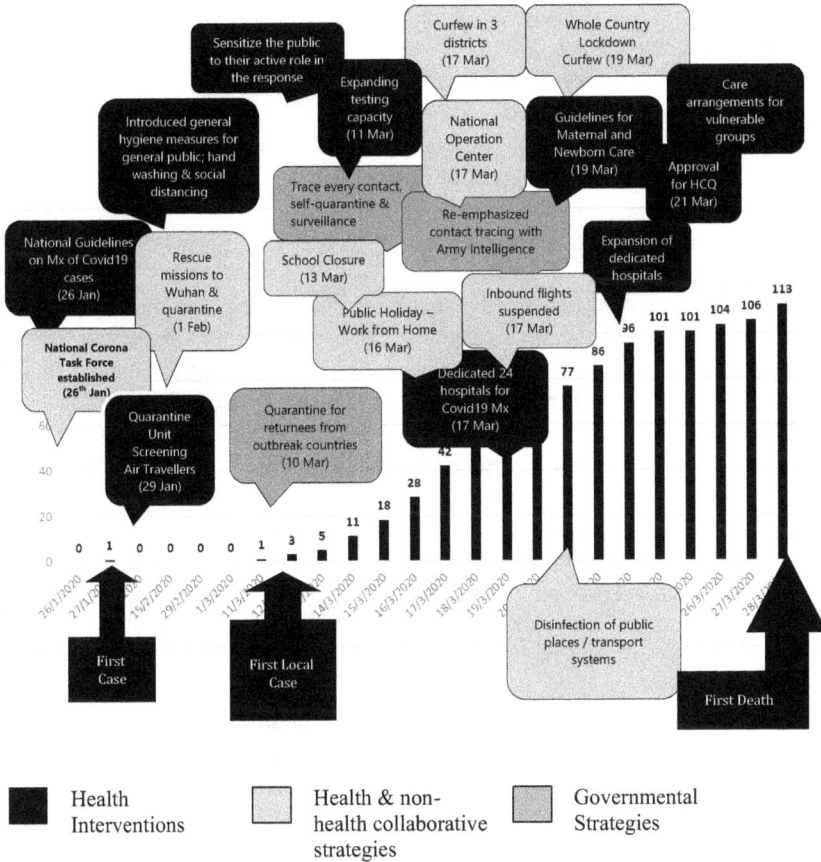

Figure 2.4 Cumulative Number of Cases and Key Interventions. Source: Author.

force of the Epidemiology Unit for active surveillance. The already established National Influenza Pandemic Preparedness Plan (Epidemiology Unit 2012) was activated immediately to provide a coordinated and effective national response in the event of an influenza pandemic in the country. Standard Operational Procedures were formulated with expert involvement. Active case search, contact tracing, and follow-up for early case detection were coordinated through an Emergency Operation Cell established at the Epidemiology Unit. The network of regional epidemiologists based in all health districts was guided through an effective communication system to ensure a flawless liaison. The Epidemiology Unit under the guidance of the administrative hierarchy of the Ministry of Health maintained its activities in monitoring and evaluating and its role of advocacy to contain the epidemic from progressing into a community transmission stage (Widanapathirana et al 2020).

Another prominent modality was the well-organized quarantining process. Initially, the tri forces—Army, Navy, and Air Force—maintained 58 quarantine centers to accommodate 3,000 people. This was later expanded to seventy-two centers. Overseas returnees were also offered "pay and stay" hotels. In combination, quarantine centers catered to more than 10,000 people. Special quarantine centers were established for healthcare workers and other categories in operation for COVID-19 cases (Prathapan & Arambepola 2020).

The country also had its Chemical, Biological, Radioactive, and Nuclear (CBRN) preparedness and response strengthened by improving the Disaster Management Centre.

Identification of cases depended on real-time PCR testing. Ramping up country-level testing capacity has been a challenge for all countries. Sri Lanka was one of the first countries in the region to focus on increasing testing capacity. That resulted in the establishment of a central real-time PCR testing laboratory for COVID-19 at the Medical Research Institute in Colombo. The laboratory was amply supported by the Department of Microbiology of the Faculty of Medical Sciences, University of Sri Jayewardenepura that deployed its full capacity to support the national testing effort. Today there is a network of nearly thirty laboratories, ranging from laboratories in hospitals in the Ministry of Health, Medical Faculties in Universities, to private hospitals that are capable of fulfilling the entire testing demand of the country. In addition, a laboratory established at the international airport at Katunayake in August 2020 provided rapid testing for passengers entering the country and facilitated the opening of the airport for incoming passengers.

All suspected cases fitting into case definitions were transferred by ambulance to the closest designated hospital for confirmatory testing and management. Country-wide operative Suwaseriya Ambulance Network was deployed to transport COVID-19 suspected patients to designated COVID-19 hospitals. A unique feature of Sri Lanka's response was that when a person was found to be real-time PCR positive, irrespective of whether the person was symptomatic or asymptomatic, that person was admitted to a designated COVID-19 treatment hospital. This required rapid scaling up of treatment capacity. The main infectious disease hospital—the National Institute for Infectious Diseases at Angoda near Colombo—and several other hospitals were designated to treat COVID-19 patients. A separate hospital was designated to care for pregnant women suspected of COVID-19. Expanding treatment facilities including intensive care capacity and mobilization of health staff meaningfully with all safety measures were done with coordination at the highest level. All treatments were provided free of charge.

One of the key measures in Sri Lanka's response was the quarantine process implemented flawlessly by the public health teams and armed forces. Once a case was identified, the public health teams backed by the law enforcement agencies responded rapidly to ensure that all contacts were identified, real-time PCR tested, and isolated either at home or in quarantine centers. This included enforcing strict lockdowns in certain areas and evacuating residents to quarantine centers when they failed to comply.

Maintenance of healthcare services without interruption was high on the agenda of the response. A well-thought plan was implemented to provide services to non–COVID-19 patients in the government sector. Caregivers were trained on safety measures, given personal protective equipment, and a risk-free patient and caregiver interphase was created.

Highly vulnerable populations amidst this type of a pandemic are pregnant women and children. Maintenance of normal Maternal and Child Health (MCH) services was a challenge. Family Health Bureau, the focal point of the Ministry of Health for MCH, formulated and circulated evidence-based interim guidelines on the implementation of the essential services related to MCH for both curative and preventive settings following the reporting of the first local case in the country. Actions were taken to establish maternal and newborn care facilities in the isolation centers of designated hospitals for COVID-19. Instructions were given to relevant regional-level health staff on the provision of domiciliary care, field clinic care, referral criteria for specialized care, protective measures, managing logistics, and creating community awareness. Site visits were carried out to assess the ground situation of curative care for pregnant mothers who are suspected and confirmed with COVID-19 with the collaboration of experts in clinical specialties. Telephone interviews were conducted among disadvantaged pregnant and postpartum mothers to enable uninterrupted services. Pregnant mothers were allowed to use their pregnancy record as a curfew pass for traveling during the lockdown period (De Silva et al 2020).

The deployment of digital tools facilitated continuing care for non–COVID-19 patients. The ministry of health launched its own app—My Health Sri Lanka—and other tele-health services that provided tele-health connectivity to patients with doctors, hospitals, and pharmacies and delivery of medicines to homes of patients with chronic disorders who needed continuous supply of medicines. At hospital levels too, there was quick improvisation and adoption of digital technologies to ensure the safety of patients and healthcare workers and continuity of care for all patients. Only a few healthcare workers contracted the disease, and there were no fatalities among healthcare workers.

Risk Communication

The country identified the importance of an effective risk communication modality to ensure the trust of people, credibility, and transparency of information on controlling COVID-19 well ahead of reporting of the first patient in Sri Lanka. A larger chunk of the credit of success of Sri Lanka's COVID-19 control goes to efficiently launched risk communication strategy. Risk communication involves the exchange of real-time information, advice, and opinions between experts and the general public facing threats to their health, economic, or social well-being. Such a mechanism will empower communities at risk to take informed decisions to safeguard themselves and their relatives (WHO 2017, WHO 2019).

The Health Promotion Bureau (HPB), as the focal point of risk communication in the country, formulated a risk communication plan. The plan covered strategies for each stage of transmission; preparation and initial response phase of risk communication targeted for zero cases/few sporadic cases, crisis communication for cluster transmission stage with lockdown status, and cluster transmission stage with a gradual exit from lockdown as a guide for action. HPB also revamped and strengthened the already established rumor monitoring, reporting, verification, and mitigation systems.

Liaising with Government Information Department opened a gateway to government media and all mass media networks. A social media network including an official Facebook page with blue tick verification and the HPB's official trilingual website were capitalized to convey messages. Behavior changes were targeted at different settings at the community level, e.g., village, hospital, workplace, school, preschool. The preparedness and response activities in the risk communication system were continuously updated and optimized according to community feedback through behavior surveillance and public response (Ranasinghe et al 2020).

Maintaining the Psychological Well-Being

Psychological impacts on entire strata of the general public due to an epidemic of this nature are immense: Fear of infection and losing loved ones, restricted movements, confined to home, staying quarantined, prolonged curfew with social isolation, losing livelihood, closure of schools, and social stigma are the main psychosocial issues (Inter-Agency Standing Committee 2020). The Directorate of Mental Health in the Ministry of Health took steps to integrate Mental Health and Psycho-Social Support within the country's COVID-19 response. Collaborations were maintained to provide psychological support for defined target audiences with several government and non-government key stakeholders (Wickramasinghe et al. 2020).

Non-Health Measures

The non-health measures contributed to the success were the early closure of entry points to the country; closure of schools, training centers, and universities; and an early strong lockdown strategy which resulted in the imposition of an island-wide curfew for the most part of the month of March 2020 and the entire month of April 2020. The police were strict in checking compliance with the curfew and legal action was taken against curfew violators. In addition, social distancing measures as well as wearing face masks were made compulsory. The compliance of the general public with social distancing measures, wearing face masks and the curfew was at a very high level. Inter-district movement was also restricted. There were people-friendly intermittent relaxations of the curfew.

The curfew necessitated work-from-home protocols for both government and private sectors. Online education programs were introduced. The mobile operators in the country provided strong support for these measures by introducing low-cost data packages that facilitated rapid adoption of online working and online learning.

Measures were taken to strengthen supportive mechanisms such as the availability of food and essential medicines, economic packages for all sectors affected, and special care for financially vulnerable families. In short, both the health services and social services were mobilized to respond to the special situation.

With the emergence of a cluster from a Navy base, the President appointed a Special Presidential Task Force (PTF) to ensure health security at military camps in April 2020. This was for the purpose of taking prompt and swift measures to prevent the transmission of Coronavirus among the tri forces in Sri Lanka. Detailed instructions and guidelines were sent to all service commanders regarding the prevention of the pandemic. Members of the PTF visited inspecting military establishments of tri forces and ensured that such sites were complying with already issued health safety measures on the prevention of COVID-19 epidemic.

All these non-health measures were backed by a strong media campaign that was launched with the objective of educating the general public for better compliance. Print and electronic media strongly supported the health and law enforcement authorities to ensure that their messages reached the public.

The Exit Strategy

As Sri Lanka came out of the lockdown, the focus was on a smooth and effective exit strategy that could be implemented in a staggered manner taking into consideration the evolving dynamics of the epidemic. The objectives of the strategy were maintaining the caseload well below the country's health system capacity, returning to near normal public life, and economic recovery. To facilitate this, the Ministry of Health issued guidelines covering almost all sectors and all aspects of public life. Implementation of the guidelines and adherence to them were strictly monitored (Jayaratne et al 2020b). The curfew was relaxed gradually over two months after assessment on the risk level of each district, but a night-time curfew was maintained across the island much longer till late June 2020 when it was lifted completely.

In the first phase, government and private sector offices were reopened with half the staff and at different time intervals. Public transport systems were started while restricting inter-district movement. People were allowed to go out of their home only for pre-identified requirements and on designated days of the week based on their national identity card number. Hospitals were reopened and community health services such as immunization programs were resumed. The universities opened for examinations and schools were opened for higher grades.

The government was under public pressure for repatriation of Sri Lankans stranded in overseas countries. Repatriation flights began to operate in late April 2020. There were about 48,000 persons requesting repatriation and so far, more than 30,000 persons have been repatriated.

The scheduled parliamentary elections had to be postponed indefinitely due to the COVID-19 outbreak just after obtaining nominations in mid-March 2020. A special challenge as Sri Lanka came out of the lockdown was the need to conduct the general elections. The health and the elections authorities coordinated their efforts at the highest level to ensure that all health safety measures were maintained. The elections were successfully conducted on August 5, 2020.

Challenges

The response was not without any challenges. The main challenges encountered were: initial difficulties in logistics supply for real-time PCR testing; communities with irresponsible behavior not complying with guidelines; conflicting messages on wearing face masks; food supply chain management in the early days of the lockdown due to sudden imposition of the curfews; financial difficulties faced by the daily-waged labor force; compromised care for the non–COVID-19 patients; controversy over disposal of dead bodies due to cultural sensitivities of different ethnic groups; unexpected clusters originating from a navy camp and a rehabilitation center with an exponential increase of cases; and the continuous influx of imported cases. Being located next to India, which is currently reporting the second largest outbreak in the world, Sri Lanka should not underestimate its very high vulnerability for frequent waves of COVID-19.

The Current Situation

The day-to-day life in the country has returned to normalcy, more than a month has passed since the last case was detected in the country. All cases reported now are those detected at the airport or on ships. Therefore, strict measures are in place now to prevent reintroduction of COVID-19 to the country. All those arriving in the country through both airports and harbors are tested by real-time PCR on arrival and 5 days after arrival. They also have to undergo 14 days of mandatory quarantine at a designated quarantine center followed by 14 days of mandatory self-isolation at home and be certified by public health authorities prior to integration into society. However, the threat is not yet over. Potential for a community leak of COVID-19 exists from returnees from overseas, attending staff at airlines and airports, army personnel handling the quarantine process and quarantine center or hotel staff caring for returnees. A solid surveillance system is needed for the rapid and early detection of COVID-19 cases among overseas returnees and to prevent any spill over that may lead to community transmission. The existing, severe acute respiratory infection (SARI) and Influenza-like illness (ILI) surveillance has been expanded to capture COVID-19 cases as well. The Epidemiology Unit of the Ministry of Health, Sri Lanka Army and supporting triforces and State Intelligence Services are in full alert to avert a possible leakage.

Summary

This manuscript was aimed at documenting some of the essential elements of Sri Lanka's response to the COVID-19 pandemic. It is safe to say that Sri Lanka has come out strongly through its response to the COVID-19 pandemic during the past few months baring for the economic fallout. Sri Lanka's success so far lies on the reliance on suppression of the pandemic curve by implementing multi-faceted, multi-stakeholder, and society-oriented strategies with leadership from health and law enforcement authorities backed by the highest level of political commitment. Sri Lanka has also shown that the basic public health measures and technology were both vital to face a situation such as this. The country has reaped the benefits of its long-standing investment and reliance on a strong system of public health coupled with the appropriate use of modern technology in its response to the COVID-19 pandemic. Strong high-level political will, top-down approach, and judicious interventions contributed to controlling the virus on the island.

References

Central Bank of Sri Lanka, Annual Report, 2019. Retrieved on Sept, 9th 2020 from: https://www.cbsl.gov.lk/en/publications/economic-and-financial-reports/annual-reports/annual-report-2019

De Silva C, Batuwanthudawe R, Lokubalasooriya A et al, 2020. Continuing Maternal and Child Health (MCH) Services During COVID-19: Activities, Challenges and the Lessons Learnt. *Journal of the College of Community Physicians of Sri Lanka*, 2020, 26 (Special Edition on COVID-19).

Epidemiology Unit, Ministry of Health, Sri Lanka 2020, Coronavirus (COVID-19) Sri Lanka - Analytics Dashboard. Retrieved on Jan, 7th 2022 from: https://covid.iq.lk/, https://www.epid.gov.lk/web/

Epidemiology Unit. National Influenza Pandemic Preparedness Plan - 2012. Epidemiology Unit, Ministry of Health. Retrieved on Sept, 02nd 2020 from: https://www.epid.gov.lk/web/images/pdf/ Influenza/completed_nipp_2013-03-20.pdf

Fernando, D, 2000. An overview of Sri Lanka's Healthcare System. *Journal of Public Health*, 22(1), 14–20.

Inter-Agency Standing Committee, 2020. *Interim Briefing Note Addressing Mental Health and Psychosocial Aspects of COVID-19 Outbreak*. Retrieved on Sept, 02nd 2020 from: https://interagencystandingcommittee.org/iasc-reference-group-mental-health-and-psychosocial-support-emergency-settings/interim-briefing.

Jayaratne K, Arambepola C, Prathapan S et al, 2020a. Flattening the Epidemic Curve of COVID –19 in Sri Lanka: The Public Health Response. *Journal of the College of Community Physicians of Sri Lanka*, 26(1), 56. 10.4038/jccpsl.v26i1.8311

Jayaratne K, Arambepola C, Prathapan S et al, 2020b. Exit Strategy of COVID-19 Epidemic in Sri Lanka: Recommendations of the College of Community Physicians of Sri Lanka. *Journal of the College of Community Physicians of Sri Lanka*, 2020, 26 (Special Edition on COVID-19).

Maddumage KS, 2020. Lines of Operation of the Military, Police and State Intelligence. *Journal of the College of Community Physicians of Sri Lanka*, 1; Nov 2020.

Ministry of Health—Sri Lanka, Annual Health Statistics 2018. Retrieved on Sept, 02nd 2020 from: http://www.health.gov.lk/moh_final/english/public/elfinder/files/publications/AHB/2020/Final%20AHS%202018.pdf

Ranasinghe PD, Karunapema P, Balasingham S and Gunathilaka N, 2020. Response to COVID-19 Through Risk Communication: Sri Lankan Experience. *Journal of the College of Community Physicians of Sri Lanka*, 2020, 26 (Special Edition on COVID-19).

Wickramasinghe EP, Ratnayake R and Ellawala Y, 2020. Mental Health and Psychosocial Support Response in Sri Lanka During Pandemic COVID-19. *Journal of the College of Community Physicians of Sri Lanka*, 2020, 26 (Special Edition on COVID-19).

Widanapathirana N, Gamage D, Hemachandra C et al, 2020. Facing up to COVID-19: Role of the Epidemiology Unit in Surveillance During the Outbreak Response in Sri Lanka. *Journal of the College of Community Physicians of Sri Lanka*, 2020, 26 (Special Edition on COVID-19).

World Health Organization (WHO), 2017. *Communicating Risk in Public Health Emergencies: A WHO Guideline for Emergency Risk Communication (ERC) Policy and Practice*. Geneva: WHO. Retrieved from: https://www.who.int/risk-communication/guidance/download/en/.

World Health Organization (WHO), 2019. *Risk Communication Strategy for Public Health Emergencies in the WHO South-East Asia Region: 2019–2023*. New Delhi: Regional Office for South-East Asia.

World Health Organization (WHO), 2020. *Covid19 Strategy Update*. Geneva: WHO.

3 COVID-19 in Pakistan

Challenges and Responses

Khuram Iqbal

Introduction

During the formative years of security studies (SS), the discipline was dominated by a singular focus on causes and prevention of war. The traditional approach towards security was state centric and only considered the response to threat against the military and political survival of state.[1] A paradigm shift occurred in the immediate aftermath of the Second World War when intellectual capital was dedicated to answering more specific and technical questions such as nuclear proliferation and avenues of conflict and cooperation between the Capitalist and Socialist blocks. But as the Cold War ended in 1989–1990, a new debate started within security studies' scholars and practitioners about the nature of security. The proponents of non-traditional security advocated for a more comprehensive definition of security to look beyond the threats emanating from non-military sources such as environmental degradation, famines, poverty, water scarcity, societal issues, natural calamities, and public health hazards.[2]

The non-traditional approach towards security was pioneered by Barry Buzan and the Copenhagen School of security studies. They defined security as "freedom from threat and the ability of states and societies to maintain their independent identity and their functional integrity against forces of change which they see as hostile," while such threats that "warrant emergency action and exceptional measures, including the use of force" are considered as security threats.[3] Another non-traditional definition of security, termed as "human security" by the United Nations Development Programme (UNDP) in its Human Development Report 1994, is "It means, first, safety from such chronic threats as hunger, disease and repression. And second, it means protection from sudden and hurtful disruptions in the patterns of daily life-whether in homes, in jobs or in communities."[4] The inclusion of economic, societal, environmental, and human concerns, apart from traditional military-political concerns, into the framework of security, is also sometimes termed comprehensive security.

As the world moved from an orthodox to a more inclusive and comprehensive approach to security, many countries in the third and developing world including Pakistan remained glued to the military aspect of security, committing little or no resources to other aspects of human and comprehensive security including public

DOI: 10.4324/9781003291909-4

health. In the recent history of the country, there has been an expansion of scope of national security and a range of internal security, political, and societal threats have also been securitized.[5] With the expansion of scope of national security, steps have been taken which suggest arrangements in the health sector so as to prevent any existential threat or emergency situation.

In April 2010, the national assembly of Pakistan passed the 18th Amendment to the Constitution of Pakistan. Among many other steps taken to decentralized power, resources, and issues, the operation and strategic planning for health was also made a provincial subject. The federal government only remained responsible for the coordination and regulation of health. In 2013, the Ministry of National Health Services, Regulation and Coordination (NHSRC) was created to oversee health services in the country. Consequently in 2016, the government of Pakistan announced a National Health Vision 2016–2025 which set the provision of universal healthcare access to affordable quality health services as its goal.

In 2015, Pakistan also volunteered to undergo Joint External Evaluation (JEE) by the World Health Organization (WHO) in order to achieve compliance with WHO International Health Regulations (2005). Pakistan was the first country to undergo JEE in WHO's Eastern Mediterranean region, and the fourth in the world. The JEE identified nineteen technical areas which required three to five priority actions in each area.[6] Consequently, a five-year National Action Plan for Health Security (NAPHS) was formed to work on the identified issue areas as well as to achieve the common goal of providing universal health care in accordance with National Health Vision.[7]

Pakistan has also worked on epidemiology and epidemic management with WHO with regard to seasonal dengue fever outbreaks, which intensified in the past few years and the most recent of which came in 2019. As per the requirements of International Health Regulations (2005), Pakistan kept reporting to WHO on the dengue outbreak, which had reached 52,485 patients and 91 deaths until December 2019. An Emergency Operations Center was created at National Institute of Health to monitor the situation of dengue outbreak on a daily basis which coordinated information with provinces, federation, and other support organizations like WHO.[8]

Despite these constitutional and institutional reforms, Pakistan's response to public health hazards remained unmethodical. Take for instance the government's response to the H1N1 (Swine Flu) in 2010. Nishtar concluded that due to the lack of epidemiological surveillance, a large number of viral cases went under-reported. Additionally, the ongoing counter-terrorism efforts, law and order situation, medical facilities in rural areas, and issues of energy security made effective transport of medicine and vaccines difficult. The study concluded Pakistan is vulnerable to systematic constraints and unprepared for pandemic management.[9] The state of epidemiology in Pakistan continues to deteriorate due to the state's under-investment in the public health sector. It was in this context that Pakistan was hit by the modern plague, known as COVID-19.

The Pandemic (Scaling the Threat)

The recent COVID-19 (also generally called coronavirus) pandemic has brought about a huge challenge to health security across the globe. Several countries around the globe have locked down to prevent the spread of infection. The global economy has seen a major slowdown and disruption of supply chains around the world. There have also been diverse societal and traditional security implications as well as impacts on the environment.

At the outset of the global pandemic, Pakistan faced hard choices as two of the country's four neighbors, China and Iran, were hit hardest by the virus. Due to geographic, cultural proximity, and economic interdependence, people-to-people contact among Pakistan, China, and Iran has always remained very high, thus increasing the risk of imported infections manifolds. Pakistan was reported on February 26, 2020, after the twenty-two-year-old Yahya Jaffry was reported positive after his return from a pilgrimage in Iran.

The total number of infections did not exceed 100 until March 15, 2020,[10] with most of the infections emerging among Pakistanis returning from Iran, Saudi Arabia, Europe, and America. However, during the month of April, the number of outside infected cases fell down and a trajectory of local infection transmission started. By the time of writing of this chapter, the total number of confirmed cases stood at 116,189, out of which 1,433 have been diagnosed in Zaireen coming from outside the country and 92,550 cases have been locally transmitted.[11]

According to WHO's COVID-19 situation report on 2020, the fatality rate in Pakistan was 2.06% with 1935 deaths. While in neighboring Iran the fatality rate was 4.87% in total number of 157,156 cases, in India mortality rate was 2.81% with 236,657 cases, while in Afghanistan mortality rate was 1.67% with 19,551 cases.[12] The reason for comparatively lesser infection and low mortality rate in Pakistan during the early phase of the pandemic was because of timely emergency measures by the government, which announced to lockdown the country on March 23, 2020.[13] However, the situation started to change after the lockdown was lifted on May 09, 2020.[14] A Reuters report concluded that around 20,000 COVID-19 cases were reported in three weeks before lifting the lockdown, while the number of new cases was more than double after the lockdown was lifted.[15] The sudden increase in the number of cases was largely because of increased commercial and consumer activity around Eid, during which preventive measures were not carefully observed among the public. Similarly, hundreds of thousands of Pakistani Shias flocked to attend religious gatherings on "Yuam-e-Ali" a few days prior to Eid, in complete violation of the government's ban on such gatherings.

In most of the countries including South Korea, Spain, China, and Italy, the fatality rate due to COVID-19 was highest among the age groups of seventy to seventy-nine years and eighty plus years.[16] However, in Pakistan, the fatality rate is highest in age groups of fifty to fifty-nine years and sixty to sixty-nine years, while the distribution across other age groups was also comparatively more uniform.[17] This, along with comparatively lesser mortality rate, may indicate a development towards herd immunity in the country. However, the idea of herd immunity being successful is not certain, as was indicated in the Reuters report.[18]

COVID-19 and Economic Security of Pakistan

The COVID-19 pandemic also brought about severe global economic repercussions. According to the International Monetary Fund (IMF), the global economic growth can fall up to –3% starting 2020 onwards.[19] This will be even more severe than the Global Financial Crisis of 2009 and will be the worst economic slowdown after the Great Depression of the 1930s. It also brought global supply chains at a halt as demand fell sharply after lockdowns across the world. Oil prices hit twenty-one year low globally, and oil prices in the US fell to a negative value for the first time in history going to as low as –$37 US dollars.[20]

In the face of ongoing global recession, Pakistan is also set to face severe economic issues during the COVID-19 pandemic. Pakistan's GDP growth is expected to fall to –2% in 2020 according to IMF estimates. Pakistan's economy is largely reliant on exports and the services sector. Foreign remittances also make up an important part of Pakistan's economy standing at USD $21 billion in 2018–2019, almost equivalent to Pakistan's exports.[21] In such a scenario, any significant impact to the national economy can raise the threat to security level. The coming part looks into how the economic situation has developed so far for Pakistan and what Pakistan is doing to contain it.

The exports sector of Pakistan started to dwindle as early as March 2020, as the global supply chains were disturbed, demand fell, and countries started entering lockdowns. In the same month, a managing director of a Lahore based textile factory told in an interview that 90% of their orders were on hold by the customers. CEO of another supply chain management firm noted that "the apparel export in 2020 could overall drop by 30 percent to 40 percent compared to 2019."[22] Even though exports of Pakistan during the first three quarters of fiscal year 2019–2020 increased slightly by 2.23%, it was expected that even this nominal rate will not continue in the last quarter.

The decline in global oil prices also impacted Pakistan's foreign remittances, most of which came from oil-exporting Gulf Cooperation Council (GCC) countries.[23] According to Special Assistant to Prime Minister (SAPM) on Overseas Pakistanis and Human Resource Development Zulfikar Bukhari, around 17,743 Pakistani workers were laid off from jobs in United Arab Emirates (UAE) alone, while 1,245 workers were laid off in Saudi Arabia, 691 in Qatar, and 600 in Oman. Despite early lay-off of workers, Saudi Arabia also issued a decree forbidding companies to further lay off their employees and ensured that they receive full salaries for at least the next three months.[24] This number is dramatically increase after the oil-rich gulf countries seek to reset their economies hit by low oil prices.

The agriculture sector, which is the mainstay of Pakistan's economy, contributes 19 percent to the country's GDP and employs 39 percent of the country's labor force. The lockdown during the COVID-19 pandemic resulted in disruption of food supply chains by creating constraints for labor during the harvesting season. While the government allowed agriculture-related machinery to move even during the lockdown, many farmers were not able to operate their machines as the workshops to carry seasonal repairs were closed. Due to issues in food supply chain management, one food security expert noted that "We may witness food surplus in one place and demand somewhere else for which we should be prepared."[25]

During the pandemic, unemployment became another major economic issue for Pakistan. The informal sector of the country's economy makes up around 18% to 71% of the national economy according to various estimates, and employs around 27.3 million workers.[26] This sector of the country's economy was affected the most by the pandemic. According to estimates from Pakistan Institute for Development Economics (PIDE), 3 million jobs are to be lost in the ongoing initial phase of COVID-19. While 18 million people may become unemployed in the overall situation, and the number of people living below the poverty line may double up to 125 million due to the COVID-19 pandemic.[27]

In order to contain this economic crisis, the government of Pakistan had taken measures that included social protection relief, stimulus package to the industry, and tax relaxation. Just at the start of the lockdown, the government announced a 900-billion-rupee ($5.66 billion) relief package.[28] The package included 200 billion rupees ($1.25 billion) for the low-income groups, 280 billion rupees ($1.76 billion) for wheat procurement, and 100 billion rupees ($63 million) for small industries and the agriculture sector. The relief to low-income groups included a bracket of 10 million people in three categories.[29] By end of March 2020, the government had also cut taxes on the import of food items and food suppliers to government-owned stores, and additional customs duty on oils had also been exempted. The government also elevated the construction sector to the status of "industry" and provided various incentives to the new industry in order to boost economic activity and employment.[30]

In addition to these steps to contain the economic fallout by the government, Pakistan also received foreign aid and loans to deal with emergency measures. $1.386 billion zero-interest loan was received under IMF's Rapid Financing Instrument. World Bank and Asian Development Bank also provided loans of $500 million and $800 million, respectively, for emergency financial assistance to Pakistan.[31]

China also provided considerable aid to Pakistan. According to the National Disaster Management Authority (NDMA) of Pakistan, China's assistance accounted for around 80% of foreign anti-pandemic assistance received by Pakistan. The Chinese Embassy and various non-profit organizations also made large donations to Pakistan, including protective equipment amounting to ¥4.56 million Chinese Yuans in value from the Red Cross Society of China. While in late April 2020, a group of Chinese doctors also arrived in Pakistan along with medical personal protective equipment (PPE) to train Pakistani medical professionals in dealing the COVID-19 pandemic.[32]

With these internal and external efforts, the government of Pakistan attempted to contain the economic crisis that came about amid the COVID-19 pandemic.

Impacts on Societal Security

Societal security is concerned with protection of different identities within a state and society without any conflict or tensions that may threaten the normal interaction between those identities. In Pakistan, the societal security issues that were observed during the COVID-19 pandemic related mostly to a communal debate between Shia pilgrims returning from Iran and Tablighi Jamat, a missionary organization of Sunni Deobandi sect.

The communalization of the pandemic started when the earliest cases of COVID-19 were reported in Zaireen (pilgrims), belonging to Shia-Muslim sect, coming from Iran.[33] Until April 2020, a large number of COVID-19 cases in Pakistan remained to be those having a recent travel history to Iran.[34] The communal debate intensified when forty cases of COVID-19 were also detected among the members of Tableeghi Jamaat who had attended annual gathering of around 250,000 people connected to Tableeghi Jamat before the lockdown.[35] In later days a communal debate intensified on social media each group accusing the other for spreading Corona virus. This argument, however, soon vanished into thin air without culminating into violence.

The COVID-19 outbreak also exposed inter-provincial fault lines on the issue of distribution of resources. Since the start of the pandemic, there have also been tensions between the federal government and provincial governments, particularly the Sindh government, ruled by the Pakistan Peoples' Party. According to the 18th Amendment to the Constitution of Pakistan, provinces were made autonomous and various federal ministries, including the ministry of health, came under provincial jurisdiction. After initial cases were reported from Sindh, the Sindh government immediately announced strict measures to contain the outbreak of COVID-19. However, the federal government hesitated to put the country on lockdown in order to prevent socio-economic downfall. In order to improve coordination between all provinces, a National Command and Control Center (NCOC) was also established with representation from all provinces and different stakeholders.[36] The debate of either having strict lockdown or more lenient "smart" lockdown continued between Sindh and federal governments, with Sindh favoring the former and federal favoring the latter option.[37]

In the meanwhile, another debate on the 18th Amendment started when Federal Information Minister declared the Amendment a hurdle in fighting COVID-19.[38] The issue of the 18th Amendment has been a subject of debate between ruling and opposition parties. The Sindh government's Pakistan Peoples' Party introduced the Amendment in 2010 and is strictly against any change to it. This further increased the tensions between federal and provincial governments. And the first session of the National Assembly which was convened after the COVID-19 pandemic was occupied more with debate on the 18th Amendment rather than on the COVID-19 crisis.[39] However, the debate subsided when the Supreme Court of Pakistan criticized both provincial and federal governments and ordered to lift lockdown restrictions, which left health implications regarding the ongoing COVID-19 situation uncertain for the governments.[40]

COVID-19 and Extremism and Terrorism

Terrorist and extremist groups always attempt to find opportunities in crises. The COVID-19 crisis was not an exception to the trend. Even though the UN Secretary General Antonio Gueterres appealed for a universal ceasefire during the ongoing pandemic, terrorist groups in the region intensified their activities despite the COVID-19 pandemic. Among them, the most prominent was ISIS-K (Khorasan), the Afghanistan wing of Islamic State in Iraq and Syria, which attacked the maternity ward in a Kabul hospital and a funeral in Nangarhar province recently.[41] Similarly, the number of terrorist attacks in Pakistan's border region adjoining Afghanistan also increased.

In Pakistan, the province of Balochistan remained a center of focus for Baloch separatist extremist and terrorist groups. During March and April 2020, most of their activities centered on social media activism and propaganda. Some separatist groups declared COVID-19 as a hoax and even attempted to run a Twitter trend #Covid19PakBioWeaponAgainstBaloch, but the trend failed to generate any impressions and died away.

However, in the month of May 2020, the incidents of violent terrorist attacks saw an increase in Balochistan. On May 8, 2020, six personnel including an officer of the Pakistan Army were martyred in an IED blast in the Kech district of Balochistan. In two more separate attacks on May 19, 2020, seven soldiers were martyred.[42] Balochistan Liberation Army (BLA) claimed responsibility for all the attacks. Even though violent attacks from Baloch separatist groups are carried out whenever they find any space. The recent mix of social media propaganda along with resurgence of violent activity shows that the terrorists in Balochistan might exploit the COVID-19 situation to achieve their goals.

Impacts on Environmental Security

In the wake of the global pandemic, the environment has been the only component which has become more secure rather than facing any challenges. According to satellite imaging, nitrogen dioxide levels significantly dropped across the globe, owing to closure of large-scale industries as well as transport and other fossil fuel emissions.[43]

In Pakistan too, there was a significant reduction in pollution with decreased nitrogen dioxide concentration and decreased number on PM2.5 index, which measures the concentration of particles having less than two and a half micrometer size in the air. According to a study, huge changes were observed in levels of nitrogen dioxide across major cities of Pakistan due to a decrease in economic activity and urban traffic.[44] An Environment Protection Agency (EPA) official in an interview also reported a decrease in PM2.5 index from 90 to 11 microns.[45] These indicators showed an overall improvement in the environmental security of Pakistan.

In addition to this natural improvement of the environment, the government of Pakistan also sought to turn these crises into an opportunity to restore the country's eco-system. The incumbent government introduced a "green stimulus" amid the economic crisis during lockdown in order to provide employment while improving the environment. The government hired 63,600 unemployed farmers and laborers to plant trees in designated areas. In the second phase of "Green Stimulus," the government envisaged creating 600,000 jobs in the sector. This initiative was also intended to compliment the government's 10 Billion Tree Tsunami project, which seeks to secure the environment by increasing the forest cover of Pakistan.[46] According to WWF, forests cover only 6% of the total area in Pakistan, making it a "forest poor" country. From 1998 to 2018, Pakistan has also faced an estimated 150 extreme weather events.

However environmental experts have suggested to go beyond these measures to ensure more environmentally sustainable development amid the COVID-19 pandemic. One study noted that tree plantation is only sustainable if "human-planted forests are maintained for decades before their benefits as carbon sequesters and wildlife sanctuaries are realized. More often than not, they are cut down before then to clear land for farming."[47]

COVID-19 and Conventional Security of Pakistan

Pakistan's conventional security has always been threatened by its eastern neighbor, India. During the pandemic, Indian strategic posturing became even more aggressive, with a dramatic increase in the number of ceasefire violations, Israeli-style military suppression of Kashmiris' struggle for self-determination, supplanted by a dramatic increase in Indian defense expenditures. Tensions increased when Indian Army Chief MM Naravane was quoted by a news source alleging that Pakistan was sending terrorists to India during the COVID-19 pandemic.[48] While Foreign Office of Pakistan rejected the Indian allegation and said that baseless allegations from India are aimed at diverting the attention from increasing human rights violation across India, particularly in Indian-occupied Kashmir.[49]

Increasing ceasefire violations by India were also highlighted by the Director General of Inter-Services Public Relations (ISPR), Pakistan Army's public relations department, in a press conference on April 24. It was told that India committed 848 ceasefire violations in 2020, among which 392 were carried out from January to February 26, while 456 violations were carried out after the detection of the first COVID-19 case in Pakistan on February 26.[50] By May 21, the number has risen to 1,102 ceasefire violations with 710 violations happening during the COVID-19 crisis which started on February 26. New Delhi was seen to be flexing its muscles simultaneously against three of its neighbors (Nepal, Pakistan, and China) to divert attention from a massive economic fallout due to COVID-19. Unemployment rate in India increased from 8% to a staggering 26%, leaving 140 million workers unemployed. Goldman Sachs estimated India's economy to contract by 5% in 2020.

Despite this severe impact on the economy, India increased its military expenditure, owing to its increasing ambitions in the Indian Ocean region as well as an increasingly aggressive policy towards Pakistan and China. India's military expenditure grew by 6.8 percent to $71.1 billion making it the third largest military spender in the world after US and China, according to a report from Stockholm International Peace Research Institute (SIPRI).[51]

Even in the economic slump due to the ongoing COVID-19 pandemic, India might not like to cut down its military expenditure. Therefore, in its bid to continue the expansion of military expenditure, India may adopt an even more aggressive posture by securitizing a threat from Pakistan and then using it to justify its ballooning defense spending. Such efforts may even include a false flag operation, as indicated by the Prime Minister of Pakistan recently.[52]

Conclusion

The COVID-19 pandemic has impacted economic, societal, human, and environmental spheres and has brought about a huge change in how we view security. It has given a renewed priority to non-traditional security threats, especially in the public health sector. The global scale of death and destruction caused by this pandemic may also cause a shift in the global security agenda and how security policy and strategy is planned.

Pakistan will also have to rapidly revamp its security strategy by incorporating both traditional and non-traditional aspects in its national security policy after the COVID-19 pandemic due to the threats it poses to both traditional and non-traditional security areas. In order to achieve this, Pakistan needs to incorporate disease control and counter-epidemic exercises in military strategy, as well as improve civil-military cooperation for disease control.

In this regard, Pakistan can also learn from China's military-civilian cooperative emergency response to disease prevention and control, which incorporates various laws mandating military-civilian cooperation, information sharing, and joint operations to prevent and control infectious diseases.[53] Chinese cooperation framework also mandates China's People's Liberation Army (PLA) to initiate the emergency research mechanism in case of any health emergency or infection outbreak.

In view of Indian strategic posturing during the pandemic, it is unlikely that Pakistan may witness any paradigm shift in its security agenda. National security calculation will continue to be dominated by the traditional threat of Indian hegemonic design, perceived or real. Given a weak economy, Islamabad can ill-afford a "tit-for-tat" response to New Delhi's growing defense expenditure. Rather, cooperation on dealing with non-traditional security threats such as COVID-19 will offer a rare window of opportunity to partner in a noble mission to protect billions of South Asians against the modern plague.

Notes

1 Stephen M. Walt, "The Renaissance of Security Studies," *International Studies Quarterly* 35, no. 2 (June 1991): 211, https://doi.org/10.2307/2600471.
2 For a detailed discussion on the debate, see: Barry Buzan, Ole Waever, and Jaap de Wilde, *Security: A New Framework for Analysis* (Lynne Rienner Publishers,

1998), 2–4; Keith Krause and Michael C. Williams, "Broadening the Agenda of Security Studies: Politics and Methods," *Mershon International Studies Review* 40, no. 2 (October 1996): 229, https://doi.org/10.2307/222776.

3 Barry Buzan, "New Patterns of Global Security in the Twenty-First Century," *International Affairs (Royal Institute of International Affairs 1944-)* 67, no. 3 (July 1991): 431–51, https://doi.org/10.2307/2621945.

4 UNDP, ed., *Human Development Report 1994* (New York: Oxford Univ. Press, 1994), http://hdr.undp.org/sites/default/files/reports/255/hdr_1994_en _complete_nostats.pdf.

5 Syed Najeeb Ahmad, "Pakistan's National Security: A Cross-Sectoral Discourse Analysis of Securitization Process" (PhD Dissertation, Islamabad, National Defence University, 2017), 70, https://pdfs.semanticscholar.org/d4aa/30f55ac 158273b84236ccdab6e56993a2224.pdf.

6 Malik Safi et al., "Development of a Costed National Action Plan for Health Security in Pakistan: Lessons Learned," *Health Security* 16, no. S1 (December 2018): S-25-S-29, https://doi.org/10.1089/hs.2018.0072.

7 "Pakistan National Action Plan for Health Security (NAPHS)" (Islamabad: Ministry of National Health Services, Regulation and Coordination, 2018), http://phkh.nhsrc.pk/sites/default/files/2019-06/National%20Action %20Plan%20for%20Health%20Security%20%E2%80%93%20Pakistan%202018 .pdf.

8 "Outbreak Update – Dengue in Pakistan," WHO EMRO, December 3, 2019, http://www.emro.who.int/pandemic-epidemic-diseases/dengue/outbreak -update-dengue-in-pakistan-1-december-2019.html.

9 Sania Nishtar, "H1N1 Outbreak in Pakistan: Lessons Learnt," Working Paper, NTS Working Paper Series (Singapore: RSIS Centre for Non-Traditional Security (NTS) Studies, December 2010), http://www.heartfile.org/pdf/NTS_Working _Paper4.pdf.

10 "A Month on, Pakistan's COVID-19 Trajectory from Patient Zero to 1,000 and Beyond," Dawn, March 30, 2020, https://www.dawn.com/news/1543683.

11 "COVID-19 Live Dashboard – Pakistan," Government of Pakistan, accessed June 6, 2020, http://covid.gov.pk/stats/pakistan.

12 "Coronavirus Disease (COVID-19) Situation Report – 138," Situation Report, COVID-19 Situation Report (World Health Organization, June 6, 2020), https://www.who.int/docs/default-source/coronaviruse/situation-reports /20200606-COVID-19-sitrep-138.pdf?sfvrsn=c8abfb17_4.

13 "Pakistan Announces Lockdown of Major Provinces to Curb COVID-19 Spread," Xinhua Net, March 24, 2020, http://www.xinhuanet.com/english /2020-03/24/c_138910694.htm.

14 Mumtaz Alvi, "Lockdown Eases from Tomorrow," The News, May 8, 2020, https://www.thenews.com.pk/print/655448-lockdown-eases-from-tomor- row.

15 Charlotte Greenfield and Umar Farooq, "After Pakistan's Lockdown Gamble, COVID-19 Cases Surge," *Reuters*, June 5, 2020, https://www.reuters.com/ article/us-health-coronavirus-pakistan-lockdown-idUSKBN23C0NW.

16 Max Roser et al., "Mortality Risk of COVID-19 - Statistics and Research," Our World in Data, accessed June 7, 2020, https://ourworldindata.org/mortality -risk-covid.

17 "COVID-19 Live Dashboard – Pakistan."

18 Greenfield and Farooq, "After Pakistan's Lockdown Gamble, COVID-19 Cases Surge."

19 Gita Gopinath, "The Great Lockdown: Worst Economic Downturn Since the Great Depression," *IMF Blog*, April 14, 2020, https://blogs.imf.org/2020

/04/14/the-great-lockdown-worst-economic-downturn-since-the-great
-depression/.

20 Lora Jones Palumbo Daniele and David Brown, "Coronavirus: A Visual Guide to
the Economic Impact," *BBC News*, April 30, 2020, sec. Business, https://www
.bbc.com/news/business-51706225.

21 Arhama Siddiqa, "Pakistan and the Foreign Remittance Sector," *Asia Dialogue*
(blog), March 23, 2020, https://theasiadialogue.com/2020/03/23/pakistan
-and-the-foreign-remittance-sector/.

22 Tara Donaldson, "Pakistan Lockdown Idles Factories—Where Orders Had
Shriveled Up," *Sourcing Journal* (blog), March 26, 2020, https://sourcing-
journal.com/topics/sourcing/pakistan-coronavirus-lockdown-garment-factories
-closed-synergies-worldwide-levis-202444/.

23 Haris Ahmed, "Pakistan's Economy in Deep Trouble," The Express Tribune,
April 27, 2020, https://tribune.com.pk/story/2207551/2-pakistans-economy
-deep-trouble/.

24 Saima Shabbir, "Over 21,000 Pakistani Expats from Gulf Region Laid off amid
COVID-19 – Zulfi Bukhari," Arab News, April 25, 2020, https://arab.news/
yh54f.

25 Sana Jamal, "How Will COVID-19 Affect Pakistan Farmers, Food System?,"
Gulf News, May 1, 2020, https://gulfnews.com/world/asia/pakistan/how
-will-COVID-19-affect-pakistan-farmers-food-system-1.71196910;   Aamir
Latif and Shuriah Niazi, "COVID-19 Lockdown Sparks Harvest Crises in
Pakistan, India," Anadolu Agency, April 10, 2020, https://www.aa.com.tr/
en/asia-pacific/COVID-19-lockdown-sparks-harvest-crises-in-pakistan-india
/1799536.

26 "COVID-19 Pandemic | UNDP in Pakistan," UNDP, accessed May 20, 2020,
https://www.pk.undp.org/content/pakistan/en/home/coronavirus.html.

27 Nadir Guramani, "3 Million Jobs Likely to Be Lost Due to Pandemic, Finance
Ministry Tells Senate," Dawn, June 5, 2020, https://www.dawn.com/news
/1561492; Mehtab Haider, "Economic Fallout of COVID-19 in Pakistan: People
under Poverty Line May Double to 125 Million," The News, March 27, 2020,
https://www.thenews.com.pk/print/635146-economic-fallout-of-COVID-19
-in-pakistan-people-under-poverty-line-may-double-to-125-million.

28 Aamir Latif, "COVID-19: Pakistan Unveils Economic Relief Package," Anadolu
Agency, March 24, 2020, https://www.aa.com.tr/en/asia-pacific/COVID-19
-pakistan-unveils-economic-relief-package/1777961.

29 "Rs12,000 to Be given per Family via Ehsaas Emergency Cash Programme: Dr
Sania," Pakistan Today, March 24, 2020, https://www.pakistantoday.com.pk
/2020/03/24/ehsaas-emergency-cash-programme-benefit-10m-corona-affect-
ees-dr-sania/.

30 "Pakistan: Tax Developments in Response to COVID-19," KPMG, May 14,
2020,   https://home.kpmg/xx/en/home/insights/2020/04/pakistan-tax
-developments-in-response-to-COVID-19.html.

31 Raphaël Cecchi, "Pakistan: External Support and Debt Relief to Face the COVID-
19 Crisis," Credendo, April 28, 2020, https://www.credendo.com/country-risk
-monthly/pakistan/pakistan-external-support-and-debt-relief-face-COVID-19
-crisis.

32 "China's Support to Pakistan on COVID-19 Reflects Deep-Rooted Friendship,"
The News, April 21, 2020, https://www.thenews.com.pk/print/647477-china
-s-support-to-pakistan-on-COVID-19-reflects-deep-rooted-friendship;   Aamir
Latif, "Chinese Doctors to Join Pakistan's COVID-19 Battle," Anadolu Agency,
April 24, 2020, https://www.aa.com.tr/en/asia-pacific/chinese-doctors-to-join
-pakistans-COVID-19-battle/1817676.

33 "Pakistan Confirms First Two Cases of Coronavirus," France 24, February 26, 2020, https://www.france24.com/en/20200226-pakistan-confirms-first-two-cases-of-coronavirus.

34 Saima Shabbir, "46% Pakistanis with Coronavirus Have Travel History to Iran — WHO," Arab News PK, April 4, 2020, https://www.arabnews.pk/node/1653006/pakistan.

35 Suddaf Chaudry, "Coronavirus: Pakistan Quarantines Tablighi Jamaat Missionaries," Middle East Eye, April 4, 2020, http://www.middleeasteye.net/news/coronavirus-pakistan-tablighi-jamaat-missionaries-quarantined.

36 "Command & Control Center Set up for Inter-Provincial Coordination on COVID-19: FM," The Nation, March 28, 2020, https://nation.com.pk/28-Mar-2020/command-control-center-set-up-for-inter-provincial-coordination-on-COVID-19-fm.

37 Syed Irfan Raza, "Centre Assails Sindh Govt over 'stricter' Lockdown Measures," Dawn, April 16, 2020, https://www.dawn.com/news/1549621; Tahir Siddiqui, "Sindh Entering Second Phase of Lockdown with 'Some Extra Restrictions', Says Murad," Dawn, May 9, 2020, https://www.dawn.com/news/1555630.

38 Kalbe Ali, "Info Minister Terms 18th Amendment Hurdle in Fight against COVID-19," Dawn, May 2, 2020, https://www.dawn.com/news/1553906.

39 Rizwan Shehzad, "18th Amendment Overshadows COVID-19 in NA Session," The Express Tribune, May 12, 2020, https://tribune.com.pk/story/2219542/1-18th-amendment-overshadows-COVID-19-na-session/.

40 Asif Shehzad, "Coronavirus 'not a Pandemic in Pakistan' Says Top Court, Ordering Curbs Lifted," *Reuters*, May 18, 2020, https://www.reuters.com/article/us-health-coronavirus-pakistan-lockdown-idUSKBN22U2NV.

41 "'Islamic State' Responsible for Deadly Afghanistan Bombings, Says US," Deutshe Welle, May 15, 2020, https://www.dw.com/en/islamic-state-responsible-for-deadly-afghanistan-bombings-says-us/a-53444892.

42 Ali Hussain and Fazal Sher, "6 Soldiers, Driver Martyred in Balochistan," Business Recorder, May 20, 2020, https://www.brecorder.com/2020/05/20/598933/six-soldiers-driver-martyred-in-balochistan/.

43 "COVID-19: Nitrogen Dioxide over China," European Space Agency, March 19, 2020, https://www.esa.int/Applications/Observing_the_Earth/Copernicus/Sentinel-5P/COVID-19_nitrogen_dioxide_over_China; "Coronavirus Lockdown Leading to Drop in Pollution across Europe," European Space Agency, March 27, 2020, https://www.esa.int/Applications/Observing_the_Earth/Copernicus/Sentinel-5P/Coronavirus_lockdown_leading_to_drop_in_pollution_across_Europe.

44 Sunil Dahiya and Dawar Butt, "Air Quality before and after National Lockdown during Coronavirus Disease (COVID-19) Outbreak across Pakistan," *Centre for Research on Energy and Clean Air* (blog), April 24, 2020, https://energyandcleanair.org/air-quality-before-and-after-national-lockdown-during-coronavirus-disease-COVID-19-outbreak-across-pakistan/.

45 "Virus Curfew Leads to Clearer Skies in Pakistan," Arab News, April 13, 2020, https://www.arabnews.pk/node/1658161/pakistan.

46 Rina Saeed Khan, "COVID-19: Pakistan's 'green Stimulus' Scheme Is a Win-Win for the Environment and the Unemployed," World Economic Forum, April 30, 2020, https://www.weforum.org/agenda/2020/04/green-stimulus-pakistan-trees-coronavirus-covid10-enviroment-climate-change/.

47 Sara Hayat, "Pakistan Needs to Go beyond Tree Planting to Thrive after COVID-19," Dawn, June 3, 2020, https://www.dawn.com/news/1561024.

48 "'India Exporting Medicines While Pak…': Army Chief's Stinging Takedown of Islamabad," Hindustan Times, April 17, 2020, https://www.hindustantimes

.com/india-news/we-are-fighting-COVID-19-pakistan-is-only-exporting-terror -says-army-chief/story-YVINlgRrzy0zM40adQwZeN.html.
49 Naveed Siddiqui, "FO Blasts Indian Army Chief for 'irresponsible, False' Allegations against Pakistan," Dawn, April 17, 2020, https://www.dawn.com/ news/1549989.
50 "Saffronisation of Indian Army amid Coronavirus Crisis Sad Spectre, Says ISPR," The Express Tribune, April 24, 2020, https://tribune.com.pk/story/2205967 /1-attempt-india-link-coronavirus-pakistan-muslims-failed-dg-ispr/.
51 Shaurya Karanbir Gurung, "India Third Largest Military Spender in World, after US and China," The Economic Times, April 27, 2020, https://economictimes .indiatimes.com/news/defence/global-military-spending-saw-largest-increase -in-decade-in-2019-china-india-in-top-3-study/articleshow/75404166.cms.
52 Syed Irfan Raza, "India May Conduct False Flag Operation, Says Imran," Dawn, May 18, 2020, https://www.dawn.com/news/1557912.
53 Hui Ma et al., "Military-Civilian Cooperative Emergency Response to Infectious Disease Prevention and Control in China," *Military Medical Research* 3, no. 1 (December 30, 2016): 5, https://doi.org/10.1186/s40779-016-0109-y.

Bibliography

Ahmad, Syed Najeeb, 2017. "Pakistan's National Security: A Cross-Sectoral Discourse Analysis of Securitization Process." PhD Dissertation, National Defence University. Retrieved on Sept, 02nd 2020 from: https://pdfs.semanticscholar.org /d4aa/30f55ac158273b84236ccdab6e56993a2224.pdf.

Ahmed, Haris, 2020. "Pakistan's Economy in Deep Trouble." *The Express Tribune*, Retrieved on April 27, 2020 from: https://tribune.com.pk/story/2207551/2 -pakistans-economy-deep-trouble/.

Ali, Kalbe, 2020. "Info Minister Terms 18th Amendment Hurdle in Fight against COVID-19." *Dawn*, Retrieved on May 2, 2020 from: https://www.dawn.com /news/1553906.

Alvi, Mumtaz, 2020. "Lockdown Eases from Tomorrow." *The News*, Retrieved on May 8, 2020 from: https://www.thenews.com.pk/print/655448-lockdown -eases-from-tomorrow.

Arab News, 2020. "Virus Curfew Leads to Clearer Skies in Pakistan." Retrieved on April 13, 2020 from: https://www.arabnews.pk/node/1658161/pakistan.

Buzan, Barry, 1991. "New Patterns of Global Security in the Twenty-First Century." *International Affairs* (Royal Institute of International Affairs 1944–) 67, no. 3 (July 1991): 431–51. https://doi.org/10.2307/2621945.

Buzan, Barry, Ole Waever, and Jaap de Wilde. 1998. *Security: A New Framework for Analysis*. Lynne Rienner Publishers.

Cecchi, Raphaël, 2020. "Pakistan: External Support and Debt Relief to Face the COVID-19 Crisis." *Credendo*, Retrieved on April 28, 2020 from: https://www .credendo.com/country-risk-monthly/pakistan/pakistan-external-support-and -debt-relief-face-COVID-19-crisis.

Chaudry, Suddaf, 2020. "Coronavirus: Pakistan Quarantines Tablighi Jamaat Missionaries." *Middle East Eye*, Retrieved on April 4, 2020 from: http://www .middleeasteye.net/news/coronavirus-pakistan-tablighi-jamaat-missionaries -quarantined.

"Coronavirus Disease (COVID-19) Situation Report – 138." Situation Report. COVID-19 Situation Report, 2020. World Health Organization, Retrieved on

June 6, 2020 from: https://www.who.int/docs/default-source/coronaviruse/situation-reports/20200606-COVID-19-sitrep-138.pdf?sfvrsn=c8abfb17_4.

Dahiya, Sunil, and Dawar Butt, 2020. "Air Quality before and after National Lockdown during Coronavirus Disease (COVID-19) Outbreak across Pakistan." *Centre for Research on Energy and Clean Air* (blog), Retrieved on April 24, 2020 from: https://energyandcleanair.org/air-quality-before-and-after-national-lockdown-during-coronavirus-disease-COVID-19-outbreak-across-pakistan/.

Dawn. "A Month on, Pakistan's COVID-19 Trajectory from Patient Zero to 1,000 and Beyond." 2020. Retrieved on March 30, 2020 from: https://www.dawn.com/news/1543683.

Deutshe Welle, 2020. "'Islamic State' Responsible for Deadly Afghanistan Bombings, Says US." Retrieved on May 15, 2020 from: https://www.dw.com/en/islamic-state-responsible-for-deadly-afghanistan-bombings-says-us/a-53444892.

Donaldson, Tara, 2020. "Pakistan Lockdown Idles Factories—Where Orders Had Shriveled Up." *Sourcing Journal* (blog), Retrieved on March 26, 2020 from: https://sourcingjournal.com/topics/sourcing/pakistan-coronavirus-lockdown-garment-factories-closed-synergies-worldwide-levis-202444/.

European Space Agency, 2020. "Coronavirus Lockdown Leading to Drop in Pollution across Europe." Retrieved on March 27, 2020 from: https://www.esa.int/Applications/Observing_the_Earth/Copernicus/Sentinel-5P/Coronavirus_lockdown_leading_to_drop_in_pollution_across_Europe.

European Space Agency, 2020. "COVID-19: Nitrogen Dioxide over China." Retrieved on April 4, 2020 from: https://www.esa.int/Applications/Observing_the_Earth/Copernicus/Sentinel-5P/COVID-19_nitrogen_dioxide_over_China.

France 24, 2020. "Pakistan Confirms First Two Cases of Coronavirus." Retrieved on February 26, 2020 from: https://www.france24.com/en/20200226-pakistan-confirms-first-two-cases-of-coronavirus.

Gopinath, Gita, 2020. "The Great Lockdown: Worst Economic Downturn Since the Great Depression." *IMF Blog* (blog), Retrieved on April 14, 2020 from: https://blogs.imf.org/2020/04/14/the-great-lockdown-worst-economic-downturn-since-the-great-depression/.

Government of Pakistan, 2020. "COVID-19 Live Dashboard - Pakistan." Retrieved on June 6, 2020 from: http://covid.gov.pk/stats/pakistan.

Greenfield, Charlotte, and Umar Farooq, 2020. "After Pakistan's Lockdown Gamble, COVID-19 Cases Surge." *Reuters*, Retrieved on June 5, 2020 from: https://www.reuters.com/article/us-health-coronavirus-pakistan-lockdown-idUSKBN23C0NW.

Guramani, Nadir, 2020. "3 Million Jobs Likely to Be Lost Due to Pandemic, Finance Ministry Tells Senate." Retrieved on June 5, 2020 from: https://www.dawn.com/news/1561492.

Gurung, Shaurya Karanbir, 2020. "India Third Largest Military Spender in World, after US and China." *The Economic Times*, Retrieved on April 27, 2020 from: https://economictimes.indiatimes.com/news/defence/global-military-spending-saw-largest-increase-in-decade-in-2019-china-india-in-top-3-study/articleshow/75404166.cms.

Haider, Mehtab, 2020. "Economic Fallout of COVID-19 in Pakistan: People under Poverty Line May Double to 125 Million." *The News*, Retrieved on March 27, 2020 from: https://www.thenews.com.pk/print/635146-economic-fallout-of-COVID-19-in-pakistan-people-under-poverty-line-may-double-to-125-million.

Hayat, Sara, 2020. "Pakistan Needs to Go beyond Tree Planting to Thrive after COVID-19." Retrieved on June 3, 2020 from: https://www.dawn.com/news /1561024.

Hindustan Times, 2020. "'India Exporting Medicines While Pak...': Army Chief's Stinging Takedown of Islamabad." Retrieved on April 17, 2020 from: https:// www.hindustantimes.com/india-news/we-are-fighting-COVID-19-pakistan -is-only-exporting-terror-says-army-chief/story-YVINlgRrzy0zM40adQwZeN .html.

Hussain, Ali, and Fazal Sher, 2020. "6 Soldiers, Driver Martyred in Balochistan." *Business Recorder*, Retrieved on May 20, 2020 from: https://www.brecorder.com /2020/05/20/598933/six-soldiers-driver-martyred-in-balochistan/.

"India's Economy Has Suffered Even More than Most, 2020." *The Economist*, Retrieved on May 23, 2020 from: https://www.economist.com/asia/2020/05 /23/indias-economy-has-suffered-even-more-than-most.

Jamal, Sana, 2020. "How Will COVID-19 Affect Pakistan Farmers, Food System?" *Gulf News*, Retrieved on May 1, 2020. https://gulfnews.com/world /asia/pakistan/how-will-COVID-19-affect-pakistan-farmers-food-system-1 .71196910.

Khan, Rina Saeed, 2020. "COVID-19: Pakistan's 'green Stimulus' Scheme Is a Win-Win for the Environment and the Unemployed." *World Economic Forum*, Retrieved on April 30, 2020 from: https://www.weforum.org/agenda/2020 /04/green-stimulus-pakistan-trees-coronavirus-covid10-enviroment-climate -change/.

KPMG, 2020. "Pakistan: Tax Developments in Response to COVID-19." Retrieved on May 14, 2020 from: https://home.kpmg/xx/en/home/insights/2020/04/ pakistan-tax-developments-in-response-to-COVID-19.html.

Krause, Keith, and Michael C. Williams, 1996. "Broadening the Agenda of Security Studies: Politics and Methods." *Mershon International Studies Review* 40, no. 2 (October 1996): 229. https://doi.org/10.2307/222776.

Kuchay, Bilal, 2020. "Why Arabs Are Speaking out against Islamophobia in India." *Al Jazeera*, Retrieved on April 30, 2020 from: https://www.aljazeera.com/news /2020/04/arabs-speaking-islamophobia-india-200423112102197.html.

Latif, Aamir, 2020a. "Chinese Doctors to Join Pakistan's COVID-19 Battle." *Anadolu Agency*, Retrieved on April 24, 2020 from: https://www.aa.com.tr/en/ asia-pacific/chinese-doctors-to-join-pakistans-COVID-19-battle/1817676.

———, 2020b. "COVID-19: Pakistan Unveils Economic Relief Package." *Anadolu Agency*, Retrieved on March 24, 2020 from: https://www.aa.com.tr/en/asia -pacific/COVID-19-pakistan-unveils-economic-relief-package/1777961.

Latif, Aamir, and Shuriah Niazi, 2020. "COVID-19 Lockdown Sparks Harvest Crises in Pakistan, India." *Anadolu Agency*, Retrieved on April 10, 2020 from: https:// www.aa.com.tr/en/asia-pacific/COVID-19-lockdown-sparks-harvest-crises-in -pakistan-india/1799536.

Ma, Hui, Ji-Ping Dong, Na Zhou, and Wei Pu, 2016. "Military-Civilian Cooperative Emergency Response to Infectious Disease Prevention and Control in China." *Military Medical Research* 3, no. 1 (December 30, 2016): 5. https://doi.org/10 .1186/s40779-016-0109-y.

"National Biodefense Strategy, 2018." Washington, DC: White House. Retrieved on September 8, 2018 from: https://www.whitehouse.gov/wp-content/uploads /2018/09/National-Biodefense-Strategy.pdf.

Nishtar, Sania, 2010. "H1N1 Outbreak in Pakistan: Lessons Learnt." Working Paper. NTS Working Paper Series. Singapore: RSIS Centre for Non-Traditional Security (NTS) Studies, December 2010. http://www.heartfile.org/pdf/NTS_Working_Paper4.pdf.

"Novel Coronavirus (2019-NCoV) Situation Report, 2020." Situation Report. COVID-19 Situation Report. World Health Organization, Retrieved on January 21, 2020 from: https://www.who.int/docs/default-source/coronaviruse/situation-reports/20200121-sitrep-1-2019-ncov.pdf?sfvrsn=20a99c10_4.

"Pakistan National Action Plan for Health Security (NAPHS), 2018." Islamabad: Ministry of National Health Services, Regulation and Coordination. http://phkh.nhsrc.pk/sites/default/files/2019-06/National%20Action%20Plan%20for%20Health%20Security%20%E2%80%93%20Pakistan%202018.pdf.

Pakistan Today, 2020. "Rs12,000 to Be given per Family via Ehsaas Emergency Cash Programme: Dr Sania." Retrieved on March 24, 2020 from: https://www.pakistantoday.com.pk/2020/03/24/ehsaas-emergency-cash-programme-benefit-10m-corona-affectees-dr-sania/.

Palumbo, Lora Jones, Daniele, and David Brown, 2020. "Coronavirus: A Visual Guide to the Economic Impact." *BBC News*, Retrieved on April 30, 2020, sec. Business. https://www.bbc.com/news/business-51706225.

Rana, Muhammad Amir, 2020. "Terrorism under COVID-19." Retrieved on May 17, 2020 from: https://www.dawn.com/news/1557728.

Raza, Syed Irfan, 2020. "Centre Assails Sindh Govt Over 'Stricter' Lockdown Measures." Retrieved on April 16, 2020 from: https://www.dawn.com/news/1549621.

———. "India May Conduct False Flag Operation, Says Imran, 2020." Retrieved on May 18, 2020 from: https://www.dawn.com/news/1557912.

Roser, Max, Hannah Ritchie, Esteban Ortiz-Ospina, and Joe Hasell, 2020. "Mortality Risk of COVID-19 - Statistics and Research." *Our World in Data*, Retrieved on June 7, 2020. from: https://ourworldindata.org/mortality-risk-covid.

Safi, Malik, Kashef Ijaz, Dalia Samhouri, Mamun Malik, Farah Sabih, Nirmal Kandel, Mohammad Salman, et al, 2018. "Development of a Costed National Action Plan for Health Security in Pakistan: Lessons Learned." *Health Security* 16, no. S1 (December 2018): S-25–S-29. https://doi.org/10.1089/hs.2018.0072.

Shabbir, Saima, 2020a. "46% Pakistanis with Coronavirus Have Travel History to Iran — WHO." *Arab News PK*, Retrieved on April 4, 2020 from: https://www.arabnews.pk/node/1653006/pakistan.

———, 2020b. "Over 21,000 Pakistani Expats from Gulf Region Laid Off Amid COVID-19 – Zulfi Bukhari." *Arab News*, Retrieved on April 25, 2020 from: https://arab.news/yh54f.

Shehzad, Asif, 2020. "Coronavirus 'Not a Pandemic in Pakistan' Says Top Court, Ordering Curbs Lifted." *Reuters*, Retrieved on May 18, 2020 from: https://www.reuters.com/article/us-health-coronavirus-pakistan-lockdown-idUSKBN22U2NV.

Shehzad, Rizwan, 2020. "18th Amendment Overshadows COVID-19 in NA Session." *The Express Tribune*, Retrieved on May 12, 2020 from: https://tribune.com.pk/story/2219542/1-18th-amendment-overshadows-COVID-19-na-session/.

Siddiqa, Arhama, 2020. "Pakistan and the Foreign Remittance Sector." *Asia Dialogue* (blog). https://theasiadialogue.com/2020/03/23/pakistan-and-the-foreign-remittance-sector/.

Siddiqui, Naveed, 2020. "FO Blasts Indian Army Chief for 'Irresponsible, False' Allegations against Pakistan." Retrieved on April 17, 2020 from: https://www .dawn.com/news/1549989.

Siddiqui, Tahir, 2020. "Sindh Entering Second Phase of Lockdown with 'Some Extra Restrictions', Says Murad." Retrieved on May 9, 2020 from: https://www.dawn .com/news/1555630.

The Express Tribune, 2020. "Saffronisation of Indian Army amid Coronavirus Crisis Sad Spectre, Says ISPR." Retrieved on April 24, 2020 from: https://tribune.com .pk/story/2205967/1-attempt-india-link-coronavirus-pakistan-muslims-failed -dg-ispr/.

The Nation, 2020. "Command & Control Center Set up for Inter-Provincial Coordination on COVID-19: FM." Retrieved on March 28, 2020 from: https://nation.com.pk/28-Mar-2020/command-control-center-set-up-for-inter -provincial-coordination-on-COVID-19-fm.

The News, 2020. "China's Support to Pakistan on COVID-19 Reflects Deep-Rooted Friendship." https://www.thenews.com.pk/print/647477-china-s-support-to -pakistan-on-COVID-19-reflects-deep-rooted-friendship.

Ujjan, Ikram Din, Bikha Ram Devrajani, Akbar Ali Ghanghro, and Syed Zulfiquar Ali Shah, 2020. "The Clinical and Demographical Profile of Coronavirus Illness: The Tale of Tablighi Jamaat and Zaireen in Quarantine / Isolation Center at Sukkur and Hyderabad." *Pakistan Journal of Medical Sciences* 36, no. COVID19-S4 (May 18, 2020). https://doi.org/10.12669/pjms.36.COVID19-S4.2829.

UNDP, ed, 1994. *Human Development Report 1994.* New York: Oxford Univ. Press. http://hdr.undp.org/sites/default/files/reports/255/hdr_1994_en_complete _nostats.pdf.

UNDP, 2020. "COVID-19 Pandemic | UNDP in Pakistan." Retrieved on May 20, 2020 from: https://www.pk.undp.org/content/pakistan/en/home/coronavirus .html.

Walt, Stephen M., 1991. "The Renaissance of Security Studies." *International Studies Quarterly* 35, no. 2 (June): 211. https://doi.org/10.2307/2600471.

World Health Organization, 2020a. "WHO Coronavirus Disease (COVID-19) Dashboard." Retrieved on May 23, 2020. from: https://covid19.who.int/ ?gclid=EAIaIQobChMIjdSGzLHK6QIV2JrVCh3mYgXXEAAYASAAEgJMFPD _BwE.

World Health Organization, 2020b. "WHO Director-General's Opening Remarks at the Media Briefing on COVID-19–11 March 2020." Retrieved on April 4, 2020 from: https://www.who.int/dg/speeches/detail/who-director-general-s -opening-remarks-at-the-media-briefing-on-COVID-19---11-march-2020.

WHO EMRO, 2019. "Outbreak Update – Dengue in Pakistan." Retrieved on December 3, 2019 from: http://www.emro.who.int/pandemic-epidemic -diseases/dengue/outbreak-update-dengue-in-pakistan-1-december-2019.html.

Xinhua Net, 2020. "Pakistan Announces Lockdown of Major Provinces to Curb COVID-19 Spread." Retrieved on March 24, 2020 from: http://www.xinhuanet .com/english/2020-03/24/c_138910694.htm.

4 Terrorism in Pakistan during COVID-19

Muhammad Amir Rana

Introduction

Pakistan lifted the COVID-19 related lockdown on August 10, 2020 after having employed strict to smart lockdown strategies for about five months. During these months, the security landscape of Pakistan did not witness any major shift. However, the frequency and intensity of terrorist attacks slightly increased from May to July, particularly in the North Waziristan district of Khyber Pakhtunkhwa and the restive southwestern province of Balochistan. Meanwhile, violent Sindhi nationalist groups launched a number of attacks against the security forces in Sindh. Similarly, in June, Balochistan Liberation Army (BLA) militants attacked the Pakistan Stock Exchange (PSX) building in Karachi, where law enforcement personnel were alert enough to kill all four attackers; three security guards and one police officer also lost their lives before the attack was successfully foiled. Hizbul Ahrar, a breakaway faction of militant group Jamaatul Ahrar, has recently perpetrated two attacks in Rawalpindi district of Punjab.

However, linking this relative increase in terrorist attacks with the pandemic is difficult. But it certainly indicates that the terrorist groups continue to demonstrate the capacity to plan and conduct attacks from the tribal belt to Karachi, despite the government's claims of counter-terrorism successes. At the same time, terrorists could be eying the opportunities created by the pandemic, but they are, apparently, yet waiting to take any major action in that regard. To fully reactivate their operational networks, they would have to reconnect to their support bases in the country, besides increasing recruitment and fund-raising efforts.

Though the nature of the Baloch insurgency is different from religiously motivated terrorism, the Baloch insurgent groups can also capitalize on the pandemic-related opportunities. That makes it imperative for the government and the security forces to not let their guards down in the counter-terrorism campaign. In recent years, the Baloch groups have not only intensified their attacks but also expanded the outreach of their terrorist violence beyond Balochistan. The foiled BLA attack on PSX Karachi on June 29, 2020, as cited earlier, created the intended impact in terms of raising the group's profile and highlighting its cause. In a related attack in November 2018, the BLA terrorists, including one wearing

DOI: 10.4324/9781003291909-5

a suicide vest, attacked the Chinese consulate in Karachi, but the security forces managed to kill all three attackers (Khan, 2018).

The developments in Afghanistan could also affect the security landscape of Pakistan. Since the US and the Afghan Taliban signed a peace deal on February 29, 2020, the Afghan Taliban have gained political legitimacy without giving up their reliance on the use of force. As the intra-Afghan talks begin, their relationship with foreign militant groups, including Al-Qaeda and the Pakistani Taliban, will bear security consequences for Pakistan.

Experts agree that COVID-19 has increased vulnerabilities on the level of state and society and violent extremists could exploit those, mainly with the purpose of adding instability and insecurity by carrying out terrorist attacks. Secondly, in a way, that would also serve the militants' purpose by adding to people's anti-government grievances. Pakistan is managing a significant number of Afghan refugees as well as Internally Displaced Persons (IDPs), whose vulnerability to COVID-19 disease is relatively higher due to a lack of available facilities in camps. Militants since the past have been exploiting the grievances of the marginalized groups including those living in camps. Therefore, the threat could have multiple aspects, ranging from the possibility of the spread of the disease to recruitment for the militants.

Against this backdrop, this report focuses on the key challenges related to terrorism in Pakistan and its interface with the COVID-19 pandemic situation. The first part consisting of a review of the terrorist groups' activities since March 2020 is aimed at studying changes in their operational targets, strategies, and tactics, as well as how they are using the coronavirus pandemic for propaganda purposes. The second part focuses on the Afghan Taliban's nexus with foreign terrorist groups and its implications for Pakistan. The last part looks into state responses to all emerging threats, and offers an analysis of the responses in the context of the COVID-19 pandemic.

Pakistan's Security Landscape (March 1 to August 10, 2020)[1]

A total of sixty-one terrorist attacks have happened in Pakistan since the outbreak of coronavirus in Pakistan, or from March 1 to August 10, 2020, to be precise. These attacks caused 79 deaths and left another 195 injured. Apart from the terrorist attacks, twenty anti-militant operational strikes and four incidents of clashes between the security forces and the militants claimed all eighty-seven lives (see Table 4.1).

Khyber Pakhtunkhwa (KP)

Over 52 percent of the total terrorist attacks reported from across Pakistan since March 1 to August 10 concentrated in KP. As data from intelligence, the highest number of terrorist attacks for any one KP district was reported from North Waziristan, where militants perpetrated fifteen terrorist attacks out of the total thirty-two attacks reported from the province (Table 4.2).

Table 4.1 Overall Violent Incidents and Casualties in Pakistan (Mar 1 to Aug 10, 2020)

Nature of Incidents	No. of Incidents	Killed	Injured
Terrorist attacks	61	79	195
Clashes between security forces and militants	4	15	6
Operational attacks by security forces	20	72	10
Plot/foiled terror attempt	8	0	0
Targeted attacks [not specific if terrorist]	7	10	1
Total	**100**	**176**	**212**

Source: Author.

Table 4.2 Violent Incidents in KP (Mar 1 to Aug 10, 2020)

Nature of Incidents	No. of Incidents	Killed	Injured
Terrorist attacks	32	32	52
Clashes between security forces and militants	4	15	6
Operational attacks by security forces	14	54	9
Plot/foiled terror attempts	7	0	0
Targeted attack (not specified as terrorist)	6	10	0
Total	**63**	**111**	**67**

Source: Author.

Table 4.3 Targets of the Terrorists in KP (Mar 1 to Aug 10, 2020)

Targets	No. of Attacks	Killed	Injured
Security forces/law enforcement	21	25	31
Tribal elders	1	0	0
Civilians	5	5	6
Shia religious scholars/community	2	1	15
Political leaders/workers	2	0	0
Health/polio workers, security escorts	1	1	0
Total	**32**	**32**	**52**

Source: Author.

As many as twenty-one terrorist attacks in KP, or 65 percent of the total attacks recorded in the province, targeted personnel of security forces and law enforcement agencies, which caused twenty-five deaths and inflicted injuries on thirty-one others. Five attacks hit civilians killing five and injuring six persons. Two attacks hit Shia community, and one attack targeted immunization workers (Table 4.3).

Militants are apparently expanding their areas of presence and operations in merged districts of KP. While North Waziristan has been witnessing terrorist violence for many months now, four violent incidents were reported from Bajaur tribal district in July alone including two terrorist attacks, one cross-border attack from Afghanistan, and one foiled terror plot in which at least twelve IEDs planted on a hill pass were defused by security forces (PIPS, 2020). The growing cross-border activities of the Pakistani Taliban militants in merged districts also validated a recent UN report that claimed that "[t]he total number of Pakistani foreign terrorist fighters in Afghanistan, posing a threat to both countries, is estimated at between 6,000 and 6,500, most of them with the TTP" (Iqbal, 2020).

The situation in Afghanistan—especially after the US signed a peace deal with the Afghan Taliban—could also impact the militant landscape and militancy of the Khyber Pakhtunkhwa, mainly of the bordering districts. The government and security agencies should be ready to confront and counter these and similar threats.

Balochistan

In Balochistan, Baloch nationalist insurgents perpetrated thirteen terrorist attacks since March, which caused twenty-three deaths. Baloch insurgent groups including BLA, BLF, United Baloch Army (UBA), and Lashkar-e-Baluchistan (LeB) perpetrated all of these attacks. The religiously motivated militant groups, including the Pakistani Taliban groups and factions of Sunni and Shia violent sectarian groups, are still active in the province, and were responsible for four attacks from March 1 to August 10, 2020. Thus, in all, seventeen terrorist attacks happened in Balochistan during these five months, which is a slight declining trend comparing with the first two months of the year, when a combined number of eight attacks had killed thirty-five people. Improved security measures could be a cause for that.

However, in May 2020, BLA and United Baloch Army militants carried out, separately, two major attacks against security forces, in Kech and Bolan, respectively. These attacks claimed the lives of six army soldiers, six Frontier Constabulary (FC) personnel, and one civilian. Such attacks against security forces, although sporadic and less frequent, indicate that the Baloch separatists still pose a potent threat. To their operational advantage, they have also established networks in areas closer to the Pak-Iran border (Table 4.4).

Apparently, the provincial government of Balochistan appears vigilant of the emerging situation in the aftermath of the coronavirus pandemic. According to

Table 4.4 Violent Incidents in Balochistan (Mar 1 to Aug 10, 2020)

Nature of Incidents	No. of Incidents	Killed	Injured
Terrorist attacks (by nationalist insurgents)	13	23	34
Terrorist attacks (by religiously inspired) militants	4	8	33
Operational attacks by security forces	4	9	1
Total	**21**	**40**	**68**

Source: Author.

Table 4.5 Targets of the Terrorists in Balochistan (Mar 1 to Aug 10, 2020)

Targets	No of Attacks	Killed	Injured
Security forces/law enforcement agencies	11	29	49
Tribal elders	1	0	2
Civilians	5	2	16
Total	**17**	**31**	**67**

Source: Author.

Minister for Home and Tribal Affairs Mir Ziaullah Langove, with proper efforts by law enforcement agencies, the law and order situation in Balochistan is being maintained adequately amid the coronavirus outbreak (*Dawn*, 2020). Still, one cannot rule out the possibility of the militants' exploitation of the situation mainly in areas closer to Iranian border, where security forces are mainly focused on addressing the situation arising out of the spread of coronavirus.

Eleven terrorist attacks in Balochistan, during the period under review, targeted personnel of security forces, which caused twenty-nine deaths and injuries to forty-nine others. Six attacks hit civilians including one attack on tribal elders (see Table 4.5).

The Active Terrorist Groups

In early 2020, four religiously inspired militant and seven separatist nationalist groups were active in Pakistan, and they all together perpetrated sixty-one terrorist attacks across the country as shown in Table 4.6.

Table 4.6 Terrorist Attacks Claimed/Perpetrated by Terrorist Groups (Mar 1 to Aug 10)

Organization	Balochistan	KP	Punjab	Sindh	Total
Tehreek-e-Taliban Pakistan (TTP)	2	16	-	-	18
Jamaatul Ahrar	-	1	-	-	1
Local Taliban	-	7	-	-	7
United Baloch Front (UBA)	1	-	-	-	1
Balochistan Liberation Army (BLA)	5	-	-	1	6
Balochistan Liberation Front (BLF)	2	-	-	-	2
Balochistan Republican Army (BRA)	2	-	-	-	2
Lashkar-e-Balochistan	1	-	-	-	1
Sindhu Desh Liberation Front (SDLF)	-	-	-	1	1
Sindhu Desh Revolutionary Army	-	-	-	5	5
Rival Sectarian group	-	2	-	-	2
Hizbul Ahrar	-	-	2	-	2
Unspecified militants and Baloch insurgents	4	5	1	3	13
Total	**17**	**31**	**3**	**10**	**61**

Source: Author.

Tehreek-e-Taliban Pakistan (TTP)

The TTP was the major actor of instability during the last five months. It was found involved in eighteen terrorist attacks, out of which sixteen were reported from KP province and two from Balochistan. The small militant groups in KP and its tribal districts, described as the local Taliban, carried out seven terrorist attacks since March 1, 2020.

Hizbul Ahrar

Hizbul Ahrar carried out two terrorist attacks in Rawalpindi district of Punjab in which one person was killed and twenty others were injured. It is also believed to be involved in target killing of at least three policemen in the city, which were reported by media as acts of crime. Its parent organization, i.e., Jamaatul Ahrar, also perpetrated one attack in KP.

Islamic State (IS)

The killing of Abu Bakr Al-Baghdadi in October 2019 was a big blow for the Islamic State (IS) and its chapters across the world including its Khorasan chapter for Afghanistan and Pakistan. Though the group had announced a separate chapter for Pakistan in 2019 (Gul, 2019), so far it has failed to show its presence in the country and has not perpetrated any attack this year (2020). The credit for this may also go to the law enforcement agencies, who dismantled a few cells of the group during the last few months (*Dawn*, 2020a). For one, the counter-terrorism department (CTD) of Punjab province also claimed success against the banned IS after killing four of its suspected terrorists in an intelligence-led operation in Bahawalpur district (*Express Tribune*, 2020).

AQIS

Though Al-Qaeda in the Indian Subcontinent (AQIS) was not found involved in any terrorist attack in Pakistan over the last few years, law enforcement departments still considered it a potent threat. An appraisal by police's counter-terrorism department (CTD) noted in 2019 that the banned AQIS was regrouping in Karachi, apparently to carry out some major attacks (Ali, 2019). Karachi has remained a hub of jihadist, sectarian, and criminal violence and there is a possibility that their remnants are still there. The COVID-19 pandemic has overstretched the law enforcers, yet they need to remain vigilant enough to not allow the militants any opportunity to initiate a new wave of violence in the provincial metropolis.

Baloch Insurgent Groups

Around seven Baloch insurgent groups are active in Balochistan but the BLA and BLF are the major groups, which represent the new generation of insurgents, mainly coming from urban backgrounds. BLA perpetrated six terrorist attacks since March 2020, including five in Balochistan and one in Karachi that targeted the Karachi Stock Exchange. BLF and BRA perpetrated two attacks each in Balochistan. Meanwhile, one attack was claimed by each of the UBA and Lashkar-e-Balochistan groups. The UBA claimed an attack after a long time in which, according to a statement by ISPR, six FC soldiers including a Junior Commissioned Officer (JCO) and a civilian driver embraced martyrdom in Pir Ghaib, Mach (Bolan district) on May 19 (*The News*, 2019).

Sindhi Insurgent Groups

The terrorist activities of Sindh-based separatist groups have increased since the coronavirus pandemic started in Pakistan. They have managed six attacks since March 1, 2020. The Interior Ministry banned the JSQM-A, Sindhudesh Liberation Army (SDLA), and Sindhudesh Revolutionary Army (SDRA) under the Anti-Terrorism Act 1997, arguing that "there are reasonable grounds to believe that the organisations are engaged in terrorism" in Sindh province (Syed, 2020).

The SDLA is an underground militant outfit linked with Shafi Burfat-led Jeay Sindh Muttahida Mahaz (JSMM), the only nationalist group to have announced its planned armed struggle. In 2013, the Interior Ministry banned the JSMM for its involvement in province-wide violence and placed Burfat, who lives in Europe in self-exile, on its list of wanted people. A few years back, Syed Asghar Shah, an SDLA leader hailing from Jamshoro district, abandoned the SDLA after developing differences with Burfat over funds and leadership, and formed his own outfit, the SDRA. In the beginning, both militant outfits were carrying out attacks on law enforcement personnel, railway tracks, gas pipelines, and electricity pylons as well as undertaking targeted killing on the basis of ethnicity. "But since the start of China Pakistan Economic Corridor (CPEC)-linked development projects, the group has started attacking the Chinese nationals using roadside improvised explosive devices (IEDs) in the province." Luckily, no Chinese national has died in the attacks in the province so far (Rehman, 2020).

Shift in Targets and Tactics?

A little variation has been witnessed in the tactics of the terrorists during the coronavirus pandemic, but it is difficult to directly link this variation with the changing situation. In thirty-five terrorist attacks, the terrorists employed IED blasts including some vehicle-born improvised explosive devices (VB-IEDs) mostly in form of motorcycle blasts. A few years back, that was a pertinent attack tactic employed by the Baloch insurgents. But now it seems some other groups, including the Taliban, are tending to rely on the tactic, which is apparently easier to perpetrate and involves less reliance on suicide bombers while having a similar impact.

Target killing in North and South Waziristan was also on the rise. While there is no evidence to say these killings are terrorist attacks, locals suspected that some militant groups could be involved in these incidents with the aim of making a comeback. In such high-profile killing, on May 1, 2020, Pashtun Tahafuz Movement (PTM) leader Arif Wazir received bullet injuries when unidentified persons opened fire on him near his house in South Waziristan. A day after, he succumbed to his injuries at the Pakistan Institute of Medical Sciences (PIMS) in Islamabad (*The News*, 2020).

Afghanistan and Terrorism in Pakistan

The Afghan Taliban surprised the world when they said that Al-Qaeda did not exist in Afghanistan (Joscelyn, 2020). The Taliban has a history of employing the "denial" as a war tactic, but denying the presence of Al-Qaeda in Afghanistan reflects on the Taliban's political compulsions, which may bring them at a crossroad. Reacting to the Taliban statement, the US Central Command's top general, Marine Gen. Kenneth F. McKenzie, had warned that he would not recommend a full withdrawal of US troops from Afghanistan unless the Taliban demonstrate that they no longer support Al-Qaeda forces there (Tolo News, 2020).

The Taliban have been using the "denial strategy" effectively against friends and foes since they first came into power during the late 1990s. For instance, the terrorists of violent sectarian group Lashkar-e-Jhangvi (LeJ) were running their training camps in Afghanistan. However, quite surprisingly, whenever Pakistan demanded the extradition of these terrorists, the Taliban denied their presence on the Afghan soil. Even now the Afghan Taliban do not publicly acknowledge their close bond with the Pakistani militant groups including the TTP. A recent report from the UN's Analytical Support and Sanctions Monitoring Team has indicated that Pakistani militant groups, mainly the TTP, are operating inside Afghanistan with the permission and support of the Afghan Taliban. In many instances, they remain reluctant to take action against the TTP and its affiliates despite Pakistan's apprehensions. The same report claimed that the Afghan Taliban regularly consulted with Al-Qaeda during negotiations with the US, and Al-Qaeda gave a nod to the deal.

The Taliban have also given the impression that severing ties with Al-Qaeda is in process, but there is no proof of it. Five hundred to 600 members of Al-Qaeda are known to still be in Afghanistan, and have become a strategic burden for the Taliban, who believe they have secured the best possible deal with the US. Many believe that the Taliban's continuing ties with Al-Qaeda could sabotage the peace process.

Three points need to be considered. First, if the Taliban have consulted with Al-Qaeda during their talks with the US, it is not possible that the US would not have been aware of it. If Al-Qaeda guarantees that it has no intention to launch terrorist assaults on NATO members, the US can tolerate the group though it would be difficult to guarantee this.

Secondly, the Taliban were ousted from power in 2001 because of Al-Qaeda, and it may be considered against their political and ideological code to disconnect with the group for whom they had sacrificed their government and fought a long war. Thirdly, breaking with Al-Qaeda may also cause an internal crisis within the rank and file of the Taliban. The two groups have also built strong family bonds through inter-marriages.

In that context, denial seems a good option for the Taliban, but their similar attitude toward the TTP and other Pakistani militant groups may have other factors behind it as well. Apart from the prevailing theory that the TTP is a strategic tool in the hands of the Afghan Taliban against Pakistan, the Afghan Taliban have engaged the Pakistani Taliban in their war. The fact that the TTP has carried out terrorist activities in Pakistan may cast doubt on such observations. However, when it comes to power-sharing in Afghanistan, the Pakistani Taliban might be seen as contenders too as they served during the Taliban regime in the 1990s. If that happens, Afghanistan and the Afghan Taliban will become prime attractions for madressah graduates in Pakistan, particularly in the country's border regions, revealing a nightmare scenario for Pakistan (Rana, 2020).

The Policy Challenges and Responses

Amnesty for TTP?

The government is also facing the dilemma about what to do with the Pakistani Taliban militants who are sheltered across the border and may want to relocate to their native towns in tribal districts. A BBC report quoted the defense analyst Brigadier (Retd.) Mehmood Shah to claim that about 9,000 Taliban militants wanted to come back to their native towns in Khyber Pakhtunkhwa after seeking a forgiveness and promising to quit violence. Local accounts from North and South Waziristan have been claiming that they have seen some of those in their areas who had remained in the past attached to militant groups (BBC Urdu, 2020). However, not all the Taliban in these areas were attached to the TTP, nor the Taliban are currently so strong to challenge the writ of the state as they used to do before the operation Zarb-e-Azab was launched in 2014. Still, the government and local administration will have to develop a policy on how to deal with the militants, including those operating discreetly in tribal districts and those living in Afghanistan and willing to come back.

FATF and Curbing Terror Financing

The Financial Action Task Force (FATF) in June 2018 put Pakistan on its "gray list" or in list of countries described by FATF as the ones with inadequate control over curbing money laundering and terrorism financing. Pakistan is currently working with the global money laundering and terrorist-financing watchdog to comply with twenty-seven-point Action Plan.

The coronavirus pandemic has provided some relief to Pakistan in fulfilling the provisions of the Action Plan it has agreed with the FATF; Pakistan has submitted its due-in-June compliance report in September. Pakistan's case was also not taken up at FATF's last meeting held in Paris on June 24, 2020. However, Pakistan will have to show "significant and sustainable progress" to get off the gray list (*Dawn*, 2020b).

In one of his briefings to the Prime Minister, Federal Interior Minister Ijaz Shah claimed that Pakistan has met most of the conditions set by the FATF (*Express Tribune*, 2020a). The minister also stated that his ministry had frozen 976 movable and immovable properties of proscribed outfits, and taken over several schools, colleges, hospitals, dispensaries, ambulances, etc. of the proscribed organizations into government's control.

The Pakistan government has taken some initiatives to meet the requirements of the FATF. First, Federal Interior Ministry has set up a single-template database to curb money laundering and terror financing, which will also facilitate the provincial efforts for countering terrorism and terror financing. Secondly, an Interior Ministry cell, which was established to implement the FATF recommendations, has been activated again. The cell functions were temporarily suspended because of the coronavirus. Thirdly, the lower and upper houses of Parliament have approved the United Nations Security Council (UNSC) Amendment Bill, 2020 and the Anti-Terrorism Act Amendment Bill, 2020, in an effort to fulfill the FATF requirements (*Express Tribune*, 2020b).

On the other side, the anti-terrorism courts have sped up the process of hearing the terror financing cases. In June 2020, anti-terrorism courts have sentenced top Jamaatud Daawa (JuD) leadership including its head Hafiz Saeed and his brother-in-law Abdul Rehman Makki, among others, in cases of terrorist financing (*The Nation*, 2020). It is essential that these actions against banned groups are sustained and developed into a strong resolve of the state because they don't merely relate to FATF provisions but are indeed integral to Pakistan's national security interests.

In a related development on curbing terror financing, the Federal Investigative Agency (FIA) took control of five properties of Afghan Taliban chief Mullah Akhtar Mansour, who was killed in a drone strike along the Pakistan-Iran border on May 21, 2016, had purchased these properties, including plots and houses for auction in Karachi (Sahoutra, 2020).

There are multiple areas and factors, which make Pakistan vulnerable to terrorist financing. At the same time, there are challenges related to governance and law enforcement, which affect the state's responses to curb terrorism financing. These challenges and vulnerabilities, both transactional and structural, raise the risk profile of Pakistan. They have also "led [among other factors] the FATF to put Pakistan on 'grey list'; [and] the country also holds the critical risk of being blacklisted" (NIOC, 2020). Experts assert that the "approach and plan of eradicating terrorist financing needs to be developed beyond FATF," and should entail sustained policy endeavors (NIOC, 2020).

Security Challenges during the Pandemic

Pakistan's internal security landscape is complicated due to both internal and external threats. The internal security dimension not only includes threats from hardcore radical and sectarian terrorist groups but also from groups that promote religious extremism and intolerance. The latter pose a different sort of critical challenge because such groups can mobilize their support bases to cause more damage to the economy, the social cohesion of society, and the global image of the country.

The pandemic has created space for sectarian and radical groups, who tend to spread hate including in cyberspace. In the beginning of the pandemic, while Sunni extremists and activists blamed the Shia pilgrims returning from Iran for the spread of the COVID-19 infection in Pakistan, the Shia activists accused the Tablighi Jamaat tours and gatherings for the spread of the virus. Posts and messages rife with sectarian hate speech also went viral on social media platforms.

The Wall Street Journal (WSJ) recently reported about the removal of a significant number of names of suspected violent actors from the terrorism watchlist maintained by the National Counter-Terrorism Authority (NACTA) of Pakistan. Pakistan Annual Security Report 2019, prepared by Pak Institute for Peace Studies (PIPS), had also highlighted the need for developing a National Databank (NDB) synchronized with the police departments of the country, National Database and Registration Authority (NADRA), NACTA, FIA, and State Bank of Pakistan. The report recommended that the Databank should have the following features:

- A synchronized National Red Book, containing updated information about the wanted, suspected, and arrested terrorists and their groups.
- The national databank could be divided into two categories, one for public consumption, which would include details about terrorists and their activities, and the second dedicated for the police and law enforcement agencies containing details of bank accounts, financial transactions data, property, and other assets of the suspected and active terrorists whose names had been placed under the Fourth Schedule.
- A common website can be developed under the supervision of NACTA and all police and relevant authorities could be bound to provide updates/information on weekly or monthly bases.
- There is a need that all provinces have their forensic labs linked with National Forensic Laboratory (NFL) in Islamabad.
- Capacity building training programs for the counter-terrorism departments needed to be developed and they must know the best practices around the world to avoid any mishandling of the sensitive issues.

As noted earlier in the report, COVID-19 has increased vulnerabilities of people in terms of provision of health, shelter, food, and other amenities of life. Similarly, a sense of insecurity could increase due to economic deprivation and the state's failure to provide adequate social safety nets; preoccupation of the security, particularly due to police force's pandemic-related duties; and restriction of mobility to maintain the demand and supply of things, etc. Violent extremists could try to exploit these vulnerabilities, mainly with the purpose to add to instability and insecurity by carrying out terrorist attacks. In a way, that would also serve the militants' purpose by adding to people's anti-government grievances.

The government will have to adopt a clear policy not only against non-violent extremist groups. The National Action Plan (NAP) had put some pressure on religious extremists including those propagating hate speech, but in recent years, its implementation has been faltering. As of now, it appears as if the government has abandoned the country's first counter-terrorism and counter-extremism plan. The government should revamp its focus on NAP besides enhancing counter-terrorism vigilance and action.

Note

1 Most statistics used in this report are based on PIPS database on conflict and security incidents: www.pakpips.com/app/database

References

Ali, Imtiaz. 2019. "CTD says splinter group of outlawed AQIS reorganizing in Karachi." *Dawn*, October 15th.

BBC Urdu. 2020. April 16th. <https://www.bbc.com/urdu/pakistan-52305891>

Dawn. 2020. "Security situation in Balochistan reviewed." April 1st. <https://www.dawn.com/news/1545469/security-situation-in-balochistan-reviewed>

Dawn. 2020a. "Police arrest 'IS militant' on extortion, terrorism charges." May 31st. <https://epaper.dawn.com/print-textview.php?StoryImage=31_05_2020_113_002>

Dawn. 2020b. "Pakistan case not taken up at FATF meeting: FO." June 27th. <https://www.dawn.com/news/1565473/pakistans-case-not-taken-up-at-fatf-meeting-fo>

Express Tribune. 2020. "Four IS terrorists killed in Bahawalpur: CTD." May 17th. <https://tribune.com.pk/story/2223338/1-four-terrorists-killed-bahawalpur-ctd>

Express Tribune. 2020a. "Pakistan meets major FATF conditions: Shah." June 11th. <https://tribune.com.pk/story/2240041/1-pakistan-meets-major-fatf-conditions-shah>

Express Tribune. 2020b. "Senate unanimously approves UNSC ATA amendment bills." July 30th. <https://tribune.com.pk/story/2257377/senate-unanimously-approves-unsc-ata-amendment-bills>

Gul, Ayaz. 2019. "Islamic state announces 'Pakistan province'." *VOA*, May 15th. <https://www.voanews.com/south-central-asia/islamic-state-announces-pakistan-province>

Iqbal, Anwar. 2020. "6,500 terrorists still active in Afghanistan: UN." *Dawn*, July 26th.

Joscelyn, Thomas. 2020. "Taliban falsely claims Al-Qaeda does not exist in Afghanistan." *The Long War Journal*, June 15th. <https://www.longwarjournal.org/archives/2020/06/taliban-falsely-claims-al-qaeda-doesnt-exist-in-afghanistan.php>

Khan, Faraz. 2018. "Terrorist hit Chinese consulate in Karachi, target Friday bazaar in Orakzai: 39 die in twin terror attacks." *The News*, November 24th. <https://www.thenews.com.pk/print/397403-terrorists-hit-chinese-consulate-in-karachi-target-friday-bazaar-in-orakzai-39-die-in-twin-terror-attacks>

NIOC (National Initiative against Organized Crime). 2020. "Strategic policy options to curb terrorism financing in Pakistan." June 17th. <https://nioc.pk/article/777>

PIPS (Pak Institute for Peace Studies). 2020. "Pakistan monthly security report: July 2020." August 7th. <http://pakpips.com/app/reports/793>

Rana, M. Amir. 2020. "Afghan Taliban's strength." *Dawn*, June 28th. <https://www.dawn.com/news/1565703>

Rehman, Ziaur. 2020. "The crackdown intensified." *The News on* Sunday, June 7th. <https://www.thenews.com.pk/tns/detail/668374-the-crackdown-intensifies>

Sahoutra, Naeem. 2020. "Court seizes slain Taliban chief's properties for auction." *Dawn*, May 8th. <https://www.dawn.com/news/1555423/court-seizes-slain-taliban-chiefs-properties-for-auction>

Syed, Azaz. 2020. "Daily Jang." May 8th. <https://e.jang.com.pk/05-08-2020/pindi/pic.asp?picname=510.png>

The Nation. 2020. "4 JUD leaders convicted for terror financing." June 19th. <https://nation.com.pk/E-Paper/islamabad/2020-06-19/page-12/detail-6>

The News. 2019. "Seven soldiers martyred in two separate incidents in Balochistan." May 19th. <https://www.thenews.com.pk/latest/660544-seven-soldiers-martyred-in-two-separate-incidents-in-balochistan>

The News. 2020. "PTM leader Arif Wazir dies from injuries." May 3rd. <https://www.thenews.com.pk/print/653594-ptm-leader-arif-wazir-dies-from-injuries>

Tolo News. 2020. "US Gen: If Al-Qaeda remains, US troops should not fully withdraw." June 11th. <https://tolonews.com/afghanistan/us-gen-if-al-qaeda-remains-us-troops-should-not-fully-withdraw>

5 COVID-19 in India

Threat and Response

Adil Rasheed

Introduction

India's response to the COVID-19 crisis has been like the three-dimensional chess game played in the television series "Star Trek"—with "health," "economy," "social," and "political" fronts panning out at separate levels and yet interconnected to a grand strategy.[1] In order to score a decisive victory, the Indian central and state governments have had to not only consider the pros and cons of their coordinated actions but keep tabs on an unknown and unpredictable adversary—the elusive coronavirus. Again, as in the game of chess, some of the best-laid plans have tended to go awry and have not necessarily delivered the intended results.

The challenge and the costs involved for India in fighting the pandemic—both in humanitarian as well as in economic terms—have been enormous. For a nation with 1.3 billion people—of which 275 million (22 percent) live below the poverty line—the big question has been whether the overstretched administrative machinery and weak public healthcare system could prevent a pandemic from causing a major humanitarian crisis.

Enormity of the Challenge

The first case of COVID-19 reported in India came from the state of Kerala on January 30, 2020, which rose to three cases by February 3, as all were students who had returned home for a vacation from Wuhan University in China.[2]

By June 18, India's Ministry of Health and Family Welfare (MoHFW) confirmed 366,946 cases, 194,325 recoveries (including 1 migration), and 12,237 deaths in the country.[3] Having the largest number of confirmed cases in Asia, India had the fourth highest number of cases in the world, even though the fatality rate was relatively lower at 2.8 percent against the global 6.13 by June.[4] Six big Indian cities—Delhi, Mumbai, Ahmedabad, Chennai, Pune, and Kolkata—accounted for almost half of all reported cases in the country.[5]

More problematic than being the second most populous country in the world is that India has a huge population density of 464 people/km². Compare this figure with the population density of other countries that have been badly affected

DOI: 10.4324/9781003291909-6

by the pandemic such as Italy with a population density of 206 people/km², Spain 91, Iran 52, and the USA 36.[6] India may have the second largest population after China, but its population density far exceeds it (455/km² as opposed to 148/km²).[7]

Thus, the dreaded prospect of the pandemic proliferating out of control is multiplied many times, given the potential for its spread. Social distancing in Indian cities with overcrowded and fetid shanty towns has proven to be a near impossibility. As over 160 million Indians still have no access to clean water to wash their hands, the prospect of a geometric progression of the pandemic has given sleepless nights to policymakers.[8] The prevalence of diabetes and hypertension among Indian adults—diseases that are said to worsen COVID-19 outcomes—is as high as 10% and 25%, respectively. The high rates of tuberculosis and pneumonia vex an already critical situation. Further, India's poor (who constitute 22% of its population and live below the official poverty limit of earning less than $1.25 per day) have little access to health care.[9]

About 90 percent of this population has no form of private or government health insurance (shows data from India's largest national survey on social consumption, conducted between July 2017 and June 2018),[10] making them incapable of availing any decent healthcare treatment. There has also been a shortage of doctors and healthcare personnel,[11] in addition to the dearth of hospital beds, testing kits, personal protective equipment (PPE), N95 masks, ventilators, gloves, goggles, gowns, aprons, and face shields as India imports about 80 percent of its medical device requirement.[12]

According to a COVID-19 SWOT analysis report by Niti Ayog,[13] a premier policy think tank of the Government of India, the doctor-to-patient ratio in the country stands at an alarming 1:1445, hospital beds to people ratio at 0.7:1000, and ventilators to population ratio at 40,000 to 1.3 billion. The Indian government also faces the twin challenge of containing the virus even as the economy is undergoing a major slowdown.

Salient Features of Government Response

The Indian government has undertaken several initiatives to safeguard the country against the COVID-19 pandemic. According to the Information and Broadcasting Ministry, India's response to COVID-19 has been "pre-emptive, pro-active and graded."[14] Since the time of the outbreak, it has put in place a "comprehensive response system" at the borders of the country, much before the World Health Organization (WHO) declared the coronavirus as a public health emergency of international concern on January 30.[15]

The government claims its response has focused on divesting leadership in its fight against the pandemic at various administrative levels—from the federal to provincial, municipal, block, and down to village levels—and has involved various ministries to work in a synchronized manner to implement a grand strategy against the spread of the pandemic.[16] Its approach has also sought to involve and engage with the international community "not only in sending shipments of essential medical supplies to various nations, including the US,"[17] but also in bringing back Indian expatriates in large numbers from various countries afflicted with the disease (such as the Vande Bharat Mission launched to bring home Indian expats from the Gulf).[18] The government's response has included spreading awareness of the pandemic to a very large population, ably led by the eloquent prime minister himself for providing right information intelligibly to the country's poor and uneducated masses without causing panic.

The Indian government campaign has used scientific evidence-based projections to guide its decision making and has used state-of-the-art technology in its fight against the disease, such as the launch of Aarogya Setu, a "contact tracing, syndromic mapping and self-assessment mobile app,"[19] which tells how many COVID-19 positive cases are likely in a radius of 500 meters, 1 kilometers, 2 kilometers, 5 kilometers, and 10 kilometers from the mobile user. It used the right kind of legislative and law-enforcement measures to ensure the disease did not spread, has involved private sector and civil society organizations in its campaigns, and launched a specific fund to fight the disease—The PM CARES Fund—to receive domestic and foreign donations for further availability of quality treatment of the patients infected by COVID-19.[20]

The aforementioned measures come within the ambit of the Indian government's phased strategy to fight the COVID-19 pandemic, which covers the initial preventive stage, the subsequent containment phase, and the final mitigating phase.

The Preventive Stage (Late January to Mid-March 2020)

In this stage, India sought to control ingress of the virus from abroad. The country began thermal screening of passengers arriving from China on January 21 at seven airports, which was subsequently expanded to twenty airports toward the end of that month.[21] All visas were suspended on March 13, barring a few diplomatic and official visas.[22] Thereafter, government ordered seven ministries—Home, Labor, Defense, Aviation, Railways, Tourism, and Minorities Affairs—to set up additional treatment and quarantine facilities across the country. In early March, The Ministry of Consumer Affairs, Food and Public Distribution was instructed to ensure the availability of essential goods and food items throughout the country, The Ministry of Textiles was instructed to ensure the availability of protective and medical materials, and The Department of Pharmaceuticals took steps to ensure that essential medicines were available.[23]

The government also formulated a plan to create greater public awareness about the COVID-19 threat, while avoiding panic in society. Central and state governments set up helpline numbers and a COVID-19 Economic Response Task Force was formed around the third week of March.[24] On March 15, the Ministry of Culture closed all monuments and museums under Archeological Survey of India.[25] Over the course of the month, several Indian states started closing educational institutions (schools and colleges), as well as public places like shopping malls, gyms, cinema halls, and other public places to check the pandemic from spreading.

The Containment Stage (World's Largest Lockdown)

However, measures taken in the preventive stage did not stop the COVID-19 infection from spreading in the country. By March 22, the number of confirmed cases rapidly neared the 500-mark, with eight deaths. The Indian government decided that the best way to flatten the rising curve of infection and fatalities and avoid large-scale community transmission was to buy time for ramping up the health infrastructure and to achieve social distancing was to impose a nation-wide lockdown. This was a difficult decision for the government, as the country's economy had been struggling before the outbreak of the pandemic, and fear that the shutdown could cause massive job losses in economy where over 90 percent of the workforce is employed in the informal sector.[26]

Taking the cue from China, Spain, and Italy, the Indian government opted for a nationwide lockdown and rejected the "herd immunity" approach initially employed in the UK, or that of "voluntary social distancing" as used in Sweden or merely restricting itself to aggressive testing, contact tracing, and isolation as practiced by South Korea. The Indian prime minister used a highly emotive pop-ular Hindi idiom (*"Jaan Hai toh Jahaan Hai,"* which can be roughly translated as "life comes first and then the world"[27]) to convey the point that the safety of the life of people should take precedence over the state of the national economy, as a justification for the national lockdown.

On March 19, Prime Minister Narendra Modi addressed the nation on televi-sion and asked all citizens to observe a one-day "Janta Curfew" ("people's cur-few") on Sunday, March 22. Following the successful completion of the curfew, the Prime Minister made another televised address on March 23, wherein he announced a nationwide lockdown (the largest and one of the most stringent lockdowns in the world over 1.3 billion people) from midnight of that day, for a period of twenty-one days. "Jahan Hai, Wahan Rahain" (stay where you are) was his new catchphrase this time.[28]

Phase I of the Lockdown lasted 21 days from March 25 to April 14. As a result, people were prohibited from stepping out of their homes, all shops and services were closed (except grocery shops, pharmacies, hospitals, banks, and other essential services), and there was closure of commercial and private establishments as well as all educational, training, and research institutions. In addition, all places of worship were closed, non-essential public and private transport suspended, and all social, political, sports, entertainment, academic, cultural, and religious activities were prohibited. During this phase, the police were very strict and made arrests in all the states of the country for violating lockdown restrictions, such as people coming out on the streets for no reason, opening their shops or businesses, and driving on roads, highways unless in an emergency.

To mitigate the economic impact of the lockdown on the poor, Finance Minister Nirmala Sitharaman announced Rs 1.7 trillion (US $24b) worth of relief package[29] on March 26 to provide food security for poor families through direct cash transfers, free grains, and free cooking gas for three months. On March 27, the Reserve Bank of India announced several measures to mitigate the economic impact of the lockdown.

Toward the end of the Phase I lockdown (21 days), the spread of COVID infections seem to have been checked significantly, with the rate of doubling every three days registered before the lockdown slowing down to doubling every eight days by April 18. Reputed Indian journalist Shekhar Gupta noted the benefit of the lockdown then with some measure of satisfaction: "India isn't going through a picnic, but our drains aren't filled with bodies, hospitals haven't run out of beds, crematoriums and graveyards not out of wood or space."[30]

Phase II of the Lockdown (from April 14 to May 3): At the end of the 21-day lockdown, Prime Minister Modi delivered another televised address to the nation and claimed that India was doing better with his government's "timely decision" of enforcing a national lockdown and a "holistic approach" in comparison with other countries. He claimed the lockdown slowed down the disease's spread that allowed for labs to come up with vaccinations and beds to increase and said that "more than 600 hospitals are working for coronavirus treatment. These facilities are being added every day."[31]

However, Prime Minister Modi announced the extension of the lockdown for twenty more days (from April 14 to May 3), as India still needed to curtail the pandemic as there were already 100,000 confirmed cases and over 300 deaths across various states by April 14. The premier announced a conditional relaxation in some places where the spread had been contained. A new classification of areas was announced on April 16, wherein hotspots with high rate of infection were branded as "red zones," areas with relatively fewer cases were tagged as "orange zones," while places with no infections—where restrictions could be eased—were classified as "green zones."[32]

The government also allowed relaxations for agricultural businesses (including dairy, aquaculture, and plantations), banks, small retail shops (with half the staff), public works programs, and cargo transportation vehicles to operate. However, social distancing norms had to be strictly adhered to and the wearing of masks in public places, slums, and shanty towns was made mandatory.

Phase III of the Lockdown came with another extension from May 4 to 18, albeit with some relaxation spread out across Indian districts split into three zones: red zones (130 districts), orange zones (284 districts), and green zones (319 districts). Buses were allowed to operate on only 50 percent capacity in green zones, while private and hired vehicles were allowed in orange zones.

Phase IV of the Lockdown (from May 18 to 31): This was the final phase of the lockdown, announced by the National Disaster Management Authority (NDMA) and the Ministry of Home Affairs (MHA) for a period of two weeks from May 18 to 31, although it introduced additional relaxations. Unlike the previous extensions, the central government gave a larger say to states in the demarcation of Green, Orange, and Red zones and the implementation roadmap.

Unwinding the Lockdown—Unlock I (June 1–30): The growing economic problems faced by India's struggling economy under the lockdown forced the government to open the lockdown, albeit gradually all over the country. While opening the lockdown during the so-called "Unlock I" phase, the MHA states that the re-opening would "have an economic focus." It was decided that lockdown restrictions would from now only be imposed in containment zones (hotspots), while regular business would be permitted to function in other zones in a phased manner.[33] Thus, religious places, shopping malls, hotels, and restaurants were allowed to reopen from June 8 and restrictions on inter-state travel were finally lifted. In upcoming Phase II, educational institutions are scheduled to reopen in July 2020, pending consultations with state governments, while in Phase III, restrictions on international air travel, operation of metro trains and recreation (gymnasiums, cinema halls, entertainment parks, auditoriums and assembly halls) are scheduled to end in August 2020.

Cases, Deaths Shoot Up after Lockdown

Even as the lockdown continues to unwind, the success of this stringent containment measure has become a matter of contentious debate in the country, as government sources claim that the lockdown was successful in preventing a rapid rise in infections, even though it admits that a large proportion of the population still remains highly susceptible to contracting the disease. Thus, the government believes it has managed to bring down the growth in confirmed cases "from 24.3 percent in the pre-lockdown period to 3.8 percent during the current 'Unlock 1.0.'" The daily rise in cases spiked above 10,000 for several days in the second and third week of June, even as deaths topped 300 per day.

Indian opposition parties have been highly critical of the lockdown. They claim that the over two-month-long "curfew" on the country has proven to be a total failure and have questioned the effectiveness of the financial package announced to mitigate the effects of the lockdown. In a tweet, former president of the opposition Congress party Rahul Gandhi said "This is what a failed lockdown looks like," as he compared the grim Indian figures on corona-infected cases with worst-hit countries like Spain, the UK, and Italy.

Even the Indian press gradually shifted its views against the measure from its largely favorable view of the lockdown when it was enforced. Writing for the online news portal The Wire, Suvrat Raju argued that the government was unable to take advantage of the lockdown to increase its healthcare capacities and had few effective long-term measures. He wrote:

> A lockdown reduces the number of infections for a short period. In the absence of sustainable long-term measures, the pandemic will resume its original trajectory when the lockdown ends. Simple models suggest that, in such a scenario, when the pandemic has run its course, it will have extracted almost exactly the same final toll in lives as it would have without the lockdown.

The *Deccan Chronicle* newspaper highlighted the spike in COVID cases once the lockdown was lifted: "Between June 1 and 18, the country has seen a surge of 1,76,411 coronavirus infection cases with Maharashtra, Tamil Nadu, Delhi, Gujarat and Uttar Pradesh remaining among the top ten states."[34]

Economic Fallout (Major Recession Ahead)

The outbreak of the COVID-19 pandemic as well as the government's response to fight it has taken a heavy toll on the Indian economy. According to the Indian Ministry of Statistics and Programme Implementation (MoSPI), India's gross domestic product (GDP) rose by 3.1% in the Q4 of FY20 (January–March 2020), compared to 4.1% in the preceding three months.[35] At 4.2 percent, FY20's growth rate is the lowest in 11 years.[36] According to the World Bank's South Asia Economic Focus (Spring 2020) edition, COVID-19 pandemic has "magnified pre-existing risks to India's economic outlook."[37]

The World Bank report added that India may record its worst growth performance since 1991 liberalization, which may veer around 1.5 percent to 2.8 percent in 2020–2021. However, the prognosis became more dire after the May 12 Atmanirbhar Bharat: COVID-19 Special Economic Package announced pumping Rs 20 trillion stimulus package (US $260 billion) to revive the pandemic-struck economy.[38] Since then, India's GDP estimates have been reduced further by credit rating agencies, such as Moody's June 1 downgrade to a notch above junk (Baa3), which signal a deep recession ahead.[39]

While CRISIL fears that the recession, which is "already here," will be perhaps India's worse since independence and that it will be "tough for India to return to its pre-pandemic growth levels at least for the next three years,"[40] irrespective of policy support, State Bank of India research estimates that the country's economy faces a "humongous" loss in the June quarter and gross domestic product (GDP) could contract by more than 40 percent during the period.[41]

Within half a month of the lockdown, the reputed Centre for Monitoring Indian Economy (CMIE) reported unemployment figures shot up from 6.7 percent (as estimated on March 15) to over 23 percent (as of April 07, 2020), with one of its reports estimating that 140 million people lost their employment while salaries were cut for many others.[42] Over 45 percent of households in the country have reported a drop in income as compared to the previous year.[43] About 53 percent of Indian businesses have been said to be significantly hit by the pandemic fallout, while supply chains were severely disrupted by lockdown restrictions in place. Farmers who grow perishable crops also faced great uncertainty.[44]

Workers Flee Cities on Foot

Indian cities depend on a vast workforce that comes from far-flung provinces (small towns and the countryside) of the country, a poor yet aspirant population that migrates in search of opportunity to the big metropolises, leaving behind their extended families in the remote regions in the prospect of a brighter future.

This population of internal migrants, which is in the tens of millions, ends up working in small industries, construction sector, hotels, and restaurants. After the

Indian Prime Minister announced an all-India lockdown, many of these migrant workers saw their business establishments close and even their wages and puny savings fizzle away. Transport restrictions also blocked their option to return to their places of origin. As the period of lockdown extended for months, many of these migrant workers started facing starvation. Consequently, hundreds of thousands of them started walking back home, covering hundreds of kilometers, as there was no public transport available. They also had to face police action for straying into the streets and onto the highways.

It took some time for the central and state governments to view the flight of these migrant workers sympathetically, as city establishments and industry viewed the exodus of laborers as an adverse development that could impede resumption of business even after the lockdown is lifted. By mid-May, the Indian central government started providing a relief package worth $22.6 billion to ease the economic plight of about 800 million poor people.[45] However, these schemes could not stop migrant workers from leaving cities and walking back on foot to their hometowns, with their images streaming on national televisions covering stories of their exhaustion, starvation, road and railway accidents, and police high-handedness. Thus, the correct and well-meaning action of the government and law-enforcement agencies started to be misconstrued as "insensitive," and even "draconian" in the Indian and foreign media.

According to data compiled by the SaveLIFE Foundation, a road safety NGO, 198 migrant workers lost their lives in road accidents during the lockdown period.[46] The workers leaving cities that were killed while returning to their home towns and villages constituted 26.4 percent of the deaths during the lockdown, the report states.

India's Successes, Achievements, and Plaudits

The Indian government's *decisive, effective, and timely measures* for fighting the pandemic have drawn praise from various international institutions. The United Nations and the World Health Organization (WHO) hailed India's management of the COVID-19 crisis as "comprehensive and robust," and termed the decision to enforce a *nationwide lockdown an "aggressive but vital" containment measure.*[47]

The Indian government has also been praised by the WHO for increasing its healthcare capacities to prevent, contain, and mitigate the impact of the disease. WHO Representative to India Hank Bekedam hailed the Modi government by stating: "Massive efforts have been made toward prevention and containing the spread, including *strengthening surveillance, laboratory capacity, contact tracing and isolation and risk communications.*"[48]

Rapid Increase in Healthcare Facilities

The Indian government has been praised for its swift action in the wake of the crisis, evident from its screening of international passengers as early as mid-January. The nation had six COVID testing labs ready before it found its first patient with the disease. In fact, it had reportedly screened 150,000 people when just three active cases were found.[49] By April 21, India reportedly had over 21,000 round-the-clock medical institutions dedicated to fighting the disease, over 173,000 patients in isolation, and 21,000 ICU beds. Over 276 labs had conducted over 400,000 tests by that time.

Timely Relief for the Poor

In 2020, the government also drawn praise for having launched Rs 348 billion financial assistance scheme under *Pradhan Mantri Gareeb Kalyan Anna Yojana* which would use digital payment infrastructure to about 390 million people—primarily low-wage earners, farmers, senior citizens, disabled, widows, and the needy. The measure became part of the government's massive economic relief and stimulus package (under the *Atma Nirbhar Bharat Abhiyan*) worth Rs 20 trillion (US $260 billion), announced in mid-May.[50]

The scheme provides free 5 kilograms wheat/rice and 1 kilogram pulses for 800 million people for a period of three months. It also provided three free LPG cylinders to 80 million beneficiaries of Ujjwala Scheme. Nearly 200 million holders of Jan Dhan bank accounts (dedicated to the poor) have reportedly received Rs 500 each directly into their bank accounts, as 83.1 million farmers have reportedly received Rs 2,000 each as first installment under the PM-KISAN Yojana, as part of the government's relief measures. Wages for the rural unemployed under Mahatma Gandhi National Rural Employment Guarantee Act (MNREGA) have been increased to Rs 202 per day.

Criticism of Government Response

The difficult decisions the Indian government made to fight the COVID-19 pandemic, an unprecedented challenge in nature and scope, naturally drew a lot of criticism from mainly within the country.

Lockdown without Advance Notice Hurt Workers, Small Businesses

To begin with, the government was criticized in some quarters for announcing the lockdown suddenly, without allowing Indian businesses and households, particularly the poor and daily wage earners. People also remained unsure for how long the lockdown would last and that caused a lot of workers (daily wage earners), small farmers, and the poor great economic hardship, even starvation. In his weekly radio address, Prime Minister Modi himself apologized for the impact of his stay-at-home enforcement. Thus, he admitted: "Especially when I look at my poor brothers and sisters, I definitely feel that they must be thinking, what kind of prime minister is this who has placed us in this difficulty?"

However, he insisted that he had "no other way."[51] Critics argue that the Prime Minister could have alerted the population a week or a few days earlier, and point out that he repeated the mistake of keeping the nation in the dark even before declaring subsequent extensions to the lockdown.

The Shortfall in Testing

The other criticism the government faces is that it has still not prioritized and procured for more testing of the disease in the population. Opposition party leader Rahul Gandhi has ardently stressed upon the need for expanding the test base, which experience from other nations show is the key method to counter the virus. India has made progress in this regard, but even the goal of conducting 10 million tests to reach the "threshold level of one percent of the population," as former union minister Jairam Ramesh demands, remains elusive.

Lockdown Flattened the GDP Curve

Some political leaders and even industrialists like Rajiv Bajaj have called the lockdown a "draconian" measure, which ended up flattening the wrong curve—i.e., the GDP "growth curve" of the country—instead of flattening the COVID-19 spread curve.[52] Some businessmen and economists assert that while the number of coronavirus cases rise at the rate of roughly 10,000 per day after the lifting of the lockdown since June 1, businesses may take months or even years to recover from the shock dealt by the lockdown. Some experts have said that social distancing, even enforced as in a lockdown, is inconceivable in Indian cities, where people live in overcrowded buildings and shanty town tenements in large numbers.

Prognosis: Silver Lining on a Dark Horizon

By mid-June of 2020, India has become the *fourth country worst hit by the coronavirus* after the US, Brazil, and Russia.[53] Whereas the disease is on the decline in other parts of the world, the pace of coronavirus transmission in the country has started picking up dramatically after the lockdown. Authorities in the states of Maharashtra, Tamil Nadu, Delhi, Gujarat and Uttar Pradesh are fearing acute shortage of intensive care units and ventilators in the coming months. The Harvard Global Health Institute director Ashish K. Jha fears that India might become "the global epicenter" of the coronavirus pandemic and believes India has 50,000 unreported pandemics a day already, which may rise to 200,000 cases a day by August.[54]

Many experts believe the disease has already entered the stage of community transmission in the country and aver that because of the migrant workers' mass exodus the focal point of the pandemic will soon "shift from urban centres like Delhi, Mumbai, Ahmedabad to second- and third-tier cities and even district towns."[55] The grim prospect of doctors, nurses, and paramedics falling sick of the disease in large numbers is highly worrisome. It seems unlikely for the government to re-enforce lockdowns given the precarious state of the economy and it has few options other than going for aggressive testing and sequestering as well as enforcing the wearing of masks.

However, there is a silver lining amidst dark clouds hovering on the horizon. The Drug Controller General of India (DGCI) has given approval to three companies to produce their COVID-19 treatment medicines in India. The companies are Cipla, Hetero and Glenmark which are now licensed to roll out Cipremi, Covifor and FabiFlu respectively.[56] All three medicines have shown efficacious results in tests conducted so far and would slowly be made available and administered under strict medical observation. The country is also ardently hoping that a vaccine would also be produced at least by early next year so that the threat of a major humanitarian crisis is averted.

Notes

1 Sarah Farooqui, 'India Coronavirus Dispatch: Visualizing a Response Moving Forward', Business Standard, June 5, 2020
2 Mukesh Rawat, 'Coronavirus in India: Tracking country's first 50 COVID-19 cases; what numbers tell', India Today, March 12, 2020, https://www.indiatoday.in/india/story/coronavirus-in-india-tracking-country-s-first-50-COVID-19-cases-what-numbers-tell-1654468-2020-03-12 (last accessed on 19 June 2020)
3 COVID-19 India, Ministry of Health and Family Welfare, https://www.mohfw.gov.in/ (accessed on June 18, 2020)
4 Press Information Bureau of India, Twitter Account
5 'Infections over one lakh, five cities with half the cases: India's coronavirus story so far', The Week, May 19, 2020 (accessed on June 1, 2020)
6 Sagarika Kamath, Rajesh Kamath, Prajwal Salins, 'COVID-19 Pandemic in India: Challenges and Silver Linings', Post Graduate Medical Journal, 2020, https://pmj.bmj.com/content/early/2020/06/10/postgradmedj-2020-137780 (last accessed on June 3, 2020)
7 Population density (people per sq. km of land area), All Countries and Economies, The World Bank, https://data.worldbank.org/indicator/EN.POP.DNST (last accessed on June 3, 2020)
8 Sagarika Kamath, Rajesh Kamath, Prajwal Salins, 'COVID-19 Pandemic in India: Challenges and Silver Linings', Post Graduate Medical Journal, 2020, https://pmj.bmj.com/content/early/2020/06/10/postgradmedj-2020-137780 (last accessed on June 3, 2020)
9 Ibid
10 'Key Indicators of Social Consumption in India: Health', Ministry of Statistics and Programme Implementation, National Statistical Office, July 2017-June 2018, Published November 2019, http://www.mospi.gov.in/sites/default/files/NSS75250H/KI_Health_75th_Final.pdf (last accessed on June 5, 2020)
11 Banjot Kaur, 'COVID-19: Govt's survey exposes lack of preparedness across India', Down to Earth magazine, April 3, 2020, https://www.downtoearth.org.in/news/health/COVID-19-govt-s-survey-exposes-lack-of-preparedness-across-india-70221 (last accessed on June 6, 2020)
12 'Govt exempts customs duty, cess on ventilators, surgical masks, PPE, COVID-19 test kits', Economic Times, April 10, 2020, https://www.google.com/search?q=down+to+earth+india&rlz=1C1CHBD_enIN717IN718&oq=Down+to+earth+India&aqs=chrome.0.0j46j0l6.8793j1j8&sourceid=chrome&ie=UTF-8 (last accessed on June 8, 2020)

13   Arshiya Mahajan and Himanshu Agarwal, 'COVID-19: A SWOT Analysis', Niti Ayog, May 11, 2020, https://niti.gov.in/COVID-19-india-swot-analysis (last accessed on June 12, 2020)

14   'India's response to COVID-19 pre-emptive, pro-active, graded: Govt', Economic Times, March 28, 2020, https://economictimes.indiatimes.com/news/politics-and-nation/indias-response-to-COVID-19-pre-emptive-pro-active-graded-govt/articleshow/74859635.cms?utm_source=contentofinterest&utm_medium=text&utm_campaign=cppst (last accessed on May 29, 2020)

15   Ibid

16   'COVID-19: Seven ministries to set up quarantine facilities', Economic Times, March 12, 2020, https://economictimes.indiatimes.com/news/politics-and-nation/COVID-19-seven-ministries-to-set-up-quarantine-facilities/articleshow/74586054.cms?utm_source=contentofinterest&utm_medium=text&utm_campaign=cppst (last accessed on May 30, 2020)

17   'India has shown leadership in fight against COVID-19: Senior Diplomat', Times of India, May 12, 2020, http://timesofindia.indiatimes.com/articleshow/75692576.cms?utm_source=contentofinterest&utm_medium=text&utm_campaign=cppst (last accessed on May 29, 2020)

18   Vande Bharat Mission, Ministry of External Affairs, Government of India, https://mea.gov.in/vande-bharat-mission-list-of-flights.htm (last accessed on May 30, 2020)

19   Aarogya Setu Mobile App, My Gov, Government of India, https://www.mygov.in/aarogya-setu-app/

20   PM-CARES Fund (Prime Minister's Citizen Assistance and Relief in Emergency Situation Fund) https://www.pmcares.gov.in/en/

21   'Alarming Spread: On Novel Coronavirus Outbreak', Opinion (Editorial Page), The Hindu newspaper, https://www.thehindu.com/opinion/editorial/alarming-spread/article30677660.ece (last accessed on May 30, 2020)

22   Anindita Sanyal (ed.), 'India Suspends All Tourist Visas Till April 15 Over Coronavirus: 10 Facts', NDTV.com, March 12, 2020, https://www.ndtv.com/india-news/coronavirus-impact-visas-to-india-suspended-till-april-15-2193382, (last accessed on June 1, 2020)

23   Coronavirus outbreak: Govt working on a 'containment plan', Economic Times, March 6, 2020, https://economictimes.indiatimes.com/news/politics-and-nation/coronavirus-outbreak-govt-working-on-a-containment-plan/articleshow/74504048.cms?utm_source=contentofinterest&utm_medium=text&utm_campaign=cppst (last accessed on June 11, 2020)

24   'COVID-19: Task Force to Deal with Economic Challenges', DD News, March 20, 2020, http://ddnews.gov.in/national/COVID-19-task-force-deal-economic-challenges (last accessed on June 5, 2020)

25   A. Divya, 'Coronavirus: Taj Mahal, all ASI-protected monuments, museums shut till March 31', The Indian Express, March 17, 2020, https://indianexpress.com/article/india/coronavirus-all-asi-protected-monuments-museums-shut-till-march-31-govt-6317791/

26   Anjana Pasricha, 'India Extends World's Largest Lockdown till May 3rd', Voice of America, April 14, 2020, https://www.voanews.com/science-health/coronavirus-outbreak/india-extends-worlds-largest-lockdown-till-may-3rd (last accessed on May 25, 2020)

27   'Jaan Hai Toh Jahan Hai: PM Modi on India lockdown', ABP News Live, March 24, 2020, https://news.abplive.com/videos/news/india-jaan-hai-toh-jahan-hai-pm-modi-on-india-lockdown-1181631 (last accessed May 15, 2020)

28   'Coronavirus: India enters "total lockdown" after spike in cases', BBC News, March 25, 2020, https://www.bbc.com/news/world-asia-india-52024239

29 Saheli Roy Choudhary, 'India announces $22.5 billion stimulus package to help those affected by the lockdown', CNBC, March 26, 2020, https://www.cnbc.com/2020/03/26/coronavirus-india-needs-a-support-package-larger-than-20-billion-dollars.html (last accessed on June 15, 2020)

30 Shekhar Gupta, 'Covid hasn't gone viral in India yet, but some in the world & at home can't accept the truth', The Print, April 18, 2020, https://theprint.in/national-interest/covid-hasnt-gone-viral-in-india-yet-but-some-in-the-world-at-home-cant-accept-the-truth/404178/ (last accessed on June 4, 2020)

31 Niharika Sharma, 'India Extends its Nationwide Coronavirus Lockdown till May 3', Quartz India, April 14, 2020, https://qz.com/india/1836425/modi-extends-indias-nationwide-coronavirus-lockdown-till-may-3/ (last accessed on June 2, 2020)

32 Prakash K. Dutta, 'In Coronavirus Lockdown Extension, Modi Wields Stick, Offers Carrot on Exit Route', April 14, 2020, https://www.indiatoday.in/coronavirus-outbreak/story/in-coronavirus-lockdown-extension-modi-wields-stick-offers-carrot-on-exit-route-1666741-2020-04-14 (last accessed on June 4, 2020)

33 'Govt releases lockdown 5.0 guidelines: Here's what's allowed and what's not,' *The Economic Times*, May 31, https://economictimes.indiatimes.com/news/politics-and-nation/centre-extends-lockdown-in-containment-zones-till-june-30/articleshow/76109621.cms?utm_source=contentofinterest&utm_medium=text&utm_campaign=cppst (last accessed on June 14, 2020)

34 'Amid Unlock 1.0, India adds over 1.76 lakh COVID-19 cases in just 18 days', *Deccan Herald*, June 18, 2020, https://www.deccanchronicle.com/nation/current-affairs/180620/amid-unlock-10-india-adds-over-176-lakh-COVID-19-cases-in-just-18-d.html (last accessed on June 20, 2020)

35 Pallavi Nahata, 'India Q4 GDP: Growth Falls To 3.1% As Covid Pain Begins,' Bloomberg/Quint, May 29, 2020, https://www.bloombergquint.com/business/india-q4-gdp-growth-falls-to-31-as-covid-pain-begins (last accessed on June 6, 2020)

36 'India's GDP Grows 3.1% in Fourth Quarter, 4.2% in FY20', *The Week*, May 29, 2020, https://www.theweek.in/news/biz-tech/2020/05/29/indias-gdp-grows-31-in-fourth-quarter-42-in-fy20.html (last accessed on June 20, 2020)

37 'The Cursed Blessing of Public Banks', South Asia Economic Focus, The World Bank, Spring 2020, http://documents.worldbank.org/curated/en/551641586789758259/pdf/South-Asia-Economic-Focus-Spring-2020-The-Cursed-Blessing-of-Public-Banks.pdf (last accessed on June 15, 2020)

38 COVID-19 Special Economic Package – Atmanirbhar Bharat, Rajras, May 14, 2020, https://www.rajras.in/index.php/covid19-special-economic-package-atmanirbhar-bharat-part-2/ (last accessed on June 19, 2020)

39 'Moody's Downgrades India's Country Ceilings for Foreign Currency Debt to Ba2/Not-Prime; Long-Term Foreign Currency Bank Deposits to Ba3; and Assigns Ba2/Not-Prime Ratings to Government of India's Domestic Currency Debt', Moody's Investor Service, https://www.moodys.com/research/MOODYS-DOWNGRADES-INDIAS-COUNTRY-CEILINGS-FOR-FOREIGN-CURRENCY-DEBT-TO--PR_20277

40 'India's worst ever recession is here, says CRISIL', CNBC, May 27, 2020, https://www.cnbctv18.com/economy/indias-worst-ever-recession-is-here-says-crisil-6005021.htm

41 'Economy may contract by over 40% in Q1: SBI Research', Economic Times, May 27, 2020, https://economictimes.indiatimes.com/news/economy/indicators/economy-may-contract-by-over-40-in-q1-sbi-research/articleshow/76022260.cms?utm_source=contentofinterest&utm_medium=text&utm_campaign=cppst (last accessed on June 15, 2020)

42   Mahesh Vyas, 'Unemployment Rate over 23 percent", Center for Monitoring Indian Economy Pvt. Ltd., April 7, 2020, https://www.cmie.com/kommon/bin /sr.php?kall=warticle&dt=2020-04-07%2008:26:04&msec=770, (last accessed on May 24, 2020)

43   'How has India's lockdown impacted unemployment rates and income levels?' Scroll.in e-magazine, April 22, 2020, https://scroll.in/article/959756/pod-cast-how-has-indias-lockdown-impacted-unemployment-rates-and-income-levels (last accessed on June 14, 2020)

44   Biman Mukherjee, 'Coronavirus impact: Indian industry seeks relief measures to aid economy', Livemint, March 23, 2020, https://www.livemint.com/com-panies/news/coronavirus-impact-indian-industry-seeks-relief-measures-to-aid -economy-11584904435575.html (last accessed on June 14, 2020)

45   Nishant Sharma, 'For Workers Fleeing Indian Cities on Foot, COVID-19 Is the Least of Their Worries', Bloomberg/Quint, March 29, 2020, https://www .bloombergquint.com/coronavirus-outbreak/for-workers-fleeing-indian-cit-ies-on-foot-COVID-19-is-the-least-of-their-worries (last accessed on June 10, 2020)

46   Anisha Dutta, '198 migrant workers killed in road accidents during lockdown: Report', Hindustan Times, June 2, 2020, https://www.hindustantimes.com /india-news/198-migrant-workers-killed-in-road-accidents-during-lockdown -report/story-hTWzAWMYn0kyycKw1dyKqL.html (last accessed on June 12, 2020)

47   'COVID-19: WHO calls India's lockdown "comprehensive and robust", UN expresses solidarity', The New Indian Express, March 25, 2020, https://www .newindianexpress.com/world/2020/mar/25/COVID-19-who-calls-indias -lockdown-comprehensive-and-robust-un-expresses-solidarity-2121361.html (last accessed on June 18, 2020)

48   Ibid

49   Amit Malviya, 'India's phenomenal response to COVID-19 pandemic', The Times of India, April 21, 2020, https://timesofindia.indiatimes.com/blogs/ voices/indias-phenomenal-response-to-COVID-19-pandemic/, May 30, 2020

50   'Sajjan Jindal lauds Rs 20 lakh crore-economic package announced by PM Modi', Economic Times, May 13, 2020, https://economictimes.indiatimes.com/ news/economy/policy/sajjan-jindal-lauds-rs-20-lakh-crore-economic-package -announced-by-pm-modi/articleshow/75712301.cms?utm_source=contentof-interest&utm_medium=text&utm_campaign=cppst, (last accessed on June 10, 2020)

51   'Coronavirus: India's PM Modi seeks "forgiveness" over lockdown', BBC News, March 29, 2020, https://www.bbc.com/news/world-asia-india-52081396, last accessed on May 28, 2020

52   'India ended up flattening the wrong curve (GDP) because of a "draconian lockdown": Rajiv Bajaj', Economic Times, June 4, 2020, https://economic-times.indiatimes.com/news/politics-and-nation/india-ended-up-flattening-the -wrong-curve-gdp-because-of-a-draconian-lockdown-rajiv-bajaj/articleshow /76188830.cms?from=mdr (last accessed on June 18, 2020)

53   Murali Krishnan, 'India could have several coronavirus peaks', DW Magazine, June 15, 2020, https://www.dw.com/en/india-could-have-several-coronavirus -peaks/a-53814997, (last accessed on June 21, 2020)

54   'India Probably Has 50,000 New Infections a Day, Could Rise to 2 Lakh by August', The Wire, June 20, 2020, https://thewire.in/video/watch-india -probably-has-50000-new-infections-a-day-could-rise-to-2-lakh-by-august (last accessed on June 22, 2020)

55   Ibid

56 '3 COVID-19 treatment drugs available in India today. Check Details', India TV News Desk, June 22, 2020 https://www.indiatvnews.com/fyi/corona-virus-COVID-19-medicine-covifor-fabiflu-cipremi-treatment-drugs-in-india-628125

References

A. Divya, 2020. 'Coronavirus: Taj Mahal, all ASI-protected monuments, museums shut till March 31', *The Indian Express*, 17 March 2020, https://indianexpress.com/article/india/coronavirus-all-asi-protected-monuments-museums-shut-till-march-31-govt-6317791/.

Amit Malviya, 2020. 'India's phenomenal response to COVID-19 pandemic', *The Times of India*, 21 April 2020, https://timesofindia.indiatimes.com/blogs/voices/indias-phenomenal-response-to-COVID-19-pandemic/, (last accessed on 30 May 2020).

Anindita Sanyal (ed.), 2020. 'India Suspends All Tourist Visas Till April 15 Over Coronavirus: 10 Facts', *NDTV.com*, 12 March 2020, https://www.ndtv.com/india-news/coronavirus-impact-visas-to-india-suspended-till-april-15-2193382, (last accessed on 1 June 2020).

Anisha Dutta, 2020. '198 migrant workers killed in road accidents during lockdown: Report', *Hindustan Times*, 02 June 2020, https://www.hindustantimes.com/india-news/198-migrant-workers-killed-in-road-accidents-during-lockdown-report/story-hTWzAWMYn0kyycKw1dyKqL.html (last accessed on 12 June 2020).

Anjana Pasricha, 2020. 'India Extends World's Largest Lockdown till May 3rd', *Voice of America*, 14 April 2020, https://www.voanews.com/science-health/coronavirus-outbreak/india-extends-worlds-largest-lockdown-till-may-3rd (last accessed on 25 May 2020).

Arshiya Mahajan and Himanshu Agarwal, 2020. 'COVID-19: A SWOT Analysis', *Niti Ayog*, 11 May 2020, https://niti.gov.in/COVID-19-india-swot-analysis, (last accessed on 12 June 2020).

Banjot Kaur, 2020. 'COVID-19: Govt's survey exposes lack of preparedness across India', *Down to Earth Magazine*, 03 April 2020, https://www.downtoearth.org.in/news/health/COVID-19-govt-s-survey-exposes-lack-of-preparedness-across-india-70221(last accessed on 6 June 2020).

BBC, 2020. 'Coronavirus: India Enters 'Total Lockdown' after spike in cases', *BBC News*, 25 March 2020, https://www.bbc.com/news/world-asia-india-52024239.

Biman Mukherjee, 2020. 'Coronavirus impact: Indian industry seeks relief measures to aid economy', *Livemint*, 23 March 2020, https://www.livemint.com/companies/news/coronavirus-impact-indian-industry-seeks-relief-measures-to-aid-economy-11584904435575.html (last accessed on 14 June 2020).

'Coronavirus outbreak: Govt working on a "containment plan", 2020', *Economic Times*, 06 March 2020, https://economictimes.indiatimes.com/news/politics-and-nation/coronavirus-outbreak-govt-working-on-a-containment-plan/articleshow/74504048.cms?utm_source=contentofinterest&utm_medium=text&utm_campaign=cppst (last accessed on 11 June 2020).

COVID-19 India, Ministry of Health and Family Welfare, 2020. Retrieved from: https://www.mohfw.gov.in/ (accessed on 18 June 2020).

COVID-19 Special Economic Package, 2020. Atmanirbhar Bharat, Rajras, 14 May 2020, https://www.rajras.in/index.php/covid19-special-economic-package -atmanirbhar-bharat-part-2/ (last accessed on 19 June 2020).

Deccan Herald, 2020. 'Amid unlock 1.0, India adds over 1.76 lakh COVID-19 cases in just 18 days', *Deccan Herald*, 18 June 2020, https://www.deccanchronicle .com/nation/current-affairs/180620/amid-unlock-10-india-adds-over-176-lakh -COVID-19-cases-in-just-18-d.html.

Economic Times, 2020. 'Govt exempts customs duty, cess on ventilators, surgical masks, PPE, COVID-19 test kits', *Economic Times*, 10 April 2020, https://www .google.com/search?q=down+to+earth+india&rlz=1C1CHBD_enIN717IN718 &oq=Down+to+earth+India&aqs=chrome.0.0j46j0l6.8793j1j8&sourceid =chrome&ie=UTF-8, (last accessed on 8 June 2020).

India TV News, 2020. '3 COVID-19 treatment drugs available in India today. Check Details', *India TV News Desk*, 22 June 2020, https://www.indiatvnews.com/fyi /coronavirus-COVID-19-medicine-covifor-fabiflu-cipremi-treatment-drugs-in -india-628125.

'Jaan Hai Toh Jahan Hai: PM Modi on India lockdown', 2020. *ABP News Live*, 24 March 2020, https://news.abplive.com/videos/news/india-jaan-hai-toh -jahan-hai-pm-modi-on-india-lockdown-1181631 (last accessed 15 May 2020).

Mahesh Vyas, 2020. 'Unemployment Rate over 23 percent', Center for Monitoring Indian Economy Pvt. Ltd., 07 April 2020, https://www.cmie.com/kommon/bin /sr.php?kall=warticle&dt=2020-04-07%2008:26:04&msec=770, (last accessed on 24 May 2020).

Mukesh Rawat, 2020. 'Coronavirus in India: Tracking country's first 50 COVID-19 cases; what numbers tell', *India Today*, 12 March 2020, https://www .indiatoday.in/india/story/coronavirus-in-india-tracking-country-s-first-50 -COVID-19-cases-what-numbers-tell-1654468-2020-03-12 (last accessed on 19 June 2020).

Murali Krishnan, 2020. 'India could have several coronavirus peaks', *DW Magazine*, 15 June 2020, https://www.dw.com/en/india-could-have-several-coronavirus -peaks/a-53814997, (last accessed on 21 June 2020).

Niharika Sharma, 2020. 'India extends its nationwide coronavirus lockdown till may 3', *Quartz India*, 14 April 2020, https://qz.com/india/1836425/modi-extends -indias-nationwide-coronavirus-lockdown-till-may-3/, (last accessed on 2 June 2020).

Nishant Sharma, 2020.'For workers fleeing Indian cities on foot, COVID-19 is the least of their worries', *Bloomberg/Quint*, 29 March 2020, https://www .bloombergquint.com/coronavirus-outbreak/for-workers-fleeing-indian-cities -on-foot-COVID-19-is-the-least-of-their-worries (last accessed on 10 June 2020).

Pallavi Nahata, 2020. 'India Q4 GDP: Growth falls To 3.1% as covid pain begins,' *Bloomberg/Quint*, 29 May 2020, https://www.bloombergquint.com/business /india-q4-gdp-growth-falls-to-31-as-covid-pain-begins (last accessed on 6 June 2020).

Prakash K. Dutta, 2020. 'In coronavirus lockdown extension, Modi wields stick, offers carrot on exit route', 14 April 2020, https://www.indiatoday.in/coronavirus -outbreak/story/in-coronavirus-lockdown-extension-modi-wields-stick-offers -carrot-on-exit-route-1666741-2020-04-14, (last accessed on 4 June 2020).

Sagarika Kamath, Rajesh Kamath, Prajwal Salins, 2020. 'COVID-19 pandemic in India: Challenges and silver linings', *Post Graduate Medical Journal*, 2020, https://pmj.bmj.com/content/early/2020/06/10/postgradmedj-2020 -137780 (last accessed on 3 June 2020).

Saheli Roy Choudhary, 2020.'India announces $22.5 billion stimulus package to help those affected by the lockdown', *CNBC*, 26 March 2020 https://www.cnbc .com/2020/03/26/coronavirus-india-needs-a-support-package-larger-than-20 -billion-dollars.html (last accessed on 15 June 2020).

Sarah Farooqui, 2020. 'India Coronavirus Dispatch: Visualizing a Response Moving Forward', Business Standard, 5 June 2020.

Shekhar Gupta, 2020. 'Covid hasn't gone viral in India yet, but some in the world & at home can't accept the truth', *The Print*, 18 April 2020, https://theprint.in /national-interest/covid-hasnt-gone-viral-in-india-yet-but-some-in-the-world-at -home-cant-accept-the-truth/404178/ (last accessed on 4 June 2020).

The Economic Times, 2020. 'Govt releases lockdown 5.0 guidelines: Here's what's allowed and what's not,' *The Economic Times*, 31 May, https://economictimes .indiatimes.com/news/politics-and-nation/centre-extends-lockdown-in -containment-zones-till-june-30/articleshow/76109621.cms?utm_source =contentofinterest&utm_medium=text&utm_campaign=cppst (last accessed on 14 June 2020).

The Hindu Newspaper, 2020. 'Alarming spread: On novel coronavirus outbreak', Opinion (Editorial Page), The Hindu newspaper. 30 May 2020, https://www .thehindu.com/opinion/editorial/alarming-spread/article30677660.ece.

Vande Bharat Mission, 2020. 'Ministry of External Affairs, Government of India', https://mea.gov.in/vande-bharat-mission-list-of-flights.htm (last accessed on 30 May 2020).

6 Managing the COVID-19 Crisis in Singapore

Kenneth Yeo Yaoren

Introduction

COVID-19 has reshaped governance, business, and society. Human-to-human transmission of the coronavirus was first detected at Wuhan, China in late-December 2019.[1] Community spread in China resulted in a widespread transmission in East Asia due to the cultural proximity of the Chinese in territories such as Hong Kong, Taiwan, Singapore, South Korea, and Japan.

At the point of writing, Singapore has experienced three waves of outbreaks, and possibly a fourth. The first wave of infection was introduced by tourists and employees coming from the Chinese Wuhan province. The second wave was induced by Singaporeans repatriated from Europe and North America. The third wave of infection exploded at the migrant worker's dormitories which led to the exponential increase of infected cases in Singapore. The government then imposed a lockdown from April 2020 which was expected to terminate in early June 2020. However, fears of a potential fourth wave loomed as Singapore adopted a "three steps forward, two steps back" approach.

This chapter details the government's priorities and responses in each phase of the crisis. The core strategy of the Singapore government is to "save lives and livelihoods." However, the means to achieve the objective have changed significantly due to the dynamic situation.

Managing COVID-19 in a Globally Dependent Region: January 27 to March 10, 2020

Singapore first contracted the virus on January 27, 2020 when tourists from the Wuhan province of China visited Singapore on a tour group. This led to rapid action by the government to manage the threat. The initial strategy of managing COVID-19 was to contain the virus and maintain international confidence. Since the region depends on the globalization to survive, governments must:

(1) Identify, isolate, and treat all cases of COVID-19,
(2) Retain investor confidence in the country, and
(3) Maintain social cohesion while achieving the aforementioned objectives.

DOI: 10.4324/9781003291909-7

The core strategy is to manage the situation by preventing community spread while staying relevant to the international community. At this point in time, all governments would agree that it is meaningless to recover from the COVID-19 pandemic with an incapacitated economy and society. As such, borders are largely open, and people were advised to maintain the status quo since there was no evidence of community spread.

Preventing Community Transmission

Primary policy tools employed were aimed at identifying, isolating, and treating people who are infected. Measures such as government-sanctioned quarantine orders, stay-home notices, and contact tracing were some measures taken to isolate the infected while maintaining social cohesion. Singapore continued to be a step ahead as the government continued to be transparent about the number of infected cases through daily press releases. Additional proactive measures were enacted to detect transmission clusters and community spread. This was done by repurposing Singapore's Criminal Investigations Department (CID) to identify infected individuals and clusters,[2] and conducting random sampling at community hospitals and polyclinics.[3]

Sustained Employment

In response to the economic downturn, the Singapore government has put in place targeted packages to increase the cashflow of businesses with the main objective of retaining employees.[4] The retention of workers continued to be important as excessive unemployment would result in social hazard and community panic.[5]

The COVID-19 economic lull was also viewed as an opportunity for industrial transformation and workforce upgrading. Further economic incentives targeted at upgrading were in place to stimulate economic growth after the COVID-19 pandemic.

Availability of Essential Goods

The dynamic and constantly evolving regional developments led to panic buying in every country,[6] potentially leading to a market failure through overconsumption. Initially, the hoarding of masks and hand sanitizers was critical. As the Minister of Trade and Industry, Chan Chun Sing, explained, masks should be dedicated to healthcare workers and no production capacities could meet the demands of hoarders.[7]

The first round of panic buying occurred in convenience stalls on February 7, 2020[8] immediately after DORSCON Orange was announced.[9] The government of Singapore has addressed COVID-19 threat through by assuring the public that the national stockpile is sufficient[10] through efficient restocking of depleted products[11] while implementing purchase limits.[12]

The second round of panic buying happened on March 16, 2020 after Malaysia announced its national lockdown.[13] Here, the government once again reassured that the national stockpile remains robust and supply lines are not cut,[14] ultimately highlighting the importance of diversifying the production and import of essential products.

Through a litany of measures, governments in East Asia were generally able to contain the disease while maintaining social cohesion and relative economic stability. This can be attributed to the 2003 SARS experience, which has prompted the region to increase their healthcare capacities since then.

COVID-19 as a Global Pandemic

The World Health Organization (WHO) declared a global pandemic on March 11, 2020.[15] COVID-19 became a significant problem for the West due to their high-contact culture which facilitated the spread of the virus. This was due to the high rate of transmission as asymptomatic disease carriers had unknowingly transmitted the virus.[16] Scientists recommended social distancing measures to "flatten the curve."[17] The logic behind the strategy is to spread the consumption of healthcare services over time so as to not overwhelm them.

Social Distancing and Its Limitations

However, many countries had to take social distancing to the extreme and have implemented temporary lockdowns to curb the spread of the virus.[18] Lockdowns themselves do not solve the COVID-19 issue. It only works if the authorities are able to identify every individual infected with the virus and further isolate them. However, at that point in time, there was a global shortage of COVID-19 test kits[19] and hence there was no way to identify all virus carriers. As such, temporary lockdowns will only defer the transmission of the disease.

The most accurate explanation of the objective of a lockdown is articulated by the German Chancellor, Angela Merkel. She explained the policy as a measure to "buy time" (1) to minimize the strain on the health system, and (2) for scientists to develop and mass produce a vaccine.[20] Ultimately, containment is no longer possible, and moving forward, COVID-19 has to be dealt with like common flu.

Global Economic Impact

Extreme measures enacted globally have had severe social and economic ramifications. Firstly, social distancing has reduced international cashflows significantly despite economic stimulus in strategic sectors. At the point of writing, economists speculated the global GDP growth to be between –2% and 2.7% (as compared to 3.6% in 2019) and declared that we are undergoing a global economic recession.[21] The global economic failure as a result of COVID-19 signals the inevitable decline of the local economy.

Secondly, the global surge in demand for essential products due to panic would lead to a temporary inflation of global food prices.[22] COVID-19 has no impact on the global food supply; suppliers continue to produce at regular pace and maritime and air freight continue to operate. However, the artificially induced surge in demand due to hoarding behavior would shock the market temporarily and exhaust the stockpile of many countries. This is unlikely to affect Singapore due to the national stockpile of essential products.

Managing the Second Wave: March 11 to April 7, 2020

As the threat evolved into a global pandemic, Singapore must adopt a different strategy to manage the threat. Prime Minister Lee Hsien Loong hinted for the need to adopt "new social norms" to manage the increasing deadliness of the disease.[23] Hence, Singapore imposed its version of social distancing while retaining some level of social and economic activity.[24]

Preventing Community Spread

A common fear was the transmission of COVID-19 in Singapore due to the congestion at public transport spaces. However, the way to reduce congestion is not to increase capacity as it will only result in higher operating costs and more wasted capacity (Figure 6.1).

Hence, the government must, instead, flatten the spike in demand for public transport. Workplace measures have been implemented to reduce congestion. Firstly, work-from-home arrangements are encouraged to reduce the overall demand for public transport. Next, if work-from home arrangements are not

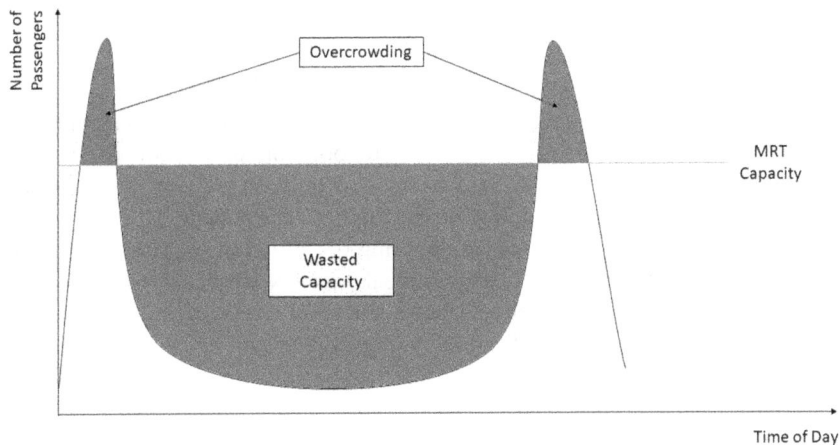

Figure 6.1 Illustration of the Status Quo of Singapore's Public Transport. Source: Author.

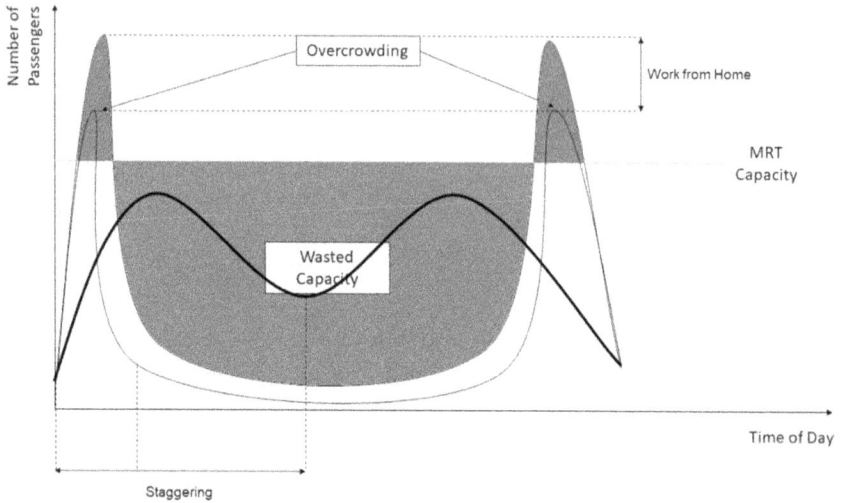

Figure 6.2 Expected Effect of Singapore's Public Transport after Workplace Distancing Measures. Source: Author.

feasible, staggering working hours would flatten the demand of public transport (Figure 6.2).

Theoretically, the effect on public transport congestion should be as reflected from the graph above. This principle could be applied to other community activities to minimize contact. However, most employers have not heeded the governmental advice and public transport continued to be congested after the announcement of the advisory.

TraceTogether Mobile App

Additionally, GovTech launched a Bluetooth enabled mobile application to facilitate contact tracing.[25] This application exchanges, records, and encrypts the contact details of individuals within the Bluetooth proximity into the mobile device.[26] This allows healthcare professionals to retrieve the encrypted contact information of every individual in close proximity to the patient.

Nonetheless, foreign critics began opposing the adoption of the mobile application due to fears of widespread state surveillance.[27] Nonetheless, local academics disagreed and argued that the mobile application can work only if there is a mandatory adoption of the application in Singapore.[28]

The Travel Ban

The Singapore travel ban on all short-term visitors was primarily to reserve healthcare facilities for Singaporeans.[29] This was implemented at a time when

East Asia began containing the COVID-19 infection while there is an outbreak globally. Drastic measures such as a blanket travel ban were implemented gradually with the principle of proportionality to avoid excessive community panic and fear.

The travel ban was implemented against the backdrop of a global lockdown.[30] This resulted in a significant reduction of traveling before the travel ban which already impacted specific industries in Singapore. As such, the travel ban would have minimal consequences to the economy of the globalization-dependent Singapore.

The travel ban was implemented to reserve Singapore healthcare resources for Singaporeans. This was to discourage medical tourism which took up the limited national healthcare resources. In the initial phases of COVID-19 in Singapore, imported cases were primarily Singaporeans returning from travels, and hence, there was no need to implement such measures. Singaporeans have since been advised to defer all non-essential travels to minimize contact with people.[31]

On March 18, 2020, the Gov.sg WhatsApp group declared that 70% of the cases were imported, most of which were Singaporeans returning from travels.[32] While the raw number of foreigners entering Singapore for medical tourism remained almost negligible, the first two deaths in Singapore included an Indonesia seeking treatment in Singapore.[33]

Overall, the travel ban is implemented primarily to reserve national healthcare resources for Singaporeans. It is only implemented now because the future economic impact to Singapore is minimal, and the number of foreign imported cases was almost negligible. Essentially, adopting the principle of proportionality to avoid unnecessary community panic.

Enacting the Circuit Breaker: April 7 to July 2, 2020

Above figures show why lockdown measures were only announced on April 3, 2020. Daily detected cases remained relatively low as most patients have imported COVID-19 from foreign countries primarily from Europe, North America and East Asia. However, the spike in community cases on March 25, 2020 might have prompted the authorities to rethink the need to implement harsher measures.

As cases continued to increase gradually, the Multi-Ministry Taskforce recommended stricter measures to curb the spread of the virus. Singapore implemented its own version of the lockdown on April 6, 2020.[34] Prime Minister Lee Hsien Loong explained that this measure would act as a circuit breaker to curb the transmission of the virus.[35] With the implementation of the circuit breaker measures, the Multi-Ministry Taskforce elevated safe distancing measures. While these measures were initially planned to cease on May 4, 2020, it was extended to June 1, 2020 to further contain community transmission.[36]

Safe distancing measures included the prohibition to dine-in at food and beverages outlets, full home-based learning for schools and institutes of higher learning,[37] and the suspension of non-essential workplaces.[38] Additionally, cloth masks were distributed to every resident through the People's Association (PA) grassroots network. Grassroot leaders used the "Supply Ally" mobile application to validate the identity of the resident, and to prevent overconsumption.

Additional measures to reduce crowding at public spaces were also implemented efficiently. Firstly, authorities repurposed non-essential civil servants from sixty-five agencies to serve as enforcement officers to ensure physical distance in public spaces. They hired members of the public and mobilized the grassroot leaders from the People's Association as Safe Distancing Ambassadors (SDAs) to supplement the manpower requirements to enforce physical circuit breaker measures.[39] The strategy of hiring SDAs also created job opportunities for freelancers or people who lost their jobs during the circuit breaker period.

Saving Lives and Livelihoods

Due to the drastic safe distancing measures, Singapore was expected to enter a recession in the year 2021 due to its dependence on the global economy.[40] The Monetary Authority of Singapore expected a –1% to –4% economic growth rate during its semi-annual review[41] while other economist forecasted the economic growth rate to be –4% to –7%.[42] Nonetheless, growth is expected in the information and communications technology (ICT), high-tech manufacturing, medical products and financial services sectors during the economic contraction.[43] This prompted various government initiatives to boost the economic outlook of the nation.

The government spared no effort in addressing both the healthcare crisis and its economic ramifications. As such, the government approved the $5.1 Billion Solidarity Budget[44] on April 6, 2020, and $33 Billion Fortitude Budget[45] on May 26, 2020 after the commencement of the circuit breaker. These budgets came on top of the $106 Billion Unity Budget[46] announced on February 18, 2020, and the $48.4 Billion Resilience Budget[47] announced on March 26, 2020. Overall, the budget used to sustain support both the healthcare deployment and employment amounted to $192.5 Billion (US$136.75 Billion).

Key initiatives for the budget include the 75% wage support with a cap of $4,600 for all employees, rental relief for small-medium enterprises (SMEs) and government tenants, and skills training for employees to pivot to sectors. Additional support on household expenses such as rebates on utility and cash payouts were made to improve the cashflow of Singaporeans.

DPM Heng Swee Keat announced the "SGUnited Jobs and Skills Package" in parliament on May 26, 2020. This initiative aimed to create jobs, apprenticeships, and training opportunities for citizens who were affected by the crisis.[48] Additional 40,000 positions in the public sector were also created in the early childhood, healthcare, and senior care sectors to meet the medium- to long-term impacts of COVID-19.[49]

The Politicization of Crisis

As measures become more drastic to curb the spread of the virus, the incumbent tends to face threats from within. Hence, the decision to implement the circuit breaker was quickly politicized by some opposition parties in Singapore. One controversial decision made by the Multi-Ministry Taskforce is the retraction of the advisory for healthy residents to not wear masks. Notably, the Singapore Democratic Party's (SDP) Secretary General, Chee Soon Juan, asserted that this is a policy reversal and a serious misstep of the government.[50] Ironically, the chair-person of SDP, Paul Ananth Tambyah, who is a professor for the department of Medicine at the National University of Singapore, was aligned with the government, who shared that masks were not required for healthy individuals along with other bold forecasts.[51]

However, governmental oversight of the migrant worker's dormitories took a big toll on Singapore's "gold standard" of managing COVID-19. It was also on April 3, 2020 when the government announced that some foreign worker dormitories became COVID-19 clusters.[52] Kristen Han, an ex-staff of the New Naratif and known government critic, published several articles criticizing the government's management of the migrant worker's dormitories.[53] International media followed suit and criticized Singapore for its management of foreign workers.[54] Both the SDP[55] and the Singapore Progress Party (PSP)[56] commented briefly on the issue and called the government out for their oversight.

The incumbent government of Singapore did not deny the oversight of the migrant worker's dormitory nor publicly accepted responsibility. This was observed when Nominated Member of Parliament, Anthea Ong, attempted to force a response from the Minister of Manpower, Josephine Teo. She asked the Minister of Manpower if she intends to apologize to the migrant workers in one of her parliamentary questions.[57] Nonetheless, Minister Josephine Teo has nei-ther made an apology nor the denied any responsibility for the issue.

Overall, the high number of foreign migrant worker infections was a stark reminder of Singapore's poor treatment of foreign migrant workers living in dormitories. Admittedly, conditions of the foreign worker's dormitories were not ideal. Infected migrant workers were a non-issue in the first two months after Singapore detected its first coronavirus case. However, the explosion of cases after April 6, 2020 signaled the discrimination between Singapore and its migrant workers. This only occurred only after Mustafa Centre was identified as a COVID-19 cluster, thereby being one of the few places where Singapore inter-acts with migrant workers socially.[58]

The migrant worker problem has been a hot topic and views on it have been divided. While there are activist groups campaigning for the rights of migrant workers in Singapore, there are others who shunned their presence. This issue was first brought to the headlines in Singapore after the Little India Riot on December 8, 2013, where 400 migrant workers rioted after a bus knocked a foreign worker after 9 pm.[59] This ignited a debate on the treatment of migrant workers where activists advocated for greater integration while the public cam-paigned for exclusion.[60]

The government of Singapore has been caught in a political gridlock for years. While gradual steps were taken to improve the conditions of foreign worker dor-mitories,[61] activists would argue that they were not aggressive enough.[62] Indeed, the living conditions of migrant workers in Singapore were not the priority of the government and more could be done to improve conditions of migrant worker dormitories.

Response to the Foreign Migrant Worker Problem

After the commencement of the circuit breaker, the authorities conducted aggressive testing on all foreign migrant workers living in dormitories.[63] At its peak, Singapore conducted 40,000 tests daily to separate the infected migrant workers from the rest.[64] This led to a spike of cases in Singapore. Figure 6.3 shows the percentage of migrant workers living in dormitories who are infected as a proportion of the total number of people infected in Singapore.

However, national statistics show that there are approximately 300,000 migrant workers living in Singapore.[65] Hence, it requires heavy investments in resources to:

(1) Relocate foreign migrant workers in suitable shelters,
(2) Redirect medical resources to care and test for cases at foreign dormitories, and
(3) Mobilize community support to support the logistic needs of the migrant workers.

After outlining the priorities, the government deployed the Singapore Armed Forces (SAF) to manage the migrant worker crisis. There are several spaces used to relocate migrant workers. Firstly, the Expo Convention Centre was converted into a medical facility for migrant workers who tested positive for COVID-19.[66] This facility was said to hold up to 15,000 migrant workers in isolation. Next,

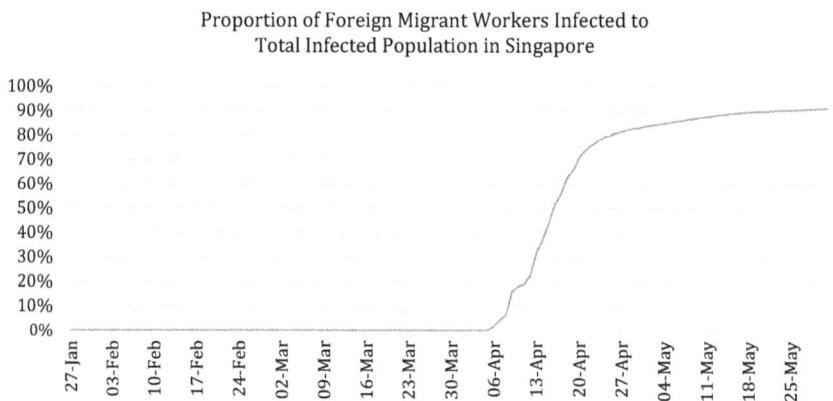

Figure 6.3 Proportion of the Infected Migrant Workers to Total Population Infected with COVID-19 in Singapore Compiled from Gov.Sg WhatsApp Daily Updates. Source: Author.

two offshore floating facilities were used to hold 500 healthy migrant workers.[67] Additionally, an unspecified number of hotels,[68] military camps,[69] and vacant HDB blocks[70] were repurposed as holding facilities for healthy migrant workers. Additionally, ex-military regulars were called back to manage existing migrant worker dormitories.[71]

Next, Singapore must redirect medical resources to serve the migrant workers. In the first phase, seventy medical personnel from the SAF were deployed to the dormitories to address health-related concerns of the migrant workers.[72] Then, healthcare workers from local polyclinics were directed to dormitories to support the medical operations.[73] Finally, the workforce was supplemented by hiring 1,500 members of the public to support healthcare operations for migrant workers such as swabbers for testing, and site supervisors.[74]

Finally, logistic support for migrant workers was conducted. First trench efforts were led by the SAF via the Forward Assurance and Support Team (FAST).[75] The team comprised logistics officers from the SAF and staff from the Ministry of Manpower and aimed to manage the migrant worker's daily needs. This included:

(1) Three meals every day,[76]
(2) Personal care equipment such as masks and hand sanitizers,[77]
(3) 5G SIM cards,[78] and
(4) Financial support.[79]

Through national platforms such as "Giving.SG" and private platforms like "GIVE.asia," the nation was able to crowdsource the above-mentioned resources rapidly. Ultimately, despite Singapore's oversight on issues pertaining to migrant worker's dormitories, both the government and society were able to mobilize both manpower and resources rapidly to address the complex issues of the dormitories.

Social Impacts of the Circuit Breaker

Apart from community transmission of the virus and a potential economic fallout, societies would face a litany of social issues when implementing lockdown measures. Singapore is no exception. Three major issues were highlighted during the circuit breaker period; domestic violence, elderly isolation, and space inadequacy.

Lockdown measures appeared to have increased domestic violence. This trend is consistent across all countries.[80] The Singapore Police Force (SPF) reported a total of 476 cases of offenses related to domestic violence between April 7 and May 6, 2020, which was a significant increase from the monthly average of 389 cases. Singapore experienced a 22% increase from the monthly average for.[81] Several explanations to this trend include prolonged interaction between the perpetrator and victims and stress from financial burdens.

Common strategy Singapore employed includes legislative tools like the Personal Protection Order (PPO) and the Domestic Exclusion Order (DEO).[82] Additionally, victims could be re-sheltered in homes operated by non-governmental organizations (NGOs) like the Singapore Council of Women's Organisation (SCWO),[83] Association of Women for Action and Research (AWARE),[84] and other family service centers (FSCs). Additionally, specialist FSCs would also conduct preventive and developmental services to decrease intervene with high-risk families.[85]

Elderly isolation became a prevalent problem as well.[86] This is particularly a problem with senior citizens living alone. Devoid from means to socialize physically, seniors living in Singapore became structurally isolated and were prone to depressive symptoms.[87] Issue of this nature was brought to light when reports of seniors dying at alone at home was reported in national media.[88]

To improve the well-being of elderly residents, various organizations have adopted telephone befriending services. The national community befriending hotline was launched to allow lonely seniors to share their stories in a safe space.[89] Notable charities which organized similar programs in Singapore include the Lions Befrienders and Fei Yue FSC. However, coordination of such services could be improved to reach out to seniors more effectively.

Finally, Singapore has issues in living spaces. While the government declared 100% home ownership of every citizen, there are vulnerable populations who choose to be homeless.[90] This could be a result of tense family relationships where it is inconvenient to live in their place of residence. The circuit breaker took a heavy emotional and physical toll on such individuals.

As such, the Ministry of Social and Family Development reported nearly 300 individuals seeking shelter during the circuit breaker period.[91] Through the Partners Engaging and Empowering Rough Sleepers (PEERS) program formed in July 2019, twenty-six public agencies, social services agencies, and community groups provided shelters and social intervention for rough sleepers.[92]

Singapore's Recovery

It is undeniable that there was some oversight from the government in managing the COVID-19 situation. Issues pertaining to the management of migrant worker dormitories and complex social problems were exacerbated during the COVID-19 crisis. Despite limitations to the esteemed Singapore foresight, the government was able to respond and react quickly to address most issues.

Intervention from the government worked. Circuit breaker measures appeared to have reduced community transmission significantly shortly after implementation. On April 12, 2020, daily community infections intersect with the weekly moving average and exhibited a declining trend. Nevertheless, authorities urged residents to exercise caution and safe distancing and good hygiene practices even after the circuit breaker period.[93]

On the healthcare sector, Singapore recovered from the initial spike in the numbers of migrant workers relatively rapidly. If we measured Singapore's healthcare capacity by the number of patients discharged, it would appear that Singapore began to dip after the proportion of patients discharged dropped from its peak at 77.78% on March 2, 2020 to 76.36% on March 3, 2020.

Singapore's healthcare system truly became overwhelmed after the enforcement of the circuit breaker where the third intersection between the actual proportions and weekly moving average between April 7 and 8, 2020 at 29.10% and 28.34%, respectively. Healthcare capacity hit its trough on May 1, 2020 as the proportion of patients discharged was only 7.85%. This can be attributed to the number of migrant workers living in dormitories who tested positive for COVID-19 as shown in Figure 6.3.

On top of that, death rates of patients suffering from COVID-19 remained almost negligible in Singapore. As of May 31, 2020, the death rates of patients infected with COVID-19 in Singapore were recorded as 0.0572%. Unfortunately, at the point of writing, there were twenty-three fatalities from COVID-19. All were above the age of sixty with pre-existing medical conditions. Some attributed the low death rates to the high proportion of migrant workers being infected as they tend to be younger and healthier.[94]

Arguably, the authorities of Singapore were able to respond swiftly to the health crisis swiftly. They took responsibility and control over the migrant worker dorms and made significant amendments to rectify their wrongs. With the gradual recovery of COVID-19, Singapore prepares to terminate the circuit breaker and psyches itself for the new normal.

The New Normal: July 2, 2020 Onwards

The Multi-Ministry Taskforce warned of an increase in community transmission if the lifting of circuit breaker measures were not calibrated. Minister Lawrence Wong explained that

> We have to do this in a very careful and calibrated manner, because we do not want to risk a flaring up of the virus again. And importantly, we do not want to sacrifice the efforts that all of us have put in over the past few weeks in controlling the outbreak.[95]

As such, recovery from the circuit breaker will occur in three phases.

The first phase, "Safe Reopening", will focus on four areas, (1) safe work, (2) safe home and community, (3) safe school, and (4) safe care.[96] The Taskforce permits the reopening of production facilities and research laboratories, but still mandates telecommuting as the main mode of work. Additionally, home visits to family members will be permitted with a limit of one visit a day with a maximum of two visitors from the same household. Other social activities such as marriage solemnization, funerals, and worship will also be permitted with restrictions on group sizes Schools will commence with a hybrid virtual-physical learning model. Lessons for institutes of higher learning will remain online. Social services will gradually reopen to serve the community.

However, authorities asserted that the reopening of facilities must be coupled with increased testing and contact tracing capacities.[97] Restrictions on movement and interactions will be upheld until the government can systematically vaccinate every citizen. This is largely dependent on the global race to develop a vaccine where it is expected to be ready in late 2020 or early 2021.[98] Till then, the authorities will maintain its position on the new normal and would tighten its policies if necessary.

Conclusion

The COVID-19 crisis is the ultimate test of our times. Lives were taken and livelihoods were lost. With that, the pandemic has ruptured our social fabric and caused widespread panic and fear; exposing the weaknesses of every society. Every nation is confronted with a Morton's fork: to break the society or risk another life. Eventually, no government withstood the pressure of another life lost and enacted some form of lockdown measure; negatively impacting business and society.

In Singapore, authorities maintained a gold standard in the management of the pandemic for an extended period of time. This is attributed to the ingenuity and prudence of the incumbent government as they contained the virus effectively by redirecting resources and manpower to critical sectors. Nonetheless, oversight from the authorities resulted in the explosion of cases in migrant dormitories, exposing the untold story of Singapore's success.

Despite its initial shock, authorities did not flinch and enacted a litany of policies to address the escalation of the threat. This included the implementation of a circuit breaker to interdict community transmission while mobilizing the whole of government and nation to aid the migrant workers' community. Within the span of two months, authorities recovered from the migrant worker crisis and prepared to lift the circuit breaker.

Authorities remained watchful about the situation and adopted a cautious approach in lifting the circuit breaker measures. They acknowledged that policies can only minimize the transmission of the COVID-19 virus and governments depend on scientists to develop a vaccine. Conclusively, Singapore's COVID-19 story is one of resilience and fortitude. The government of Singapore mobilizes the whole of society to combat COVID-19 promptly and efficiently despite some oversight. This can only be achieved by amassing political goodwill and trust between government and society over the years, one which is unique to Singapore.

Notes

1 Tony Munroe and Gerry Doyle, "Chinese officials investigate cause of pneumonia outbreak in Wuhan," *Reuters*, December 31, 2019, https://www.reuters.com/article/us-china-health-pneumonia/chinese-officials-investigate-cause-of-pneumonia-outbreak-in-wuhan-idUSKBN1YZ0GP.
2 Aqil Haziq Mahmud, "'Like an invisible criminal': How police helped find missing link between COVID-19 church clusters in a day," March 8, 2020, https://www.channelnewsasia.com/news/singapore/police-missing-link-church-clusters-covid19-coronavirus-12509492.

3 Gan Kim Yong, "Singapore conducts proactive surveillance, random sampling to detect COVID-19 cases", *Channel News Asia*, 18 February 2020, https://www .youtube.com/watch?v=3eRK2Y5jBHk.

4 Heng Swee Keat, "Singapore Budget 2020: Stabilisation and Support Package," *Singapore: Ministry of Finance (MOF)*, February 19, 2020, https://www.singa-porebudget.gov.sg/budget_2020/budget-measures/stabilisation-and-support -package.

5 Many studies of the social impact of unemployment were conducted. Among others, unemployment is found to be highly correlated to suicides. See Bijou Yang and David Lester, "The Social Impact of Unemployment," *Applied Economics Letters 1*, no. 12 (1994): 887-890. See also Eunice Rodriguez, Edward A. Frongillo, and Pinky Chandra. "Do social programmes contribute to mental well-being? The long-term impact of unemployment on depression in the United States," *International Journal of Epidemiology 30*, no. 1 (2001): 163–170.

6 Naveen Thukral, "Panic buying, lockdowns may drive world food inflation - FAO, analysts," *Reuters*, March 21, 2020, https://www.reuters.com/article/ us-health-coronavirus-food-security/panic-buying-lockdowns-may-drive-world -food-inflation-fao-analysts-idUSKBN21808G.

7 Chan Chun Sing, "Wuhan virus: Hoarding of face masks 'not appropriate', says Chan Chun Sing | Video," *Channel News Asia, January 30, 2020,* https://www .channelnewsasia.com/news/singapore/wuhan-virus-hoarding-of-face-masks -not-appropriate-says-chan-12370000.

8 Low Youjin and Alif Chandra, "The Big Read: Panic buying grabbed the head-lines, but quiet resilience is seeing Singapore through COVID-19 outbreak," *Channel News Asia*, February 17, 2020, https://www.channelnewsasia.com /news/singapore/coronavirus-COVID-19-panic-buying-singapore-dorscon -orange-12439480.

9 "Risk Assessment Raised to DORSCON Orange," *Singapore: Ministry of Health (MOH)*, February 7, 2020, https://www.moh.gov.sg/news-highlights/details/ risk-assessment-raised-to-dorscon-orange.

10 Seah Kian Peng, *Facebook*, February 7, https://www.facebook.com/ SeahKianPeng/posts/2701082116636732; Audrey Tan, "No risk of shortage of essential food, household items", *The Straits Times*, February 8, 2020, https:// www.straitstimes.com/singapore/no-risk-of-shortage-of-essential-food-house-hold-items.

11 Audrey Tan and Goh Yan Han, "Coronavirus: Calmer mood at some supermar-kets on Sunday, shelves restocked," *The Straits Times*, February 9, 2020, https:// www.straitstimes.com/singapore/health/coronavirus-calmer-mood-at-some -supermarkets-on-sunday-shelves-restocked.

12 Seah Kian Peng, *Facebook*, February 9, 2020, https://www.facebook.com/ SeahKianPeng/posts/2704923352919275; Ang Hwee Min, "FairPrice imposes purchase limits for paper products, rice and instant noodles amid coronavirus outbreak", *Channel News Asia*, February 9, 2020, https://www.channelnewsasia .com/news/singapore/coronavirus-fairprice-purchase-limits-paper-rice-instant -noodles-12412538.

13 Hazlin Hassan, "Malaysia bans travel abroad, shuts schools and businesses over coronavirus spread; lockdown till March 31", *The Straits Times*, March 16, 2020, https://www.straitstimes.com/asia/se-asia/malaysia-to-impose-lockdown-from -wednesday-to-march-31.

14 Chan Chun Sing, *Facebook*, 11.06pm, March 16, 2020, https://www.facebook .com/ChanChunSing.SG/posts/3041790732539556; "COVID-19: There's no need to rush to buy essential items," *Singapore Government*, 16 March 2020,

https://www.gov.sg/article/COVID-19-theres-no-need-to-rush-to-buy-essential-items.

15 Tedros Adhanom Ghebreyesus, "WHO announces COVID-19 outbreak a pandemic," *World Health Organisation*, March 12, 2020, http://www.euro.who.int/en/health-topics/health-emergencies/coronavirus-COVID-19/news/news/2020/3/who-announces-COVID-19-outbreak-a-pandemic.

16 Frank Diamond, "Asymptomatic Carriers of COVID-19 Make It Tough to Target," *Infection Control Today*, March 17, 2020, https://www.infectioncontroltoday.com/COVID-19/asymptomatic-carriers-COVID-19-make-it-tough-target.

17 Harry Stevens, "Why outbreaks like coronavirus spread exponentially, and how to 'flatten the curve,'" *Washington Post*, March 14, 2020, https://www.washingtonpost.com/graphics/2020/world/corona-simulator/?fbclid=IwAR09u1nH0h6_ZgevkG5mIIaxETPS_EUrqxIxaUAn9ImwDdFqjSZIYL74cLQ.

18 Holly Secon, Lauren Frias, Morgan McFall-Johnsen, "A running list of countries that are on lockdown because of the coronavirus pandemic," *Business Insider*, March 20, 2020, https://www.businessinsider.sg/countries-on-lockdown-coronavirus-italy-2020-3?r=US&IR=T.

19 Robert Kuznia, Curt Devine and Drew Griffin, "Severe shortages of swabs and other supplies hamper coronavirus testing," *CNN*, March 18, 2020, https://edition.cnn.com/2020/03/18/us/coronovirus-testing-supply-shortages-invs/index.html.

20 Angela Merkel, "Die Ansprache der Kanzlerin auf Englisch – The Chancellor's address in English," *Bundesregierung*, March 20, 2020, https://www.youtube.com/watch?v=WLxrxyk_wYo.

21 Rahul Karunakar and Shrutee Sarkar, "Global economy already in recession on coronavirus devastation: Reuters poll," *Reuters*, March 20, 2020, https://www.reuters.com/article/us-health-coronavirus-global-economy/global-economy-already-in-recession-on-coronavirus-devastation-reuters-poll-idUSKBN21702Y.

22 Naveen Thukral, "Panic buying, lockdowns may drive world food inflation - FAO, analysts," *Reuters*, March 21, 2020, https://www.reuters.com/article/us-health-coronavirus-food-security/panic-buying-lockdowns-may-drive-world-food-inflation-fao-analysts-idUSKBN21808G.

23 Lee Hsien Loong, "PM Lee: the COVID-19 situation in Singapore," *Singapore: Prime Minister Office (PMO)*, March 12, 2020, https://www.gov.sg/article/pm-lee-hsien-loong-on-the-COVID-19-situation-in-singapore-12-mar.

24 Measures include border restrictions, additionally workplace regulations, tightened regulations on public gathering, and guidelines at public venues. See Salma Khalik, "Social distancing next major line of defence in virus battle," *The Straits Times*, March 14, 2020.

25 "TraceTogether," *Singapore: Government Digital Services*, March 21, 2020, https://www.tracetogether.gov.sg/.

26 Tang See Kit and Aqil Haziq Mahmud, "Singapore launches TraceTogether mobile app to boost COVID-19 tracing efforts," *Channel News Asia*, March 20, 2020, https://www.channelnewsasia.com/news/singapore/covid19-trace-together-mobile-app-contact-tracing-coronavirus-12560616.

27 David Pierson, "Singapore says its coronavirus app helps the public. Critics say it's government surveillance," *Los Angeles Times*, March 25, 2020, https://www.latimes.com/world-nation/story/2020-03-24/coronavirus-singapore-trace-together.

28 Author cited Teo Yi-Ling, an academic from the S. Rajaratnam School of International Studies. See Navene Elangovan, "COVID-19: Governance expert says TraceTogether should be mandatory, but warns of potential 'slippery slope'

of greater surveillance," *Today Online*, May 14, 2020, https://www.todayonline .com/singapore/COVID-19-governance-expert-says-tracetogether-should-be -mandatory-warns-potential-slippery.

29 Lawrence Wong, "COVID-19: Travel restrictions for foreign visitors entering Singapore," *Singapore Government*, March 22, 2020, https://www.gov.sg/article/COVID-19-travel-restrictions-for-foreign-visitors-entering-singapore.

30 Marcin Bielecki, "In Pictures: Global lockdown to fight the coronavirus outbreak," *Al Jazeera*, March 19, 2020, https://www.aljazeera.com/indepth/inpictures/ pictures-global-lockdown-fight-coronavirus-outbreak-200319102052360.html.

31 Calvin Yang, "Singaporeans advised to defer all non-essential travel," *The Straits Times*, March 15, 2020, https://www.straitstimes.com/singapore/sporeans -advised-to-defer-all-non-essential-travel.

32 Gov.sg, "COVID-19: 18 Mar Update," *WhatsApp*, March 18, 2020.

33 Sue-Ann Tan, "Coronavirus: 64-year-old Indonesian man who died in Singapore was first hospitalised in Jakarta for pneumonia," *The Straits Times*, March 21, 2020, https://www.straitstimes.com/singapore/health/coronavirus-64-year -old-indonesian-man-dies-of-COVID-19-in-singapore.

34 "Circuit Breaker to Minimise Further Spread of COVID-19," *Singapore: Ministry of Health*, April 3, 2020, https://www.moh.gov.sg/news-highlights/details/circuit-breaker-to-minimise-further-spread-of-COVID-19.

35 Lee Hsien Loong, "PM Lee Hsien Loong on the COVID-19 situation in Singapore on 3 April 2020," *Singapore: Prime Minister's Office*, April 3, 2020, https://www .pmo.gov.sg/Newsroom/PM-Lee-Hsien-Loong-on-the-COVID19-situation-in -Singapore-on-3-April-2020.

36 "Circuit Breaker extension and tighter measures: What you need to know," *Singapore: Prime Minister's Office*, April 21, 2020, https://www.gov.sg/article/ circuit-breaker-extension-and-tighter-measures-what-you-need-to-know.

37 Ong Ye Kung, "Schools and Institutes of Higher Learning to Shift to Full Home-Based Learning; Preschools and Student Care Centres to Suspend General Services," *Singapore: Ministry of Education*, April 3, 2020, https://www.moe .gov.sg/news/press-releases/schools-and-institutes-of-higher-learning-to-shift -to-full-home-based-learning-preschools-and-student-care-centres-to-suspend -general-services.

38 Chan Chun Sing, "COVID-19 circuit breaker: Closure of workplace premises," *Singapore: Ministry of Trade and Industry*, April 3, 2020, https://www.gov.sg/ article/COVID-19-circuit-breaker-closure-of-workplace-premises.

39 Tiffany Fumiko Tay, "New roles as safe distancing ambassadors for some workers amid job disruption due to COVID-19," *The Straits Times*, April 29, 2020, https://www.straitstimes.com/singapore/workers-take-on-front-line-roles -amid-job-disruption.

40 Tang See Kit, "Singapore will enter a recession this year, 'significant uncertainty' over duration and intensity: MAS," *Channel News Asia*, April 28, 2020, https:// www.channelnewsasia.com/news/singapore/COVID-19-economy-singapore -will-enter-recession-2020-mas-review-12683096.

41 "MAS Monetary Policy Statement – April 2020," *Monetary Authority of Singapore*, March 30, 2020, https://www.mas.gov.sg/news/monetary-policy -statements/2020/mas-monetary-policy-statement-30mar20.

42 Annabeth Leow, "Singapore recession forecast for 2020 worsens to between -4% and -7%," *The Business Times*, May 26, 2020, https://www.businesstimes.com .sg/government-economy/singapore-recession-forecast-for-2020-worsens-to -between-4-and-7.

43 Ovais Subhani, "Some industries may grow even as Singapore heads for recession," *The Straits Times*, April 29, 2020, https://www.straitstimes.com/business

/economy/some-industries-may-grow-even-as-spore-heads-for-recession; Sue-Ann Tan, "Companies still hiring amid economic slump," *The Straits Times*, May 28, 2020, https://www.straitstimes.com/singapore/manpower/companies-still -hiring-amid-economic-slump.

44 "Solidarity Budget," *Singapore: Ministry of Finance*, April 6, 2020, https://www.singaporebudget.gov.sg/budget_2020/solidarity-budget.

45 "Fortitude Budget," *Singapore: Ministry of Finance*, May 26, 2020, https://www.singaporebudget.gov.sg/budget_2020/fortitude-budget.

46 "Budget 2020," *Singapore: Ministry of Finance*, February 18, 2020, https://www.singaporebudget.gov.sg/budget_2020/budget-measures.

47 "Resilience Budget," *Singapore: Ministry of Finance*, March 26, 2020, https://www.singaporebudget.gov.sg/budget_2020/resilience-budget.

48 Olivia Ho, "$2b package to create 100,000 job and training opportunities for workers hit by COVID-19 slowdown," *The Straits Times*, May 26, 2020, https://www.straitstimes.com/politics/parliament-2bn-package-to-create-40000-jobs -25000-traineeships-and-30000-skills-training.

49 Rachel Phua, "Fortitude Budget: More than 40,000 jobs to be created as part of S$2b employment, training package," *Channel News Asia*, May 26, 2020, https://www.channelnewsasia.com/news/singapore/fortitude-budget-jobs -traineeships-skills-employment-sgunited-12770508.

50 Chee Soon Juan 徐顺全, ""Do not wear mask" – 1 of 3 serious misstep leading to second crisis," *Facebook*, April 6, 2020, https://www.facebook.com/cheesoon-juan/videos/3135249036499383/?v=3135249036499383.

51 Paul Ananth Tambyah, "Part 2 of Ask Anything: Dr Tambyah says COVID-19 to disappear by June," *The Independent – Singapore*, March 2, 2020, http://theindependent.sg/part-2-of-ask-paul-anything-dr-tambyah-says-COVID-19-to -disappear-by-june/.

52 Gov.sg, "COVID-19 Situation," *WhatsApp*, April 3, 2020.

53 Kristen Han, "Singapore is Trying to Forget Migrant Workers are People," *Foreign Policy*, May 6, 2020, https://foreignpolicy.com/2020/05/06/singa-pore-coronavirus-pandemic-migrant-workers/.

54 Faris Mokhtar, "How Singapore Flipped from Coronavirus Hero to Cautionary Tale", *Bloomberg*, April 21, 2020, https://www.bloomberg.com/news/arti-cles/2020-04-21/how-singapore-flipped-from-virus-hero-to-cautionary-tale; Rebecca Ratcliffe, "Singapore's cramped migrant worker dorms hide COVID-19 surge risk," *The Guardian*, April 17, 2020, https://www.theguardian.com/world/2020/apr/17/singapores-cramped-migrant-worker-dorms-hide-COVID -19-surge-risk; Namita Bhandare, "Singapore's Coronavirus Success Story Hits a Snag," *Foreign Policy*, April 21, 2020, https://foreignpolicy.com/2020/04/21/singapore-coronavirus-response-snag/.

55 Author cited SDP secretary general, Chee Soon Juan. See Kentaro Iwamoto, "Singapore's coronavirus spike sends world a wake-up call," *Nikkei Review*, April 20, 2020, https://asia.nikkei.com/Spotlight/Coronavirus/Singapore-s-corona-virus-spike-sends-world-a-wake-up-call.

56 Progress Singapore Party, "2020 PSP May Day Message by Dr Tan Cheng Bok," *Facebook*, April 30, 2020, https://www.facebook.com/watch/?v =2725265324361638.

57 Author cited Anthea Ong's parliamentary question. See Ho Sheo Bo, "Reflections on attitude towards migrant workers," *The Straits Times*, May 13, 2020, https://www.straitstimes.com/singapore/manpower/reflections-on-attitudes-towards -migrant-workers.

58 Linette Lai, "Coronavirus: Mustafa Centre believed to be starting point for hundreds of cases," *The Straits Times*, April 10, 2020, https://www.straitstimes

.com/singapore/mustafa-centre-believed-to-be-starting-point-for-hundreds-of
-cases.

59 "What are the facts of the rioting incident at Little India on 8 Dec?," *Singapore Government*, December 13, 2013, https://www.gov.sg/article/what-are-the -facts-of-the-rioting-incident-at-little-india-on-8-dec.

60 Alfred Chua and Amanda Lee, "Views divided on how to reduce congestion at foreign worker areas," *Today*, July 4, 2014, https://www.todayonline.com/sin-gapore/views-divided-how-reduce-congestion-foreign-worker-areas.

61 Valarie Koh, "Larger dorms for foreign workers may soon need license to operate," *Today*, November 5, 2014, https://www.todayonline.com/singapore/larger-dorms-foreign-workers-may-soon-need-licence-operate; Seow Bei Yi, "Foreign workers in dormitories now have an app to alert MOM of their living conditions," *The Straits Times*, September 13, 2018, https://www.straitstimes .com/singapore/manpower/foreign-workers-in-dormitories-now-have-an-app -to-alert-mom-of-their-living.

62 Author cited Jolovan Wham, then group executive director of the Humanitarian Organization for Migration Economics (HOME). See "Go beyond COI's recommendations to better protect foreign workers: HOME," *Today*, July 2, 2014, https://www.todayonline.com/singapore/go-beyond-cois-recommendations -better-protect-foreign-workers-home.

63 The author cited the Director of Singapore's Ministry of Health, Kenneth Mak. See Aqil Haziq Mahmud and Ang Hwee Min, "COVID-19: All foreign worker dormitories to have medical teams of doctors and nurses from hospitals, polyclinics," *Channel News Asia*, April 14, 2020, https://www.channelnewsasia.com/news/singapore/COVID-19-foreign-worker-dormitories-medical-teams-doctors-nurses-12640818.

64 Wong Kai Yi, "Coronavirus: 40,000 daily tests have to be done in strategic, coordinated way, says Lawrence Wong," *The Straits Time*, May 8, 2020, https://www .straitstimes.com/singapore/coronavirus-40000-daily-tests-have-to-be-done-in -a-strategic-coordinated-way-says-lawrence.

65 The column of "Work Permit (construction)." See "Foreign workforce numbers," *Singapore: Ministry of Manpower*, April 29, 2020, https://www.mom.gov .sg/documents-and-publications/foreign-workforce-numbers.

66 Amanda Eber, "4 Singapore Expo halls occupied by COVID-19 patients, 6 more halls to be converted into isolation facilities soon: PM Lee," *Today*, April 26, 2020, https://www.todayonline.com/singapore/4-singapore-expo-halls-occu-pied-COVID-19-patients-temporary-isolation-facilities-6-more-halls.

67 "Singapore to Add Floating Accommodation to Range of Housing for Foreign Workers," *Singapore: Maritime and Port Authority*, April 11, 2020, https://www .mpa.gov.sg/web/portal/home/media-centre/news-releases/detail/6c4510c3 -0527-4dc6-b687-cc8dfc0ad001.

68 Tan Tam Mei, "Coronavirus: Hotels among lodgings being used to house foreign workers from dormitories," *The Straits Times*, April 17, 2020, https://www .straitstimes.com/singapore/coronavirus-hotels-among-lodgings-being-used-to -house-foreign-workers-from-dormitories.

69 Lim Min Zhang, "Coronavirus: 1,300 foreign workers move into SAF camps for circuit breaker period," *The Straits Times*, April 9, 2020, https://www.straits-times.com/singapore/coronavirus-1300-foreign-workers-move-into-saf-camps -for-circuit-breaker-period.

70 Yeun Sin, "Coronavirus: Diamond HDB blocks in Taman Jurong to house healthy foreign workers in essential services," *The Straits Times*, April 17, 2020, https://www.straitstimes.com/singapore/coronavirus-diamond-hdb-blocks-in -taman-jurong-to-house-foreign-workers-in-essential.

71 Wong Pei Ting, "Ex-SAF regulars called upon as 'personnel with operational experience' needed to tackle COVID-19 at dorms: MINDEF," *Today*, April 19, 2020,   https://www.todayonline.com/singapore/ex-saf-regulars-called-upon -personnel-operational-experience-needed-contain-COVID-19.

72 Zhaki Abdullah, "SAF will do more for COVID-19 fight if needed: Ng Eng Hen," *Channel News Asia*, April 9, 2020, https://www.channelnewsasia.com/ news/singapore/saf-will-do-more-for-COVID-19-fight-if-needed-ng-eng-hen -12624644.

73 Tee Zhuo, "Coronavirus: Polyclinic doctor among those helping out in dorms," *The Straits Times*, May 19, 2020, https://www.straitstimes.com/singapore/pol- yclinic-doctor-among-those-helping-out-in-dorms.

74 Hidayah Iskandar, "Interest in 1,500 temporary COVID-19 jobs including swabbers," *The Straits Times*, May 19, 2020, https://www.straitstimes.com/ singapore/coronavirus-interest-in-1500-temporary-COVID-19-jobs-including -swabbers.

75 Thrina Tham, "SAF-led fast deployment to help stabilise COVID-19 dorm situa- tion," *Singapore: Ministry of Defence: Pioneer*, April 23, 2020, https://www.min- def.gov.sg/web/portal/pioneer/article/cover-article-detail/community/2020 -Q2/23apr20_news1.

76 "Coordinated Donations to Support Our Migrant Workers More Effectively," *Singapore: Ministry of Manpower*, April 29, 2020, https://www.mom.gov.sg/ newsroom/press-releases/2020/0429-coordinated-donations-to-support-our -migrant-workers-more-effectively; Charmaine Ng, "Coronavirus: Companies donate food to migrant workers, underprivileged Singaporeans," *The Straits Times*, April 30, 2020, https://www.straitstimes.com/singapore/coronavirus -companies-donate-food-to-migrant-workers-and-underprivileged-singaporeans; Saleemah Ismail, "Care Meals for Migrant Workers," *Givng.SG*, May 4, 2020, https://www.giving.sg/campaigns/iftarformigrantworkers; Clement Yong, "200,000 migrant workers get special Hari Raya Puasa meal," *The Straits Times*, May 24, 2020, https://www.straitstimes.com/singapore/200000-migrant -workers-get-special-hari-raya-aidilfitri-meal-in-signal-of-unity-and.

77 Chew Hui Min, "Masks, hand sanitisers to be distributed to 350,000 migrant workers in dormitories," *Channel News Asia*, April 8, 2020, https://www.chan- nelnewsasia.com/news/singapore/masks-hand-sanitisers-distributed-dormitory -migrant-workers-mwc-12621826; Tee Zhuo, "1.3m reusable masks for migrant workers; over \$850k raised too," *The Straits Times*, April 20, 2020, https://www .straitstimes.com/singapore/13m-reusable-masks-for-migrant-workers-over -850k-raised-too. Red Cross Society, "Essentials Delivered to Migrant Workers," *Giving.SG*, April 23, 2020, https://www.giving.sg/singapore-red-cross-society/ edmw.

78 "StarHub Cares: Further support for Singapore's migrant worker community," *Starhub*, April 30, 2020, https://www.starhub.com/about-us/newsroom/2020 /april/starhub-cares-support-for-migrant-worker-community.html; Cheryl Tan, "Over 44,000 foreign workers receive free \$10 top-ups to their prepaid cards to call home for Hari Raya," *The Straits Times*, May 27, 2020, https://www.straits- times.com/singapore/over-44000-foreign-workers-received-free-10-top-ups-to -their-prepaid-cards-to-call-home.

79 Yuen Sin, "Coronavirus: Singaporeans donate their Solidarity payouts to chari- ties," *The Straits Times*, April 16, 2020, https://www.straitstimes.com/singapore /sporeans-donate-their-solidarity-payouts; Aw Cheng Wei, "DBS, Singtel offer- ing \$4.5m in aid to those hit by pandemic fallout," *The Straits Times*, April 17, 2020, https://www.straitstimes.com/business/companies-markets/dbs-singtel -offering-45m-in-aid-to-those-hit-by-pandemic-fallout.

80 Jeni Klugman, "Justice for Women Amidst COVID-19," *Georgetown Institute for Women, Peace and Security*, (May 2020), https://giwps.georgetown.edu/wp-content/uploads/2020/05/Justice-for-Women-Amidst-COVID-19-.pdf.

81 Jean Iau, "Coronavirus: More cases of family violence during circuit breaker; police to proactively help victims," *The Straits Times*, May 15, 2020, https://www.straitstimes.com/singapore/courts-crime/coronavirus-more-cases-of-family-violence-during-circuit-breaker-police-to.

82 "Family Protection," *Singapore: Family Justice Court*, April 13, 2020, https://www.familyjusticecourts.gov.sg/what-we-do/family-courts/family-protection; "Protection of Family", *Singapore Women's Charter Part VII paragraph 64*, last updated on June 1, 2020, https://sso.agc.gov.sg/Act/WC1961#P1VII-.

83 "Star Shelter," *Singapore Council of Women's Organisation*, n.d., https://www.scwo.org.sg/what-we-do/services/star-shelter/.

84 "What to do if you are facing family violence," *Association of Women for Action and Research*, n.d, https://www.aware.org.sg/information/dealing-with-family-violence/what-can-i-do-if-i-am-facing-family-violence/.

85 "Crisis Intervention," *Singapore: National Council of Social Service*, June 1, 2020, https://www.ncss.gov.sg/GatewayPages/Social-Services/Families/Crisis-Intervention.

86 Janice Tai, "Coronavirus: Elderly hit hard by social isolation amid circuit breaker measures," *The Straits Times*, April 11, 2020, https://www.straitstimes.com/singapore/health/elderly-hit-hard-by-social-isolation-amid-circuit-breaker-measures.

87 "Research Brief Series 4: Home Alone: Older Adults in Singapore," *Centre for Aging Research & Education – Duke NUS Medical School*, (April 2018), https://www.duke-nus.edu.sg/docs/librariesprovider3/research-policy-brief-docs/home-alone-older-adults-in-singapore.pdf?sfvrsn=6735541d_0.

88 Zhangxin Zheng, "Woman in her 30s stayed in Yishun flat with 60-year-old mother's decomposing body for 5 days," *Mothership*, May 9, 2020, https://mothership.sg/2020/05/yishun-dish-collector-death-5-days/.

89 "Community Befriending Programme | I Feel Young SG," *Singapore: Ministry of Health*, n.d., https://www.moh.gov.sg/ifeelyoungsg/our-stories/how-can-i-age-actively/volunteer/community-befriending-programme; "Introduction to Befriending Service and Neighbourhood Links," *Singapore: Agency for Integrated Care*, n.d., https://www.aic.sg/care-services/Befriending%20Services.

90 Ng Kok Hoe, "Homelessness in Singapore: Results from a nationwide street count," *Lee Kuan Yew School of Public Policy*, (2019), https://lkyspp.nus.edu.sg/docs/default-source/faculty-publications/homeless-in-singapore.pdf?fbclid=IwAR3-3FMC3W4uJ_PKecaXcjoI53J7oQ40W40koLfjsg5ewtmoCNgb6A1CAEc.

91 Goh Chiew Tong, "More seeking shelter during circuit breaker period; help for homeless to go beyond COVID-19: MSF," *Channel News Asia*, May 4, 2020, https://www.channelnewsasia.com/news/singapore/COVID-19-homeless-seek-shelter-assistance-msf-desmond-lee-12699938.

92 Tee Zhuo, "300 homeless get help from network during COVID-19 circuit breaker," *The Straits Times*, May 5, 2020, https://www.straitstimes.com/politics/300-homeless-get-help-from-network-during-circuit-breaker.

93 "End of Circuit Breaker, Phased Approach to Resuming Activities Safely," *Singapore: Ministry of Health*, May 19, 2020, https://www.moh.gov.sg/news-highlights/details/end-of-circuit-breaker-phased-approach-to-resuming-activities-safely.

94 Dewey Sim and Kok Xinghui, "Coronavirus: why so few deaths among Singapore's 14,000 COVID-19 infections?," *South China Morning Post*, April 27, 2020,

https://www.scmp.com/week-asia/health-environment/article/3081772/cor-onavirus-why-so-few-deaths-among-singapores-14000.

95   Lawrence Wong, "Full COVID-19 Press Conference by the Multi-Ministry Task Force on May 19, 2020," *Youtube (Video)*, May 19, 2020, https://www.youtube .com/watch?v=pK79uej4FKY.

96   "Safe Re-opening: How Singapore will resume activities after the circuit breaker," *Singapore Government*, May 20, 2020, https://www.gov.sg/article/safe-re -opening-how-singapore-will-resume-activities-after-the-circuit-breaker.

97   "Post-circuit breaker – when can we move on to phases 2 and 3?," *Singapore Government*, May 28, 2020, https://www.gov.sg/article/post-circuit-breaker -when-can-we-move-on-to-phases-2-and-3.

98   Author cited Dr Anthony Fauci, director of the National Institute for Allergy and Infectious Diseases. See Helen Branswell, "Anthony Fauci on COVID-19 reopenings, vaccines, and moving at 'warp speed,'" *STAT News*, June 1, 2020.

References

Abdullah, Zhaki, 2020. "SAF will do more for COVID-19 fight if needed: Ng Eng Hen". *Channel News Asia*. Retrieved on 9 April 2020 from: https://www .channelnewsasia.com/news/singapore/saf-will-do-more-for-COVID-19-fight-if -needed-ng-eng-hen-12624644.

AIC, 2020. *Introduction to befriending service and neighbourhood links*. Singapore: Agency for Integrated Care. n.d. https://www.aic.sg/care-services/Befriending %20Services.

Ang, Hwee Min, 2020. "FairPrice imposes purchase limits for paper products. rice and instant noodles amid coronavirus outbreak". *Channel News Asia*. Retrieved on 9 February 2020 from: https://www.channelnewsasia.com/news/singapore/ coronavirus-fairprice-purchase-limits-paper-rice-instant-noodles-12412538.

Aw, Cheng Wei, 2020. "DBS. Singtel offering $4.5m in aid to those hit by pandemic fallout". *The Straits Times*. Retrieved on 17 April 2020 from: https://www .straitstimes.com/business/companies-markets/dbs-singtel-offering-45m-in-aid -to-those-hit-by-pandemic-fallout.

AWARE, 2020. "What to do if you are facing family violence". *Association of Women for Action and Research*. n.d. https://www.aware.org.sg/information/dealing -with-family-violence/what-can-i-do-if-i-am-facing-family-violence/.

Bhandare, Namita, 2020. "Singapore's coronavirus success story hits a snag". *Foreign Policy*. Retrieved on 21 April 2020 from: https://foreignpolicy.com/2020/04 /21/singapore-coronavirus-response-snag/.

Bielecki, Marcin, 2020. "In pictures: Global lockdown to fight the coronavirus outbreak". *Al Jazeera*. Retrieved on 19 March 2020 from: https://www.aljazeera .com/indepth/inpictures/pictures-global-lockdown-fight-coronavirus-outbreak -200319102052360.html.

Branswell, Helen, 2020. "Anthony Fauci on COVID-19 reopenings, vaccines, and moving at 'warp speed'". *STAT News*. Retrieved on 1 June 2020 from: https:// www.statnews.com/2020/06/01/anthony-fauci-on-COVID-19-reopenings -vaccines-and-moving-at-warp-speed/.

Chan, Chun Sing, 2020. *COVID-19 circuit breaker: Closure of workplace premises*. Singapore: Ministry of Trade and Industry. Retrieved on 3 April 2020 from: https:// www.gov.sg/article/COVID-19-circuit-breaker-closure-of-workplace-premises.

Chee Soon Juan

Chee, Soon Juan, 2020. "'Do not wear mask' –1 of 3 serious misstep leading to second crisis". *Facebook*. Retrieved on 6 April 2020 from: https://www.facebook.com/cheesoonjuan/videos/3135249036499383/?v=3135249036499383.

Chew, Hui Min, 2020. "Masks, hand sanitisers to be distributed to 350,000 migrant workers in dormitories". *Channel News Asia*. Retrieved on 8 April 2020 from: https://www.channelnewsasia.com/news/singapore/masks-hand-sanitisers-distributed-dormitory-migrant-workers-mwc-12621826.

Chua, Alfred and Amanda Lee, 2014. "Views divided on how to reduce congestion at foreign worker areas". *Today*. Retrieved on 4 July 2014 from: https://www.todayonline.com/singapore/views-divided-how-reduce-congestion-foreign-worker-areas.

Diamond, Frank, 2020. "Asymptomatic carriers of COVID-19 make it tough to target". *Infection Control Today*. Retrieved on 17 March 2020 from: https://www.infectioncontroltoday.com/COVID-19/asymptomatic-carriers-COVID-19-make-it-tough-target.

Duke-NUS, 2018. "Research brief series 4: Home alone: Older adults in Singapore". Centre for Aging Research & Education – Duke NUS Medical School. https://www.duke-nus.edu.sg/docs/librariesprovider3/research-policy-brief-docs/home-alone-older-adults-in-singapore.pdf?sfvrsn=6735541d_0.

Eber, Amanda, 2020. "4 Singapore Expo halls occupied by COVID-19 patients. 6 more halls to be converted into isolation facilities soon: PM Lee". *Today*. Retrieved on 26 April 2020 from: https://www.todayonline.com/singapore/4-singapore-expo-halls-occupied-COVID-19-patients-temporary-isolation-facilities-6-more-halls.

Elangovan, Navene, 2020. "COVID-19: Governance expert says TraceTogether should be mandatory, but warns of potential 'slippery slope' of greater surveillance". *Today Online*. Retrieved on 14 May 2020 from: https://www.todayonline.com/singapore/COVID-19-governance-expert-says-tracetogether-should-be-mandatory-warns-potential-slippery.

Family Justic Court, 2020. *Family protection*. Singapore: Family Justice Court. Retrieved on 13 April 2020 from: https://www.familyjusticecourts.gov.sg/what-we-do/family-courts/family-protection.

Gan, Kim Yong, 2020. "Singapore conducts proactive surveillance, random sampling to detect COVID-19 cases". *Channel News Asia*. Retrieved on 18 February 2020 from: https://www.youtube.com/watch?v=3eRK2Y5jBHk.

Ghebreyesus, Tedros Adhanom, 2020. "WHO announces COVID-19 outbreak a pandemic". World Health Organisation. Retrieved on 12 March 2020 from: http://www.euro.who.int/en/health-topics/health-emergencies/coronavirus-COVID-19/news/news/2020/3/who-announces-COVID-19-outbreak-a-pandemic.

Goh, Chiew Tong, 2020. "More seeking shelter during circuit breaker period; help for homeless to go beyond COVID-19: MSF". *Channel News Asia*. Retrieved on 4 May 2020 from: https://www.channelnewsasia.com/news/singapore/COVID-19-homeless-seek-shelter-assistance-msf-desmond-lee-12699938.

Government Digital Services, 2020. *TraceTogether*. Singapore: Government Digital Services. Retrieved on 21 March 2020 from: https://www.tracetogether.gov.sg/.

Han, Kristen, 2020. "Singapore is trying to forget migrant workers are people". *Foreign Policy*. Retrieved on 6 May 2020 from: https://foreignpolicy.com/2020/05/06/singapore-coronavirus-pandemic-migrant-workers/.

Hassan, Hazlin, 2020. "Malaysia bans travel abroad, shuts schools and businesses over coronavirus spread; lockdown till March 31". *The Straits Times.* Retrieved on 16 March 2020 from: https://www.straitstimes.com/asia/se-asia/malaysia-to -impose-lockdown-from-wednesday-to-march-31.

Heng, Swee Keat, 2020. *Singapore budget 2020: Stabilisation and support package.* Singapore: Ministry of Finance (MOF). Retrieved on 19 February 2020 from: https://www.singaporebudget.gov.sg/budget_2020/budget-measures/ stabilisation-and-support-package.

Ho, Olivia, 2020. "$2b package to create 100.000 job and training opportunities for workers hit by COVID-19 slowdown". *The Straits Times.* Retrieved on 26 May 2020 from: https://www.straitstimes.com/politics/parliament-2bn-package-to -create-40000-jobs-25000-traineeships-and-30000-skills-training.

Ho, Sheo Bo, 2020. "Reflections on attitude towards migrant workers". *The Straits Times.* Retrieved on 13 May 2020 from: https://www.straitstimes.com/singapore /manpower/reflections-on-attitudes-towards-migrant-workers.

Iau, Jean, 2020. "Coronavirus: More cases of family violence during circuit breaker; police to proactively help victims". *The Straits Times.* Retrieved on 15 May 2020 from: https://www.straitstimes.com/singapore/courts-crime/coronavirus-more -cases-of-family-violence-during-circuit-breaker-police-to.

Iskandar, Hidayah, 2020. "Interest in 1,500 temporary COVID-19 jobs including swabbers". *The Straits Times.* Retrieved on 19 May 2020 from: https://www .straitstimes.com/singapore/coronavirus-interest-in-1500-temporary-COVID -19-jobs-including-swabbers.

Ismail, Saleemah, 2020. "Care meals for migrant workers". *Givng.SG.* Retrieved on 4 May 2020 from: https://www.giving.sg/campaigns/iftarformigrantworkers.

Iwamoto, Kentaro, 2020. "Singapore's coronavirus spike sends world a wake-up call". *Nikkei Review.* Retrieved on 20 April 2020 from: https://asia.nikkei.com /Spotlight/Coronavirus/Singapore-s-coronavirus-spike-sends-world-a-wake-up -call.

John Hopkins University, 2020. "Coronavirus COVID-19 global cases". *Systems Science and Engineering (CSSE) at Johns Hopkins University.* n.d. Retrieved on 22 March 2020 from: https://gisanddata.maps.arcgis.com/apps/opsdashboard/ index.html#/bda7594740fd40299423467b48e9ecf6.

Karunakar, Rahul and Shrutee Sarkar, 2020. "Global economy already in recession on coronavirus devastation: Reuters poll". *Reuters.* Retrieved on 20 March 2020 from: https://www.reuters.com/article/us-health-coronavirus-global-economy /global-economy-already-in-recession-on-coronavirus-devastation-reuters-poll -idUSKBN21702Y.

Khalik, Salma, 2020. "Social distancing next major line of defence in virus battle". *The Straits Times.* Retrieved on 14 March 2020 from: https://www.straitstimes .com/singapore/health/social-distancing-next-major-line-of-defence-in-virus -battle.

Klugman, Jeni, 2020. "Justice for women amidst COVID-19". *Georgetown Institute for Women. Peace and Security.* Retrieved on May 2020 from: https://giwps .georgetown.edu/wp-content/uploads/2020/05/Justice-for-Women-Amidst -COVID-19-.pdf.

Koh, Valarie, 2014. "Larger dorms for foreign workers may soon need license to operate". *Today.* Retrieved on 5 November 2014 from: https://www.todayonline .com/singapore/larger-dorms-foreign-workers-may-soon-need-licence-operate.

Kuznia, Robert. Curt Devine and Drew Griffin, 2020. "Severe shortages of swabs and other supplies hamper coronavirus testing". *CNN*. Retrieved on 18 March 2020 from: https://edition.cnn.com/2020/03/18/us/coronovirus-testing-supply -shortages-invs/index.html.

Lai, Linette, 2020. "Coronavirus: Mustafa Centre believed to be starting point for hundreds of cases". *The Straits Times*. Retrieved on 10 April 2020 from: https:// www.straitstimes.com/singapore/mustafa-centre-believed-to-be-starting-point -for-hundreds-of-cases.

Lee, Hsien Loong, 2020a. *PM Lee Hsien Loong on the COVID-19 situation in Singapore on 3 April 2020*. Singapore: Prime Minister's Office. Retrieved on 3 April 2020 from: https://www.pmo.gov.sg/Newsroom/PM-Lee-Hsien-Loong -on-the-COVID19-situation-in-Singapore-on-3-April-2020.

———, 2020b. *PM Lee: The COVID-19 situation in Singapore*. Singapore: Prime Minister Office (PMO). Retrieved on 12 March 2020 from: https://www.gov.sg /article/pm-lee-hsien-loong-on-the-COVID-19-situation-in-singapore-12-mar.

Leow, Annabeth, 2020. "Singapore recession forecast for 2020 worsens to between –4% and –7%". *The Business Times*. Retrieved on 26 May 2020 from: https:// www.businesstimes.com.sg/government-economy/singapore-recession-forecast -for-2020-worsens-to-between-4-and-7.

Lim, Min Zhang, 2020. "Coronavirus: 1,300 foreign workers move into SAF camps for circuit breaker period". *The Straits Times*. Retrieved on 9 April 2020 from: https://www.straitstimes.com/singapore/coronavirus-1300-foreign-workers -move-into-saf-camps-for-circuit-breaker-period.

Low, Youjin and Alif Chandra, 2020. "The big read: Panic buying grabbed the headlines. but quiet resilience is seeing Singapore through COVID-19 outbreak". *Channel News Asia*. Retrieved on 17 February 2020 from: https://www .channelnewsasia.com/news/singapore/coronavirus-COVID-19-panic-buying -singapore-dorscon-orange-12439480.

Mahmud, Aqil Haziq, 2020. "'Like an invisible criminal': How police helped find missing link between COVID-19 church clusters in a day". Retrieved on 8 March 2020 from: https://www.channelnewsasia.com/news/singapore/police-missing -link-church-clusters-covid19-coronavirus-12509492.

Mahmud, Aqil Haziq and Ang Hwee Min, 2020. "COVID-19: All foreign worker dormitories to have medical teams of doctors and nurses from hospitals. polyclinics". *Channel News Asia*. Retrieved on 14 April 2020 from: https://www .channelnewsasia.com/news/singapore/COVID-19-foreign-worker-dormitories -medical-teams-doctors-nurses-12640818.

MAS, 2020. "MAS monetary policy statement – April 2020". Monetary Authority of Singapore. Retrieved on 30 March 2020 from: https://www.mas.gov.sg/news/ monetary-policy-statements/2020/mas-monetary-policy-statement-30mar20.

Merkel, Angela, 2020. "Die Ansprache der Kanzlerin auf Englisch – The Chancellor's address in English". *Bundesregierung*. Retrieved on 20 March 2020 from: https:// www.youtube.com/watch?v=WLxrxyk_wYo.

MOF, 2020a. *Budget 2020*. Singapore: Ministry of Finance. Retrieved on 18 February 2020 from: https://www.singaporebudget.gov.sg/budget_2020/budget -measures.

———, 2020b. *Fortitude budget*. Singapore: Ministry of Finance. Retrieved on 26 May 2020 from: https://www.singaporebudget.gov.sg/budget_2020/fortitude -budget.

————, 2020c. *Resilience budget*. Singapore: Ministry of Finance. Retrieved on 26 March 2020 from: https://www.singaporebudget.gov.sg/budget_2020/resilience-budget.

————, 2020d. *Solidarity budget*. Singapore: Ministry of Finance. Retrieved on 6 April 2020 from: https://www.singaporebudget.gov.sg/budget_2020/solidarity-budget.

MOH, 2020a. *Circuit breaker to minimise further spread of COVID-19*. Singapore: Ministry of Health. Retrieved on 3 April 2020 from: https://www.moh.gov.sg/news-highlights/details/circuit-breaker-to-minimise-further-spread-of-COVID-19.

————, 2020b. *Community befriending programme | I Feel Young SG*. Singapore: Ministry of Health. n.d. https://www.moh.gov.sg/ifeelyoungsg/our-stories/how-can-i-age-actively/volunteer/community-befriending-programme.

————, 2020c. *End of circuit breaker, 2020. Phased approach to resuming activities safely*. Singapore: Ministry of Health. Retrieved on 19 May 2020 from: https://www.moh.gov.sg/news-highlights/details/end-of-circuit-breaker-phased-approach-to-resuming-activities-safely.

————, 2020d. *Risk assessment raised to DORSCON orange*. Singapore: Ministry of Health (MOH). Retrieved on 7 February 2020 from: https://www.moh.gov.sg/news-highlights/details/risk-assessment-raised-to-dorscon-orange.

MO, 2020a. *Coordinated donations to support our migrant workers more effectively*. Singapore: Ministry of Manpower. Retrieved on 29 April 2020 from: https://www.mom.gov.sg/newsroom/press-releases/2020/0429-coordinated-donations-to-support-our-migrant-workers-more-effectively.

————, 2020b. *Foreign workforce numbers*. Singapore: Ministry of Manpower. Retrieved on 29 April 2020 from: https://www.mom.gov.sg/documents-and-publications/foreign-workforce-numbers.

Mokhtar, Faris, 2020. "How Singapore flipped from coronavirus hero to cautionary tale". Bloomberg. Retrieved on 21 April 2020 from: https://www.bloomberg.com/news/articles/2020-04-21/how-singapore-flipped-from-virus-hero-to-cautionary-tale.

MPA, 2020. *Singapore to add floating accommodation to range of housing for foreign workers*. Singapore: Maritime and Port Authority. Retrieved on 11 April 2020 from: https://www.mpa.gov.sg/web/portal/home/media-centre/news-releases/detail/6c4510c3-0527-4dc6-b687-cc8dfc0ad001.

Munroe, Tony and Gerry Doyle, 2019. "Chinese officials investigate cause of pneumonia outbreak in Wuhan". *Reuters*. Retrieved on 31 December 2019 from: https://www.reuters.com/article/us-china-health-pneumonia/chinese-officials-investigate-cause-of-pneumonia-outbreak-in-wuhan-idUSKBN1YZ0GP.

NCSS, 2020. *Crisis intervention*. Singapore: National Council of Social Service. Retrieved on 1 June 2020 from: https://www.ncss.gov.sg/GatewayPages/Social-Services/Families/Crisis-Intervention.

Ng, Charmaine, 2019. "Coronavirus: Companies donate food to migrant workers. underprivileged Singaporeans". *The Straits Times*. Retrieved on 30 April 2020 from: https://www.straitstimes.com/singapore/coronavirus-companies-donate-food-to-migrant-workers-and-underprivileged-singaporeans.

Ng, Kok Hoe, 2019. "Homelessness in Singapore: Results from a nationwide street count". Lee Kuan Yew School of Public Policy. https://lkyspp.nus.edu.sg/docs/default-source/faculty-publications/homeless-in-singapore.pdf?fbclid=IwAR3-3FMC3W4uJ_PKecaXcjoI53J7oQ40W40koLfjsg5ewtmoCNgb6A1CAEc.

Ong, Ye Kung, 2020. *Schools and institutes of higher learning to shift to full home-based learning; preschools and student care centres to suspend general services.* Singapore: Ministry of Education. Retrieved on 3 April 2020 from: https://www.moe.gov.sg/news/press-releases/schools-and-institutes-of-higher-learning-to-shift-to-full-home-based-learning-preschools-and-student-care-centres-to-suspend-general-services.

Phua, Rachel, 2020. "Fortitude budget: More than 40,000 jobs to be created as part of S$2b employment, training package". *Channel News Asia.* Retrieved on 26 May 2020 from: https://www.channelnewsasia.com/news/singapore/fortitude-budget-jobs-traineeships-skills-employment-sgunited-12770508.

Pierson, David, 2020. "Singapore says its coronavirus app helps the public. Critics say it's government surveillance". *Los Angeles Times.* Retrieved on 25 March 2020 from: https://www.latimes.com/world-nation/story/2020-03-24/coronavirus-singapore-trace-together.

PMO, 2020. *Circuit breaker extension and tighter measures: What you need to know.* Singapore: Prime Minister's Office. Retrieved on 21 April 2020 from: https://www.gov.sg/article/circuit-breaker-extension-and-tighter-measures-what-you-need-to-know.

Ratcliffe, Rebecca, 2020. "Singapore's cramped migrant worker dorms hide COVID-19 surge risk". *The Guardian.* Retrieved on 17 April 2020 from: https://www.theguardian.com/world/2020/apr/17/singapores-cramped-migrant-worker-dorms-hide-COVID-19-surge-risk.

Red Cross Society, 2020. "Essentials Delivered to Migrant Workers". *Giving.SG.* Retrieved on 23 April 2020 from: https://www.giving.sg/singapore-red-cross-society/edmw.

Rodriguez, Eunice, Edward A. Frongillo and Pinky Chandra, 2001. "Do social programmes contribute to mental well-being? The long-term impact of unemployment on depression in the United States". *International Journal of Epidemiology,* 30(1): 163–170.

Secon, Holly, Lauren Frias and Morgan McFall-Johnsen, 2020. "A running list of countries that are on lockdown because of the coronavirus pandemic". *Business Insider.* Retrieved on 20 March 2020 from: https://www.businessinsider.sg/countries-on-lockdown-coronavirus-italy-2020-3?r=US&IR=T.

Seow, Bei Yi, 2018. "Foreign workers in dormitories now have an app to alert MOM of their living conditions". *The Straits Times.* Retrieved on 13 September 2018 from: https://www.straitstimes.com/singapore/manpower/foreign-workers-in-dormitories-now-have-an-app-to-alert-mom-of-their-living.

Sim, Dewey and Kok Xinghui, 2020. "Coronavirus: Why so few deaths among Singapore's 14.000 COVID-19 infections?" *South China Morning Post.* Retrieved on 27 April 2020 from: https://www.scmp.com/week-asia/health-environment/article/3081772/coronavirus-why-so-few-deaths-among-singapores-14000.

Singapore Women's Charter, 2020. "Protection of family". Singapore Women's Charter Part VII paragraph 64. Retrieved on 1 June 2020 from: https://sso.agc.gov.sg/Act/WC1961#P1VII-.

StarHub, 2020. "StarHub cares: Further support for Singapore's migrant worker community". *Starhub.* Retrieved on 30 April 2020 from: https://www.starhub.com/about-us/newsroom/2020/april/starhub-cares-support-for-migrant-worker-community.html.

Stevens, Harry, 2020. "Why outbreaks like coronavirus spread exponentially, and how to 'flatten the curve'". *Washington Post.* Retrieved on 14 March 2020 from:

https://www.washingtonpost.com/graphics/2020/world/corona-simulator/
?fbclid=IwAR09u1nH0h6_ZgevkG5mIIaxETPS_EUrqxIxaUAn9ImwDdFqjSZI
YL74cLQ.

Subhani, Ovais, 2020. "Some industries may grow even as Singapore heads for
recession". *The Straits Times*. Retrieved on 29 April 2020 from: https://www
.straitstimes.com/business/economy/some-industries-may-grow-even-as-spore
-heads-for-recession.

Tai, Janice, 2020. "Coronavirus: Elderly hit hard by social isolation amid circuit
breaker measures". *The Straits Times*. Retrieved on 11 April 2020 from: https://
www.straitstimes.com/singapore/health/elderly-hit-hard-by-social-isolation
-amid-circuit-breaker-measures.

Tambyah, Paul Ananth, 2020. "Part 2 of ask anything: Dr Tambyah says COVID-19
to disappear by June". *The Independent – Singapore*. Retrieved on 2 March 2020
from: http://theindependent.sg/part-2-of-ask-paul-anything-dr-tambyah-says
-COVID-19-to-disappear-by-june/.

Tan, Audrey, 2020. "No risk of shortage of essential food. household items". *The
Straits Times*. Retrieved on 8 February 2020 from: https://www.straitstimes.com
/singapore/no-risk-of-shortage-of-essential-food-household-items.

Tan, Audrey and Goh Yan Han, 2020. "Coronavirus: Calmer mood at some
supermarkets on Sunday, shelves restocked". *The Straits Times*. Retrieved on
9 February 2020 from: https://www.straitstimes.com/singapore/health/
coronavirus-calmer-mood-at-some-supermarkets-on-sunday-shelves-restocked.

Tan, Cheryl, 2020. "Over 44,000 foreign workers receive free $10 top-ups to their
prepaid cards to call home for Hari Raya". *The Straits Times*. Retrieved on 27
May 2020 from: https://www.straitstimes.com/singapore/over-44000-foreign
-workers-received-free-10-top-ups-to-their-prepaid-cards-to-call-home.

Tan, Sue-Ann, 2020. "Companies still hiring amid economic slump". *The Straits
Times*. Retrieved on 28 May 2020 from: https://www.straitstimes.com/singapore
/manpower/companies-still-hiring-amid-economic-slump.

———, 2020. "Coronavirus: 64-year-old Indonesian man who died in Singapore was
first hospitalised in Jakarta for pneumonia". *The Straits Times*. Retrieved on 21
March 2020 from: https://www.straitstimes.com/singapore/health/coronavirus
-64-year-old-indonesian-man-dies-of-COVID-19-in-singapore.

Tan, Tam Mei, 2020. "Coronavirus: Hotels among lodgings being used to house
foreign workers from dormitories". *The Straits Times*. Retrieved on 17 April
2020 from: https://www.straitstimes.com/singapore/coronavirus-hotels-among
-lodgings-being-used-to-house-foreign-workers-from-dormitories.

Tang, See Kit, 2020. "Singapore will enter a recession this year, 'significant uncertainty'
over duration and intensity: MAS". *Channel News Asia*. Retrieved on 28 April
2020 from: https://www.channelnewsasia.com/news/singapore/COVID-19
-economy-singapore-will-enter-recession-2020-mas-review-12683096.

Tang, See Kit and Aqil Haziq Mahmud, 2020. "Singapore launches TraceTogether
mobile app to boost COVID-19 tracing efforts". *Channel News Asia*. Retrieved
on 20 March 2020 from: https://www.channelnewsasia.com/news/singapore/
covid19-trace-together-mobile-app-contact-tracing-coronavirus-12560616.

Tay, Tiffany Fumiko, 2020. "New roles as safe distancing ambassadors for some
workers amid job disruption due to COVID-19". *The Straits Times*. Retrieved on
29 April 2020 from: https://www.straitstimes.com/singapore/workers-take-on
-front-line-roles-amid-job-disruption.

Tee, Zhuo, 2020a. "1.3m reusable masks for migrant workers; over $850k raised too". *The Straits Times*. Retrieved on 20 April 2020 from: https://www .straitstimes.com/singapore/13m-reusable-masks-for-migrant-workers-over -850k-raised-too.

———, 2020b. "300 homeless get help from network during COVID-19 circuit breaker". *The Straits Times*. Retrieved on 5 May 2020 from: https://www .straitstimes.com/politics/300-homeless-get-help-from-network-during-circuit -breaker.

———, 2020c. "Coronavirus: Polyclinic doctor among those helping out in dorms". *The Straits Times*. Retrieved on 19 May 2020 from: https://www.straitstimes.com /singapore/polyclinic-doctor-among-those-helping-out-in-dorms.

Tham, Thrina, 2020. *SAF-led fast deployment to help stabilise COVID-19 dorm situation*. Singapore: Ministry of Defence: Pioneer. Retrieved on 23 April 2020 from: https://www.mindef.gov.sg/web/portal/pioneer/article/cover-article -detail/community/2020-Q2/23apr20_news1.

Thukral, Naveen, 2020. "Panic buying, lockdowns may drive world food inflation – FAO, analysts". *Reuters*. Retrieved on 21 March 2020 from: https://www.reuters .com/article/us-health-coronavirus-food-security/panic-buying-lockdowns-may -drive-world-food-inflation-fao-analysts-idUSKBN21808G.

Wong, Kai Yi, 2020. "Coronavirus: 40,000 daily tests have to be done in strategic, coordinated way, says Lawrence Wong". *The Straits Time*. Retrieved on 8 May 2020 from: https://www.straitstimes.com/singapore/coronavirus-40000-daily -tests-have-to-be-done-in-a-strategic-coordinated-way-says-lawrence.

Wong, Lawrence, 2020a. "COVID-19: Travel restrictions for foreign visitors entering Singapore". Singapore Government. Retrieved on 22 March 2020 from: https:// www.gov.sg/article/COVID-19-travel-restrictions-for-foreign-visitors-entering -singapore.

———, 2020b. "Full COVID-19 press conference by the multi-ministry task force on May 19, 2020". Youtube (Video). Retrieved on 19 May 2020 from: https://www .youtube.com/watch?v=pK79uej4FKY.

Wong, Pei Ting, 2020. "Ex-SAF regulars called upon as "personnel with operational experience" needed to tackle COVID-19 at dorms: MINDEF". *Today*. Retrieved on 19 April 2020 from: https://www.todayonline.com /singapore/ex-saf-regulars-called-upon-personnel-operational-experience -needed-contain-COVID-19.

Yang, Bijou and David Lester, 1994. "The social impact of unemployment". *Applied Economics Letters*, 1(12): 887–890.

Yang, Calvin, 2020. "Singaporeans advised to defer all non-essential travel". *The Straits Times*. Retrieved on 15 March 2020 from: https://www.straitstimes.com/ singapore/sporeans-advised-to-defer-all-non-essential-travel.

Yeun, Sin, 2020. "Coronavirus: Diamond HDB blocks in Taman Jurong to house healthy foreign workers in essential services". *The Straits Times*. Retrieved on 17 April 2020 from: https://www.straitstimes.com/singapore/coronavirus-diamond -hdb-blocks-in-taman-jurong-to-house-foreign-workers-in-essential.

———, 2020. "Coronavirus: Singaporeans donate their solidarity payouts to charities". *The Straits Times*. Retrieved on 16 April 2020 from: https://www .straitstimes.com/singapore/sporeans-donate-their-solidarity-payouts.

Yong, Clement, 2020. "200,000 migrant workers get special Hari Raya Puasa meal". *The Straits Times*. Retrieved on 24 May 2020 from: https://www.straitstimes

.com/singapore/200000-migrant-workers-get-special-hari-raya-aidilfitri-meal-in
-signal-of-unity-and.

Zheng, Zhangxin, 2020. "Woman in her 30s stayed in Yishun flat with 60-year-old mother's decomposing body for 5 days". *Mothership*. Retrieved on 9 May 2020 from: https://mothership.sg/2020/05/yishun-dish-collector-death-5-days/.

7 COVID-19 and Thailand

Responses, Health Preparedness, and Policy Direction

Ruetaitip Chansrakaeo

Introduction

Part 1: COVID-19 Phenomenon and Thailand's Responses

The Coronavirus Disease 2019 (COVID-19) outbreak, causing new pneumonia with coronavirus (NCIP), has affected 71,429 people worldwide. The disease has originated in China and is rapidly growing in other countries. Work indicates that 2019-nCov has a remarkable genomic similarity with Extreme Acute Respiratory Syndrome (SARS) which had a pandemic past in 2002. Evidence of nosocomial spread employs a number of diligent measures to restrict its spread. The World Health Organization (WHO) has therefore established the Public Health Emergency of International Concern (PHEIC) with strategic objectives for public health for reducing its impact on the global health and economic environment (Arshad Ali et al., 2020).

Government Responses to COVID-19

COVID-19 has been declared a dangerous transmissible disease since March 1, 2020 under the 2015 Communicable Diseases Act. If anyone finds a suspected case or persons that meet the COVID-19 criteria, reporting to disease control officers within 3 hours is mandatory. Under Section 5, The Minister of public health is responsible for and oversaw the implementation of this Act and authorized to appoint officers for communicable disease control, issue Ministerial Regulations for additional acts, and issue Rules or Notifications for the implementation of this Act. Under Section 6, the Minister shall be empowered in the notifications by and with the advice of the Committee to prescribe for the purposes of preventing and regulating communicable diseases: (1) names and symptoms of dangerous communicable diseases and communicable diseases under surveillance, (2) classification of any ports of entry in the Kingdom as foreign transmissible disease control checkpoints and cancellation of international communicable disease control checkpoints; and (3) immunization (Communicable Diseases Act, B.E. 2558, 2015).

On March 8, 2020, Kingdom Thailand's Prime Minister and Minister of Defense, General Prayut Chan-O-cha, instructed the Provincial-level Internal

DOI: 10.4324/9781003291909-8

Security Operations Command to reinforce support for local public health agencies, including screening, referral, and care of disease control facilities. On March 11, 2020, Kingdom Thailand's Prime Minister and Minister of Defense, General Prayut Chan-O-cha, instructed the Provincial-level Internal Security Operations Command to reinforce support for local public health agencies, including screening, referral, and care of disease control facilities. On March 19, 2020, the government allowed governors to consider temporarily closing places at risk of COVID-19 spreading, such as bars, restaurants, entertainment spots, boxing stadiums, etc., before the situation returns to normal. The number of infected patients under investigation during March 2020 until early April 2020 was 2,169 cases with 23 deaths (Department of Disease Control, 2020).

General Prayuth Chan-O-cha, Thailand's premier and defense minister, asked the cabinet's authority to issue an emergency decree (2005) to contain the COVID-19 outbreak (Department of Disease Control, 2020). The Thai government employed "Emergency Decree on Public Administration in Emergency Situations, B.E. 2548 (2005)" as its legal measure to respond to the new emerging infectious disease. Under Section 4, the term "emergency situation" was defined as a situation, which affects or may affect the public order of the people or endangers the security of the State or may cause the country or any part of the country to fall into a state of difficulty pursuant to which it is necessary to enact emergency measures to preserve the interests of the nation, compliance with the law, the safety of the people, the normal living of the people, the protection of rights, liberties and public order or public interest, or the aversion or remedy of damages arising from urgent and serious public calamity. According to Section 9 of this decree, the Prime Minister has the power to issue the following regulations in case of need for the remediation and timely resolution of an emergency situation or for the prevention of aggravation of such a situation. The regulations under Section 9 consist of the following:

(1) to prohibit any person from departing from a dwelling place during the prescribed period, except with the permission of a competent official or being an exempted person;
(2) to prohibit the assembly or gathering of persons at any place or the commission of any act which may cause unrest;
(3) to prohibit the press release, distribution or dissemination of letters, publications or any means of communication containing texts which may instigate fear amongst the people or is intended to distort information which misleads understanding of the emergency situation to the extent of affecting the security of state or public order or good moral of the people both in the area or locality where an emergency situation has been declared or the entire Kingdom;
(4) to prohibit the use of routes or vehicles or prescribe conditions on the use of routes or vehicles;
(5) to prohibit the use of buildings or enter into or stay in any place; and
(6) to evacuate people out of a designated area for the safety of such people or to prohibit any person from entering a designated area (Emergency Decree on Public Administration in Emergency Situations, B.E. 2548 (2005), 2006).

On March 25, 2020, the government announced the Declaration of an Emergency Situation pursuant to the Emergency Decree on Public Administration in Emergency Situations B.E. 2548 (2005) by stating that the outbreak of the Coronavirus 2019 is rapidly spreading all over the world and is also affecting Thailand. In 2019 and early 2020, there is no vaccine or effective drugs that are available. The Thai government applied appropriate measures to prevent, stop, and delay the outbreak as well as to raise public awareness and understanding. It conducted daily assessments of the situation in response to new developments, information, and health recommendations of different experts, taking into account public impacts in terms of public welfare, living standards, government public health resources, and in order to prevent unnecessary panic.

All situations elevated to the point where the government was pushed to enforce additional measures at the highest level. The consequence of this declaration is that the government has additional legal means to track and control the situation. Therefore, the Government had to state an emergency situation in order to avoid any risks, thereby providing reassurance for officials and facilitating public anxiety. The declaration of an emergency situation was particularly urgent at that time. The government found appropriate ways to prevent and mitigate the spread of the disease in compliance with the medical and public health advice. As a consequence, the comfort of people will be reduced during this time, as everyone will need to change their behaviors; yet the public will usually live their lives without being robbed. As for remedial measures to alleviate the problems for those affected, they will be progressively implemented. This disease can attack people anywhere and anytime. Therefore, the situation needs to be controlled and high-level measures taken to ensure our collective survival. The emergent situation continued for a period of time, but will not exceed a duration of three months, as required by statute (Declaration of an Emergency Situation pursuant to the Emergency Decree on Public Administration in Emergency Situations B.E. 2548 (2005), 2020).

The World Health Organization announced the outbreak of Coronavirus 2019, a communicable disease, a pandemic. It asked ASEAN countries including Thailand to take stricter measures. The pandemic threatened the public order and the safety of the individual, requiring rigorous and urgent measures to prevent the disease from being broadly transmitted. There have been the housekeeping of the necessary goods to monitor and control the outbreak, to prevent and to treat the disease, to house consumer goods and essential products necessary for people's daily lives, which must be avoided in order to prevent shortages resulting in the aggravation of people's distress. Therefore, urgent measures were taken to protect the safety of the people and the peaceful living of the people (Declaration of an Emergency Situation in all areas of the Kingdom of Thailand, 2020).

In accordance with Section 5 of the Public Administration Emergency Decree B.E. 2548 (2005), the Prime Minister declared an emergency situation in all areas of the Kingdom of Thailand, after the approval of the Council of Ministers. This order became effective from March 26 B.E. 2563 (2020) to April 30 B.E. 2563 (2020). After the announcement, the number of confirmed cases during early April 2020 to June 3, 2020 was 3,081 cases with 57 deaths (Department of Disease Control, 2020).

Under the Declaration of Emergency Situation and the Regulation No. 1 issued on March 25 B.E. (2020) 2563, in order to take further measures to remedy the emergency, Section 9 of the Emergency Decree on Public Administration in Emergency Situations B.E., the Prime Minister issued an additional Regulation No. 2 as follows:

1. No person in the Kingdom shall be allowed to leave their homes from 22.00 am until 4.00 pm on the following day except, where necessary, those in the medical field, banking, transportation of consumer goods, agricultural produce, medicine, medical supplies, medical supplies, newspapers, fuel and petrol transportation, courier service, trafficking.
2. If notices or orders prohibit, alert or advise in the way in which Clause 1 paragraph 1 applies to any province, territory or place where conditions or timescales are more stringent or stricter than this Regulation, such notifications or orders shall also remain to be complied with.
3. In those cases where it is not possible to relocate people traveling outside the Kingdom, the Provincial Transmittable Disease Committees or the Bangkok Communicable Disease Committee shall, in accordance with specified conditions and times, provide an isolated site for monitoring or quarantine of such people in order to prevent the spread of the disease (Regulation Issued under Section 9 of the Emergency Decree on Public Administration in Emergency Situations B.E. 2548 (2005) No. 1).

Regarding the structure of the Centre for COVID-19 Situation Administration (CCSA), the Prime Minister, in the capacity of the Director of the Centre for COVID-19 Situation Administration, issued the order of the Prime Minister No. 6/2563 on the arrangement of the structure of the center for COVID-19 situation administration (CCSA) as follows:

(1) Office of the Secretariat, with the Deputy Secretary-General to the Prime Minister for Political Affairs, assigned by the Prime Minister as Head of the Office;
(2) Central Coordination Office, with the Secretary-General of the National Security Council as Head of the Office;
(3) Emergency Operation Centre for Medical and Public Health Issues Relating to the Communicable Disease COVID-19, with the Permanent Secretary of the Ministry of Public Health as Head of the Centre;
(4) Operation Centre for Measures on the Protection and Assistance of the Public, with the Permanent Secretary of the Ministry of Interior as Head of the Centre;
(5) Operation Centre for the Distribution of Masks and Medical Supplies to the Public, with the Permanent Secretary of the Ministry of Interior as Head of the Centre;

(6) Operation Centre for the Control of Goods, with the Permanent Secretary of the Ministry of Commerce as Head of the Centre;

(7) Operation Centre for Measures on the Entry into and Departure from the Kingdom, and the Protection of Thai Nationals Abroad, with the Permanent Secretary of the Ministry of Foreign Affairs as Head of the Centre;

(8) Operation Centre for Telecommunications and Online Social Media, with the Permanent Secretary of the Ministry of Digital Economy and Society as Head of the Centre;

(9) Operation Centre for Remedying the Emergency Situation on Security, with the Supreme Commander as Head of the Centre; and

(10) Operation Centre for Information on Measures to Remedy the Communicable Disease COVID-19 Situation, with the Permanent Secretary of the Office of the Prime Minister as Head of the Centre (Office of the Prime Minister, 2020).

It is deemed necessary to further alleviation the implementation of some measures to prevent the spread of COVID-19 in addition to earlier alleviation in order to reduce people's economic, social, and security impacts, according to the Center for Situation.

Whereas it was deemed appropriate to further alleviate the enforcement of certain measures for the prevention of the spread of the COVID-19 disease in addition to earlier alleviation in order to reduce the impact on the people in terms of the economy, society, and security, according to the situation assessment report of the Centre for the Administration of the Situation together with the suggestion from public-health officials who advised that the total number of infected people, the number of newly infected persons per day and statistical deaths in the country was decreased since early May 2020. However, the risk factors exist due to weather conditions, the number of cross-provincial travelers and international travelers and of groups of individuals neglecting and failing to comply with disease prevention measures, although the spread of the disease in other countries is still apparent, alleviation should be focused on the risk exposure of individuals, places and types of activities, subject to strict compliance of disease prevention measures and recommendations of the government. When an increasing number of people are infected or the risk of infection is raised, alleviation may be suspended or changed partially or completely.

On May 17, 2020, by virtue of Section 9 of the Emergency Decree on Public Administration in Emergency Situations B.E. 2548 (2005) and Section 11 of the State Administration Act B.E. 2534 (1991), the Prime Minister issued a regulation for the general public and guidelines for government agencies as follows:

1. Prohibition to Leave Dwelling Places: It is prohibited for any person throughout the Kingdom to leave their dwelling places from the time of 23.00 hrs to 04.00 hrs of the following day, and the exemptions to the prohibition to leave dwelling places in accordance with Regulation (No. 3) issued on April 10 B.E. 2563 (2020) shall remain in force.

2. Alleviation of the prohibition of use of buildings and premises of schools or educational institutions: The Governor of Bangkok or Provincial Governors shall have the power to consider alleviation of the prohibition of the use of buildings and premises of schools or educational institutions, only for assisting, caring, fostering, or sheltering orphans with family problems, impoverished or disadvantaged children, who may be a risk-prone group if left to live in their residences or other places, or for using such buildings and premises to carry out activities of public interest as permitted by the Governor of Bangkok or Provincial Governors. However, it is still prohibited to use such buildings and premises for the organization of education, examination, or training.

3. Alleviation of prohibitions or limitations on conducting or carrying out certain activities: In order to facilitate the people and to move forward certain activities, subject to the implementation of disease prevention measures as prescribed by the government as well as the setting up of orderly arrangements and systems, places, or activities for which the Governor of Bangkok and Provincial Governors have previously issued orders to temporarily close (Regulation Issued under Section 9 of the Emergency Decree on Public Administration in Emergency Situations B.E. 2548 (2005) No. 7, 2020).

Part 2: Thailand's Pandemic Preparedness

Healthcare professionals, lawmakers, intelligence experts, and politicians tend to fear pandemic influenza. In the previous century alone, three influenza pandemics in 1918, 1957, and 1968 led to millions of deaths and major social and economic disruptions. While pandemic influenza has therefore been recognized as a public health danger for decades, it has not always been constructed as a security threat that threatens political, economic, and social stability. Confirmation in November 2003 that a new highly virulent H5N1 strain of avian influenza began to infect humans and was gradually spreading throughout Asia provided a significant event which enabled the pandemic of influenza to step forward toward complete securitization. By 2005, persuaded by the increasing threat of H5N1 influenza, governments around the world had initiated a series of new pandemic planning and preparation activities. Therefore, the pandemic influenza threat persuaded government leaders that people were self-evident in the need for extensive pandemic preparations.

It is difficult to anticipate or avoid natural events that can promote an effective human pandemic influenza virus transmission. However, if such an event occurs, we must be prepared to react quickly and decisively. A diligent surveillance of new viruses in both the human and animal populations using appropriate diagnostics is critical to the containment of a potential infectious pandemic. The viruses should also be monitored for changes that can signal increased virulence or transmissibility. The creation and production of effective countermeasures are equally significant (Fauci, 2006).

Prevention of emergencies for public health requires the development of capacities and ongoing improvement, including frequent planning testing by exercises and developing and implementing corrective action plans. It also covers the practice of improving community health and resilience. The components of public health emergency preparedness consist of health risk assessment, legal climate, role and responsibilities, incident command system, public engagement, epidemiology functions, laboratory functions, countermeasures and mitigation strategies, mass health care, and public information and communication (Nelson, Lurie and Wasseman, 2007).

To understand how to prepare Thailand for health security, one way is to look at the performance of Thailand in the global security index (Global Security Index, 2019, 2020). With the last global security index report, Thailand is ranked no.6 in the world. Overall, Thailand scored 73.2 points. On prevention of the emergence or release of pathogens, Thailand scored 75.7 points. On early detection and reporting for epidemics of potential international concern, Thailand scored 81.0 points. On rapid response to and mitigation of the spread of an epidemic, Thailand scored 78.6 points. On sufficient and robust health system to treat the sick and protect health workers, Thailand scored 70.5 points. On commitments to improving national capacity, financing plans to address gaps, and adhering to global norms, Thailand scored 70.9 points. On overall risk environment and country vulnerability to biological threats, Thailand scored 56.4 points (Center for Health Security, 2020).

Part 3: Policy Implication

Changing National Security Approach

Inexplicably connected, as long as globalization continues, are human security, international security, and state development. The effectiveness of any international response would be dependent on the capacity of the intergovernmental organizations, NGOs, and the respective states to demonstrate interoperability and cooperation. Intervention requires bilateral collaborations, counterinsurgency actions require mutually beneficial military and humanitarian aid agencies and communication with intergovernmental organizations, and transnational corporations is essential in order to fight environmental degradation. With the myriad traditional and non-traditional challenges faced by the international community following the Cold War, the age of global and interagency cooperation is over in which challenges can be solved.

As an international community, a variety of international security issues, prioritize traditional challenges must be addressed which affect safety and not ignore non-traditional challenges such as food security or health protection, rather than address them after they have evolved into traditional safety concerns based on violence.

World politics tend to change too many powers, with the United States facing challenges from Russia and China. Thailand must proceed with a soft policy in determining positions in order to maintain the balance of relations between

Thailand and various major powers. Holistic security (Comprehensive Security) should be given priority focusing on various factors, such as human security with a focus on freedom from fear and with dignity and liberation from the basic need to maintain freedom. State security should be based on the development of the country to progress with the well-being of the people and the safety of the country by formulating policies, strategies, master plans, and action plans which focus on strengthening immunity and preparedness for threats or security issues creating fairness and reducing inequality.

The author wishes to recommend the strategic considerations regarding Thailand's national security preparedness to these new emerging infectious threats by emphasizing on the preparedness system capacity development and health security system as follows:

(a) Preparedness system capacity development

1. The continuing development of the national readiness system in the same way should be given priority by the central, provincial, local, and related sectors.
2. Regional and local agencies should prepare state staff information, resources and accounts, volunteers who are consistent with the types of mutual benefit disasters that take place in the area.
3. Developing guidelines for the integration of databases and information security networks for national preparedness and the national disaster data warehouse so that they can be used to support the management and coordination of disaster management and to exchange information for use among agencies for collaboration.
4. Courses and manuals for government agencies should be created with private and public sectors to be ready to face all forms of threats especially in risky areas.
5. Ministry of provincial administration organization should arrange training and practice within and between departments to prepare to handle all forms of threats by participation of the private and public sectors.

(b) Health security system

1. Governments should commit themselves to taking action to address health safety risks. Leaders should coordinate and monitor national health security investments in order to coordinate them with improvements to routine public health and healthcare systems.
2. Capacity in health security should be transparent and regularly measured. The results of these external assessments and self-assessments should be published every two years at least once.
3. New funding mechanisms to address epidemic and pandemic preparedness gaps are needed and should be set up urgently. They may include a new multilateral mechanism to finance global health security.

4. Thailand should at least annually test its health security capabilities and publish post-action reviews. Government must commit to a functioning system by holding annual simulation exercises.

It should be recognized that these recommendations will not succeed if the relevant factors are not met. Key success factors regarding this approach depend on announcing this preparedness as national agenda, having a plan to support the national preparedness plan by coordinating connections at all levels of government to develop a system of international preparation by having academic research, training, exchanges, and strengthening network partners, and all relevant sectors, especially the private and public sectors, participating in the national preparedness system in the form of network partners that share in making decisions.

Global Security Consideration

The concept of "soft power"—the "possibility to attract and persuade others"—often fails to capture what happens when autocrats reach abroad. We have argued that these efforts represent, instead, the exercise of "strong power," which strives to undermine freedom of expression, compromise and neutralize independent institutions, and distort the political environment. Leaders in Beijing and Moscow wanted to control over the information, images, and ideas of dissemination tools. They are not only increasing their media footprint, which is evident in foreign broadcasters like RT and CGTN, but they are also increasing their efforts to control and censor. The aim of these autocracies is to selectively make information available (Walker, Kalathil, and Ludwig, 2020).

Sharp power refers to the ability to influence others to achieve desired results not by attraction, as is the case for soft power, but by information distraction and manipulation. Government attempts to direct, buy, or coerce political influence and regulate the discussion of sensitive issues globally, frequently involve the exercise of sharp power, usually through untransparent or dubious, if not totally illegal, means. Beijing disseminates its discursive strategic stories containing elements of unliberal ideals and worldviews in many areas of soft/sharp control (Tae-Hwan, n.d.).

Following this pandemic change, the author assumes that in the post–COVID-19 era, this cycle will accelerate. The competition between the US and China is set to increase and what will shape the final results of this growing competition will increasingly focus on the question of how many Chinese and American followers are going to be in the coming years. Both powers have already committed themselves to a propaganda war against the success of the defeat.

How to Respond to China's Sharp Power? A more purposive, long-term strategy rooted in both civil society and state institutions can assist democracies in defending their security and in restoring the initiative for the long term. Such a response must reinforce the democratic principles to be protected at the most fundamental level. It should concentrate on the following objectives as indicated in Walker, Kalathil, and Ludwig's work (2020):

A. **Strengthening democratic values:** In order to protect themselves from sharp power, the leaders of these institutions need to take concrete steps to renew their commitment to democratic standards and free political expression. The identification of these standards can often be straightforward: Many of the institutions in question already formally commit to principles such as transparency, accountability, and free expression with their charters or other public declarations.

B. **Enhancing democratic unity:** Democratic lawmakers need expert knowledge about the incentives for survival that drive autocracies and the relationship between these regimes and their nominally autonomous private or "non-governmental" actors. To that end, it is important that established as well as younger democracies develop an independent capacity for monitoring and analysis of local involvement with authoritarians.

C. **Meet the technological challenge:** Democracies must articulate a comprehensive, coherent, and collective vision that takes a clear view of the challenges posed by the modern ecosystem of information and provides a framework of principles to address them. Such a framework must include innovations that allow democrats to use technological advances more effectively. Open democratic society has a key strategic advantage in that it lacks the creativity and initiative of a vibrant, pluralistic civil society that can inform, promote, and support such a vision. Democratic societies must use all their resources to meet the multifaceted authoritarian threat (Walker, Kalathil, and Ludwig, 2020).

Reference

Arshad Ali, Shajeea, Mariam Baloch, Naseem Ahmed, Asadullah Arshad Ali, and Ayman Iqbal. 2020. "The Outbreak of Coronavirus Disease 2019 (COVID-19)—An Emerging Global Health Threat." *Journal of Infection and Public Health*, 13(4): 644–646. https://doi.org/10.1016/j.jiph.2020.02.033

Center for Health Security, Johns Hopkins University. 2020. "Global Health Security Index 2019." Accessed April 6, 2020. https://www.ghsindex.org/wp-content/uploads/2019/10/2019-Global-Health-Security-Index.pdf

Communicable Disease Act B.E. 2558(2015). 2015. "Government Gazette Volume 132 Special Part 86A 8th September B.E. 2558 (2015)." Accessed May 10, 2020. http://web.krisdika.go.th/data/slideshow/File/2-TH-COMMUNICABLE.pdf

Department of Control Disease. 2020a. "The Coronavirus Situation 2019." Accessed April 6, 2020. https://ddc.moph.go.th/viralpneumonia/eng/file/situation/situation-no93-050463.pdf

Department of Control Disease. 2020b. "The Coronavirus Situation 2019." Accessed May 6, 2020. https://ddc.moph.go.th/viralpneumonia/eng/file/situation/situation-no114-260463.pdf

Department of Control Disease. 2020c. "The Coronavirus Situation 2019." Accessed May 6, 2020. https://ddc.moph.go.th/viralpneumonia/eng/file/situation/situation-no120-030563.pdf

Department of Control Disease. 2020d. "The Coronavirus Situation 2019." Accessed May 20, 2020. https://ddc.moph.go.th/viralpneumonia/eng/file/situation/situation-no128-100563.pdf

Department of Control Disease. 2020e. "The Coronavirus Situation 2019." Accessed May 20, 2020. https://ddc.moph.go.th/viralpneumonia/eng/file/situation/situation-no135-170563.pdf

Department of Control Disease. 2020f. "The Coronavirus Situation 2019." Accessed June 4, 2020. https://ddc.moph.go.th/viralpneumonia/eng/file/situation/situation-no142-240563.pdf

Department of Control Disease. 2020g. "The Coronavirus Situation 2019." Accessed June 4, 2020. https://ddc.moph.go.th/viralpneumonia/eng/file/situation/situation-no149-310563.pdf

Fauci, Anthony S. 2006. "Pandemic Influenza Threat and Preparedness." *Emerging Infectious Diseases*. https://doi.org/10.3201/eid1201.050983.

Nelson, Christopher, Nicole Lurie, and Jeffrey Wasserman. 2007. Assessing Public Health Emergency Preparedness: Concepts, Tools, and Challenges. *Annual Review of Public Health*, 28(April). Available at SSRN: https://ssrn.com/abstract=1077927

Office of the Council of the State. 2005. "Emergency Decree on Public Administration in Emergency Situation, B.E.2548 (2005)." Government Gazette Volume 122 Special Part 58A 16th July B.E. 2548 (2005). Accessed May 28, 2020. http://web.krisdika.go.th/data/slideshow/File/1-EN-EMERGENCY.pdf

Office of the Prime Minister. 2020a. "Declaration of an Emergency Situation in all areas of the Kingdom of Thailand." *Government Gazette*, 137, Special Part 69d 25th March B.E. 2563 (2020). Accessed May 10, 2020. http://web.krisdika.go.th/data/slideshow/File/02-Declaration.pdf

Office of the Prime Minister. 2020b. "Official Statement of the Office of the Prime Minister RE: Declaration of an Emergency Situation pursuant to the Emergency Decree on Public Administration in Emergency Situations B.E. 2548 (2005)." *Government Gazette*, 137, Part 24a 25th March B.E. 2563 (2020). Accessed May 10, 2020. http://web.krisdika.go.th/data/slideshow/File/01-Official_Statement.pdf

Office of the Prime Minister. 2020c. "Order of the Prime Minister No. 6 /2563 Re: Arrangement of the Structure of the Centre for COVID-19 Situation Administration (CCSA)." *Government Gazette*, 137, Special Part 72d 27th March B.E. 2563 (2020). Accessed May 10, 2020. http://web.krisdika.go.th/data/slideshow/File/4-3_165158_6_2563_Eng.pdf

Office of the Prime Minister. 2020d. "Regulation Issued under Section 9 of the Emergency Decree on Public Administration in Emergency Situations B.E. 2548 (2005) (No. 7)." *Government Gazette*, 137, Special Part 69d 25th May B.E. 2563 (2020). Accessed May 28, 2020. http://web.krisdika.go.th/data/slideshow/File/RegulationEN.pdf

Tae-Hwan, Kim. n.d. "China's Sharp Power and South Korea's Peace Initiative."

Walker, Christopher, Shanthi Kalathil, and Jessica Ludwig. 2020. "The Cutting Edge of Sharp Power." *Journal of Democracy*, 31(1): 124–37. https://doi.org/10.1353/jod.2020.0010.

8 Global Security Crisis of COVID-19

Threat and Response in Indonesia

Rachel Kumendong and Edwin Tambunan

Introduction

Within a very short time, the global pandemic resulting from coronavirus disease (COVID-19) has changed the face of the world on an unprecedented scale. At the time of writing, the World Health Organization (WHO) reported that COVID-19 has infected more than 3 million people with over 200,000 deaths across 212 countries.[1] Indonesia is one of the most infected countries in the Southeast Asia region after Singapore, reaching over 12,000 cases with more than 800 deaths and 2,100 recoveries: making Indonesia as the country with the highest COVID-19 mortality rate in Asia, of around 7–8%.[2]

President Joko Widodo announced Indonesia's first positive case on March 2, 2020. Prior to this, the government remained to affirm that not a single confirmed COVID-19 case had been reported in the country. Considering the neighboring countries had reported positive cases since January 2020, this raised the question of how Indonesia insisted it had no cases and the country's responses toward the pandemic.

Many argue that the Indonesian government had been indecisive and showed a slow initial response in the early stage of the pandemic. When other countries act to be on full alert in dealing with COVID-19, Indonesia seems to belittle the threat. The Central Bureau of Statistics of Indonesia reported that in January 2020, a total of 796,934 foreign tourists entered Indonesia through 32 international airports.[3]

The rapid transmission of COVID-19 has an enormous impact on the country's economic and social sectors. According to the International Monetary Fund (IMF), the global economy will shrink by 3% this year, far worse than the 2009 global crisis, and will put the global economy at risk of the worst recession. With that being said, Indonesia must enhance its vigilance and preparedness to anticipate the threats and their impacts.[4]

After announcing the first case of COVID-19, the government then issued several directions. However, amidst the shadow of the pandemic's devastating effects, it appears that the government remains slow in making decisions and often issues policies that contradict each other. This chapter contributes to an understanding that the indecisiveness of the Indonesian government's response

DOI: 10.4324/9781003291909-9

to pandemic threats is related to its poor efforts in dealing with the economic and social effects of the pandemic, while at the same time defending itself from political pressure and internal political discord.

The discussion begins with Indonesia's experience in dealing with outbreaks in the past whose impact was not as extensive as the current pandemic, and the government at that time had strong political support. Afterward, the presentation on the economic, social, and political threats of the COVID-19 pandemic as perceived by the government is given. The last section discusses the government's response in dealing with those threats.

Leave the Past Behind

Before dealing with the COVID-19 pandemic, Indonesia has experienced tackling severe acute respiratory syndrome (SARS), middle east respiratory syndrome (MERS), and H5N1 or avian influenza (AI) outbreaks a few years ago. At that time, the government adopted a number of policies that focused on preventing disease transmission.

SARS and MERS in Indonesia

Severe acute respiratory syndrome (SARS) and middle east respiratory syndrome (MERS) are both caused by coronavirus, and generated a viral respiratory disease. It spread across 26 countries, infecting more than 8,000 people with 774 deaths. Meanwhile, MERS was first detected in Saudi Arabia in September 2012, had spread to 27 countries, and infected 2,519 people with 866 deaths.[5]

According to WHO, Indonesia has no reported cases of SARS and MERS. On March 15, 2003, the government reported two probable suspects of SARS in the country but later it did not fulfill the case definition.[6]

The government remained to perceive these as a security threat to the country. In 2003, the Ministry of Health issued a Decree of the Minister of Health No. 424/MENKES/SK/IV/2003 on Stipulation of Severe Acute Respiratory Syndrome (SARS) to cause Outbreak as well as Guidance for Overcoming. As for the implementation, it was concluded as a list in Table 8.1.

H5N1 or Avian Influenza (AI) in Indonesia

On February 2, 2004, Indonesia first reported the case of avian influenza in poultry in 11 provinces. On July 21, 2005, Indonesia confirmed its first human case.[7] From the report of WHO 2003–2009, Indonesia has the highest number of avian influenza infections: 162 cases with 134 deaths (82.72% of the mortality rate). Meanwhile, the total cases worldwide were 468 cases with 282 deaths (60.26% of mortality rate), making Indonesia as the country most infected by avian influenza.[8]

The Minister of Health, Dr. Siti Fadilah Supari, decided to use public health approach by issuing Decree of the Minister of Health No. 1371/MENKES/SK/

Table 8.1 Government's Strategy in Overcoming SARS and MERS

SARS (2003)	MERS (2014–2016)
• Issued an appeal to be vigilant when visiting Hong Kong, China (Guangdong Province, Vietnam, Singapore, and Thailand) • Provided health alert cards for Indonesian citizens who have just returned from SARS-infected countries • Established referral hospitals in Jakarta, Surabaya, Medan, and Semarang to deal with the SARS outbreak • Requested the mask industry to increase production • Conducted quarantine at the hospital or at the home of every suspected patient	• Called for a delay in departures to a number of countries in the Middle East • Appointed 100 referral hospitals • Escalated alertness at 13 entrances in Indonesia, especially for migrants from countries in the Middle East and South Korea • Set up of body scanning system at international airports in Indonesia

Source: Author.

Table 8.2 Government's Strategy in Overcoming Avian Influenza

Period	Description
December 2005	Completion of Strategic Plan (2006–2008)
March 2006	Established the National Committee for Avian Influenza and Pandemic Influenza Preparedness
September 2006	10 Steps Refocusing Strategy formulated
March 2007	• Presidential Instruction 1/2007 on Managing and Controlling Avian Flu • National workshop on AI – 6 Steps Refocusing Strategy
August 2007	Guidelines on National Pandemic Preparedness and Response Plan
March 2008	National Pandemic Preparedness and Response Plan
August 2008	Guidelines for Managing Epicenter of Influenza Pandemic by the Ministry of Health

Source: Author.

IX/2005 on Stipulation of Avian Influenza as Disease Potential to cause Outbreak as well as Guidance for Overcoming and Decree of the Minister of Health No. 1372/Menkes/SK/IX/200S on Stipulation of Extraordinary Condition (*KLB*) of Avian Influenza.

Following are the government's prevention measures and concrete actions to deal with the pandemic (Table 8.2).

The key milestone of the strategies above was the establishment of the National Committee for Avian Influenza and Pandemic Influenza Preparedness

(Komnas Federasi Perjuangan Buruh Indonesia) that worked as a coordinating body, mapping things such as the distribution of medical, epidemiological, and veterinary expertise; domestic and international funding resources; media reporting; and vaccine sources and availability.[9] Furthermore, the government also endorsed a multisectoral approach to pandemic preparedness by pulling together a committee with members from 17 ministries, the National Planning Agency, and the army and police forces.[10]

It is evident that the ongoing pandemic requires more than what the country had prepared. Even so, the initial responses of the government toward COVID-19 outbreak are somewhat similar to how the country responds to SARS, MERS, and the avian influenza. However, considering the level of threat of the COVID-19 pandemic is far more beyond any of past outbreaks, it is obligatory for the government to provide more agile and accurate responses.

The government could not merely rely on the country's prior strategies in dealing with the outbreak because the current pandemic exhibits two distinctive challenges: COVID-19 is more widespread and its human-to-human transmission. Recently in July, the *Emerging Infectious Diseases* journal published a new study that changed the R0 (R-naught) for COVID-19 from 2.2 to 5.7.[11] The R0 (R-naught) refers to how many people a single infected person will infect in a population. The trend of new positive cases in Indonesia is rising significantly with an average increment rate pegged at 6–7%.[12] Started with only two positive cases on March 2, two months later Indonesia has confirmed having more than 12,000 positive cases.

Furthermore, COVID-19 is the first outbreak with human-to-human transmission that ever occurred in Indonesia. As the fourth most populous country in the world with over 270 million people, surely this is difficult work for the government to come up with a strategy that prevents any further transmission within the country. It is really difficult to control the virus once it establishes sustained human-to-human transmission in a new population: people can be contagious before even realizing they are infected. According to Sanche et al., 20% of transmission is driven by unidentified infected persons and high levels of social distancing efforts will be needed to contain the virus, highlighting the importance of early and effective surveillance, contact tracing, and quarantine.[13]

The unprecedented characteristics of COVID-19 and its transmission, objectively, lead the government not to rely on previous strategies in dealing with the current pandemic. However, in addition to the objective factors, a lack of proper perspective among high-level decision-makers also contributes to the government's reluctance to respond in reference to the previous strategies, which eventually lead the ruling government not to be as fast and as firm as previous governments in formulating strategies.

In the early period of the outbreak, the government was criticized for taking short-sighted measures in dealing with the issue. The government tends to rely more on an intelligence approach than on a scientific approach as the basis for policy-making. Moreover, the involvement of military figures appointed by President Joko Widodo in joining the government's fast-response team is becoming more evident.[14]

Further, clear communication and openness from the government to the public is one of the key factors in determining the policy effectivity during the crisis. However, the government opted to conceal information to prevent the public from panicking. On March 18, 2020, two weeks after the first cases were announced, the Indonesian COVID-19 Task Force finally launched the national official website of COVID-19 update in Indonesia.[15]

The government's initial responses are considered to prioritize the investment and infrastructure sector rather than the public health sector. Since the beginning of 2020, the COVID-19 outbreak had greatly impacted Indonesia's travel industry. As a response to this situation, the government offered tourism incentives (discounts up to 30%) to boost the country's tourism. According to the Minister of Tourism of Indonesia, the COVID-19 outbreak had potentially caused Indonesia to lose up to US$2.8 billion from Chinese tourists alone (with an average of 2 million travelers).[16]

The Multifront Battle against the COVID-19 Pandemic

In formulating strategies to mitigate the impact of the COVID-19 pandemic, the government should deal with threats related to economy, society, and politics. The pandemic undoubtedly causes devastating effects on trade, industry, investment tourism, and transportation. The harmful impacts of the pandemic on the economy potentially lead the society into social disharmony as unemployment increases and public disobedience arises. In politics, contradictory statements among decision-makers show the different interests and approaches among government units, the growing political pressure from outside government, and the possibility of the pandemic being used to delegitimize the government.

Economic Aspect

The development of the COVID-19 pandemic has caused extremely high uncertainty and has reduced the performance of global financial markets, depressed many world currencies, and triggered a reversal of capital to financial assets that were considered safe. The prospect of world economic growth is also declining due to the disruption of global supply chains, declining world demand, and weakening confidence in economic actors. In Indonesia, the impact of COVID-19 has been affecting the country mainly through channels of tourism, trade/export, and investment.

Trade and Investment

The domestic export performance of 2020 is predicted to be restrained due to limited global demand, reduced trade volume, and low commodity prices. The disruption of the global supply chain due to COVID-19 also affected the export performance of manufacturing corporations due to the limited production of raw

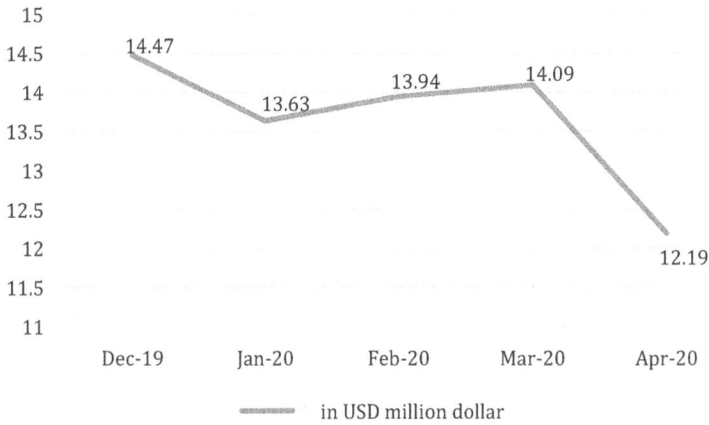

Figure 8.1 Indonesian export, December 2019–April 2020. Source: Author.

materials from other countries. In addition to goods exports, service exports are also forecasted to be on hold due to the performance of tourism-related activities which also contracted due to COVID-19 (Figure 8.1).

The Central Statistics Agency or Badan Pusat statistik (BPS) released export data in April 2020. In that period, the value of exports reached US$12.19 billion, down 7.02% from April 2019.[17]

Pressure on corporate performance occurs in all segments, including micro, small, and medium enterprises (MSMEs). The COVID-19 pandemic disrupted all sectors of the economy, especially trade, manufacturing, and services. Pressure does not merely hit corporations in the large and medium segments but also the MSME segment. MSMEs face a downward pressure on sales due to the decline in economic activity at all levels of society during large-scale social restrictions.

Tourism

Meanwhile, the country's domestic trade is affected by the difficulties of the trading corporation, which was hit due to a sharp decline in sales during the pandemic, and it also depressed the domestic tourism sector. Temporary suspension of foreign tourist visits due to fears of spreading the virus has reduced the performance of the tourism sector and other support sections including the transportation and trade activity in the tourism area.

Corporate performance related to tourism activities, such as the hospitality, aviation, entertainment industry, and food and beverage industries, and other sectors is threatened to shrink if the COVID-19 control lasts a long time.

Social Aspect

Since the business sectors, especially tourism and manufacturing, are the most affected, it resulted in the termination of employment (layoffs) or laying off workers for a while. Based on data from the Ministry of Manpower and the Social Security Body for Employment or Badan Penyelengara Jaminan Sosial (BPJS) *Ketenagakerjaan* on May 1, 2020, the number of formal sector workers who had been temporarily laid off due to the COVID-19 pandemic was 1,032,960 people and the formal sector workers laid off were 375,165 people.

While in the informal sector, workers affected by COVID-19 were 314,833 people. The total number of formal and informal sector workers affected by COVID-19 is 1,722,958 people. Moreover, there are still 1.2 million workers who are still in verification and validation stages, making the total number of affected workers to be around 3 million people.[18]

Besides, the Indonesian Migrant Workers Protection Agency (BP2MI) recorded that there were 100,094 Indonesian migrant workers (PMI) from 83 countries returning to their homeland in the last three months. Centre of Reform on Economics (CORE) Indonesia estimates that the open unemployment rate in the second quarter of 2020 will reach 8.2% with a mild scenario. While other scenarios are 9.79% in the medium scenario, and 11.47% in the severe scenario. The IMF also projects Indonesia's unemployment rate in 2020 to be 7.5%, up from 2019 which is only 5.3%.[19]

Political and Security Aspects

The development of the COVID-19 pandemic revealed the "hidden-hollow" of the country's political system and its ability to deal with the double crisis – public health disaster and economic crisis.

Lack of Cross-Government Coordination

The Jokowi administration has been criticized for the lack of transparency and poor coordination between central and local governments. The announcement of COVID-19 as a national disaster on 13 April was perceived as tardy and confusing by some of the regional governments. Along with it, many have argued that the central government did not have a clear and transparent plan for how to combat COVID-19. Thus, a number of local governments started to implement their own measures because they were losing faith in Jokowi's ability to manage the outbreak.

Some regions with a high number of cases have declared large-scale social restrictions (PSBB) before the national announcement. They are Jakarta; the municipalities of Bogor, Depok, and Bekasi; Bogor and Bekasi regencies; the municipalities of Tangerang and South Tangerang; and Tangerang regency and Pekanbaru municipality.[20]

Inconsistent regulations and contradictory statements among decision-makers in the government show the lack of coordination across ministries. The decision

of the central government to formally ban *mudik*[21] had to go through a complicated and confusing process to be dealt with. *Mudik* is believed to possess a high
risk of expanding the spread of COVID-19 across the country and could worsen
the public health crisis. On 2 April, in the exclusive meeting (*rapat terbatas*)
between the President and his ministries, Jokowi decided not to ban *mudik*
but the central government would continue to encourage people not to do it.
Later, Jokowi changed his policy to ban *mudik* effectively from April 24, 2020,
until May 31, 2020. On 6 May, Minister of Transportation, Budi Karya Sumadi
announced to re-open access to all modes of transportation starting May 7, 2020.
He conveyed that the relaxation was granted after receiving direction from the
Coordinating Minister for the Economy, Airlangga Hartarto, on the basis to
ensure the national economy would continue to run amid the pandemic.[22]

Moreover, the Katadata Insight Center (KIC) had conducted a survey of 2,437
respondents in 34 provinces in Indonesia: 12% of respondents said they would
continue going home despite the COVID-19 pandemic. By this, it is estimated
that there are 3 million people who would go home for *Lebaran*. Meanwhile, 4%
of respondents said they had gone home first.[23]

Using "Hard" Approach to the Crisis

After the declaration of COVID-19 as a national disaster, the government put
more emphasis on the country's security forces such as the National Police of
Indonesia (POLRI) and the Indonesian National Armed Forces (TNI) to be
involved in the grand strategy to deal with the pandemic. During the COVID-19
pandemic, the POLRI and TNI were involved in a number of handling efforts,
ranging from ensuring the implementation of large-scale social restrictions
(PSBB), to providing medical personnel, to guarding the country's borders.[24] In
regard to law enforcement, the police would take action related to fake news and
stockpiling of masks and foods.[25]

However, institutions of the government and security forces are also considered to have acted repressively in responding to protests on social media regarding
the handling of COVID-19 in Indonesia. In dealing with fake news or offensive
statement against the government, the police use the Criminal Code (KUHP)
Article 207 (known as "rubber provision"), which means that it could be broadly
interpreted and might tend to weaken human rights protection.[26] In addition, the
government and the parliament or Dewan Perwakilan Rakyat (DPR) were also
considered to have "taking advantage of the situation" with the discussion and
plan to ratify the Omnibus Law on Job Creation Bill, although labors and coalition of civil society had strongly rejected the bill.[27]

Furthermore, public perception of the government's performance in responding to the COVID-19 pandemic was not entirely positive. Based on the result of
the Saiful Mujani Research Consulting (SMRC) survey, the difference between
respondents who considered the government to have acted "fast/very fast" and
those who answered "slow/very slow" was not too far away, namely 52% and
41% with a margin of error of 2.9%.[28]

Politicization of the Virus

The sluggish response from the central government which seems to downplay the seriousness of COVID-19 has in fact made the issue of the pandemic become heavily politicized in Indonesia. Lack of coordination between the central government and local government had opened the way for opposition politicians to have seized the issue to score political gain against the central government.

In response to the pandemic, the tension between Jokowi and the Governor of Daerah Khusus Ibukota (DKI) Jakarta, Anies Baswedan, is evidence of a political battle between the central and local governments. On February 25, prior to the official announcement from the central government, Anies announced an instruction to increase vigilance against the coronavirus. In March, he challenged the central government's data on coronavirus cases and deaths, claiming that the situation in Jakarta was more critical that he planned to lockdown the capital city to slow the spread of the virus. To respond to this, Jokowi used emergency powers to overrule local governments' coronavirus interventions and prevent them from acting independently.[29]

This move signaled that the Governor of DKI Jakarta was more aware of the threat, which considered him a serious political threat to the Jokowi administration and that Anies, and the opposition as a whole, was politicizing the virus. Moreover, many of Jokowi's supporters saw Anies' efforts to tackle the virus as a way to bolster his chance of re-election in 2022 and the presidential election in 2024.

Government Responses towards the COVID-19 Pandemic

Defensive Responses: January–February 2020

The first phase of the government response was marked by ignorance and denial toward the crisis. The government does not seem to have a sense of crisis nor the capacity to respond to the crisis, so it tends to underestimate this disease. Many statements from the government evoked controversy. By the end of January, the Minister of Health of Indonesia, Dr. Terawan Agus Putranto, responded to the COVID-19 virus by saying that, "Prevention of corona virus is to not be panic or worried, just enjoy it, and eat well."[30] On February 7, the Minister disproved Harvard T.H.'s research Chan School of Public Health, which concluded that the coronavirus should already exist in Indonesia, but was not detected.[31] Other statements from the high rank of state officials that downplay the threat of the virus have displayed that the government is defensive in responding to the threat.

Nonetheless, the government had started to increase alertness as the virus began to spread around the world. On January 27, the Ministry of Health installed 195 thermal scanners spread across 135 national entrances and set up 100 referral hospitals to treat patients identified or infected with the coronavirus.[32] Later on, on February 2, the Indonesian government succeeded to evacuate 237 of its nationals and one foreigner living in Wuhan and quarantined them in Natuna for 14 days.[33] In an effort to tighten up security, since last February, the Indonesian government has decided to suspend all flights to and from China, as well as to halt visa waivers for Chinese travelers, to prevent the spread of a highly contagious COVID-19.[34]

STIMULUS PACKAGE

o Stimulate funds distribution via Pre-Working Card (*Kartu Pra Kerja*), which is prioritized in 3 provinces.

o Add incentives for the six-month program of Nine Kinds of Basic Needs Card.

o Add subsidized interest and housing down payment, 175,000 livable new housing units.

o Tourism industry incentives for 10 tourism destinations, discounted flights. The budget for influencers and social media is 72 billion and this allocation raises criticism from various circles.

o Provide stimulus of discounts up to 20% for 3 months for 10 tourism destinations.

o Provide aviation fuel discount for 3 months period.

o Reallocation of Special Allocation Funds (DAK) for infrastructure development in 10 Tourism Destinations.

o Hotel and Restaurant Tax Exemption in 10 Priority Tourism Destinations.

Figure 8.2 The Government's stimulus package. Source: Author.

In facing this public health crisis, the government tends to consider more the economic approach. The government seems to want to keep Indonesia's image safe and stable to convince investors. On February 25, to reduce the impact of COVID-19, the Minister of Finance, Sri Mulyani issued the first stimulus package worth Rp 10.3 trillion to the public and industrial actors particularly to the tourism, airline, and housing sectors (see Figure 8.2). The Minister also admonished that the outbreak in China, Indonesia's top trade partner and a major source of investment and tourists, could further weaken Indonesia's growth to 4.7% in 2020, from 5.02% in 2019.[35] This stimulus package aims to encourage the level of public consumption.

Initial Responses and the Rising Cases in Indonesia: March–April 2020

Since the announcement of the first COVID-19 positive cases in Indonesia on March 2, more firm but slow responses had been established by the government. On March 8, the government banned tourists from Iran, Italy, and South Korea from entering and transit in Indonesia. The policy was considered after a report

Table 8.3 Key Strategic Initial Responses of the Government of Indonesia toward COVID-19 Crisis

Date of Issued	Title of Regulation	Reference
March 13, 2020	Task Force for Rapid Response to COVID-19	Presidential Decree No. 9/2020
March 20, 2020	Refocusing of Activities, Fiscal Allocation, and Procurement of Goods and Services for the Acceleration of COVID-19 Response	President Instruction No. 4/2020
March 31, 2020	National Budgeting Policy and the Stability of Budgeting System for COVID-19 Pandemic Disaster and/or Managing Threats for National Economy and/or the Stability Budgeting System	Government Regulation in Lieu of Law No 1/2020
March 31, 2020	Declaration of Community Health Emergency Situation for COVID-19	President Decree No. 11/2020
March 31, 2020	Social Distancing on a Large Scale (PSBB) in Order to Accelerate the COVID-19 Crisis Management	Government Regulation No. 21/2020

Source: Author, compiled from various sources.

from WHO showed a significant increase in COVID-19 cases outside China, especially in three countries namely Iran, Italy, and South Korea.[36] In enhancing domestic public health infrastructure to deal with COVID-19, the government announced that they had added a number of referral hospitals which makes up to 132 hospitals; however, it is argued that there are only 49 hospitals across the country that is ready.[37] However, these responses are considered insufficient to tackle the threat of COVID-19 until March 10, and then WHO urged President Jokowi to declare a national state of emergency due to COVID-19. Since then, the response of the state had been increasing[38] (Table 8.3).

Indonesian Task Force for Rapid Response to COVID-19

It takes approximately 10 days for the government to form a coordinated response. On March 13, President Jokowi finally announced the formation of the Indonesian Task Force for Rapid Response to COVID-19 led by the head of the National Disaster Management Office or Badan Nasional Penanggulan Bencana (BNPB), General Doni Monardo, and delegated Mr. Achmad Yurianto as the Task Force spokesman. As a leading sector in dealing with the COVID-19 pandemic, this Task Force has the main task to determine, coordinate, and implement the operational plan for the acceleration of handling COVID-19 in Indonesia.[39]

From its establishment until early April, a number of efforts in dealing with COVID-19 have been carried out during the past month as follows[40]: (i) supply of medical equipment for medical workers by distributing 725,000 Personal Protecting Equipment (PPE), 13 million surgical masks, and 150,000 N95 masks; (ii) increase the COVID-19 specimen testing laboratory from three units to 78 units; (iii) increase the capacity building for government-owned hospitals and private sector hospitals. As many as 635 referral hospitals with a capacity of 1,515 isolation rooms were ready for use for severe and critical patients.

Closing Borders

Starting on March 20, 2020, the government has enacted travel restrictions in the form of a temporary ban on all arrivals and transit by foreigners in Indonesia. Free visa and visa-on-arrival (VOA) policies have been suspended for all foreign travelers (following the development of the pandemic). Furthermore, entry into Indonesia is also prohibited to people who have traveled in the last 14 days in the following countries: China, Iran, South Korea, Italy, Vatican, Spain, France, Germany, Switzerland, and UK. Exemption applies to foreigners with both limited and permanent residence permits, diplomatic officials, health workers, medical and food supplies, as well as land, air, and sea transportation crews.[41]

Economic Stimulus for Overcoming COVID-19: The Ultimate Policy?

As of March 31, the number of positive cases of COVID-19 in Indonesia has increased to 1,528 patients with a death toll reaching 136 people. Moreover, positive cases of COVID-19 have been found in 32 provinces. The perception of threats is increasing since Indonesia became the country with the worst COVID-19 mortality ratio in Asia, at 8.9%.

To respond to this situation, on March 31, President Jokowi officially declared the COVID-19 pandemic as a national disaster. He argued that the ongoing pandemic not only causes public health problems but also has broad economic implications so that many countries have to face severe challenges. Along with it, the President signed the Government Regulation in Lieu of Law No 1/2020 concerning National Budgeting Policy and the Stability of Budgeting System for COVID-19 Pandemic Disaster and/or Managing Threats for National Economy and/or the Stability Budgeting System.

This economic stimulus serves as a foundation for the government, banking authorities, and financial authorities to take extraordinary steps in efforts to ensure the public health and save the national economy and financial system stability.[42] The aforementioned stimulus spent over Rp 405.1 trillion from the state financial resources, and the budget would be allocated to several sectors: social security (Rp 110 trillion), the health sector (Rp 75 million), the economic recovery program (Rp 150 trillion), and the tax incentives and stimulus for People's Business Credit/KUR (Rp 701.1 trillion). Then, this would push the country's budget deficit past 5% (the legal threshold is 3%). The President asked the parliament for the relaxation of the deficit cap for the next three years until the end of 2022.[43]

Social security sector received the highest budget allocation around 27% as a way for the government to increase the social safety net. According to officials, it is expected that from 1.89 million to 4.89 million individuals will fall below the poverty line and 3 million to 5.23 million individuals may lose their jobs as the pandemic causes economic activity to a stalemate. This economic stimulus was released to avoid economic recession as COVID-19 hit the informal sector hard.[44]

Increase Numbers of Polymerase Chain Reaction Test

On April 13, President Jokowi instructed the COVID-19 Task Force to conduct specimen testing to detect coronavirus (COVID-19) through the polymerase chain reaction (PCR) method for 10,000 tests per day. Based on data from the Ministry of Health, the government recorded 6,663 PCR tests in the period from December 30 to March 31, while on April 1–30 the government conducted 65,658 tests. That is, the average daily examination increased from the original 204 tests per day in March 2020 to 2,189 tests per day in April 2020. Entering the midst of April, the head of the COVID-19 Task Force reported that they had conducted PCR tests ranging from 6,000 to 7,000 tests per day. The amount was also considered far from the word of massive testing, as announced by the government so far. The inability to reach the target is due to a lack of human resources in the laboratory. Meanwhile, there are still 51 referral labs from a total of 104 labs that have not been able to conduct PCR tests.[45]

Import Medical Supplies

One of the major obstacles to tackling the COVID-19 outbreak is the lack of medical equipment and public health infrastructure. Thus, Indonesia is still highly dependent on importing raw materials and medical supplies from other countries, mainly from China, accounted for 63.17% of the total value.

Indonesia has spent Rp 777.59 billion, or $50 million, on imported medical supplies since the COVID-19 outbreak began in March. The outbreak-related imports are dominated by face masks, which have totaled up to 17.1 million units. Other medical supplies being imported included 3.26 million COVID-19 testing kits, over 390,000 packs of medicine, 1.49 million hospital equipment, and 1.95 million units of PPE which included gowns, gloves, and visors.[46]

Mixed Responses: April–May 2020
Large-Scale Social Restrictions to Accelerate the Handling of COVID-19

As the COVID-19 positive cases continue to spread outside Jakarta, which is the epicenter of the pandemic in Indonesia, the government received more pressure from more local governments to implement a lockdown in their region, particularly in the capital city. However, the upheaval argument was halted when the government finally issued the government regulation concerning the implementation of large-scale social restrictions on March 31.

The President emphasized that with this regulation, local governments will no longer make their own uncoordinated rules. According to him, the lockdown option is not feasible to be implemented due to several considerations. First, locking down Jakarta will not stop the spread of the virus as it has already existed in the surrounding areas of Jakarta and even other provinces. Second, there is the need for an adequate supply of staple food. Mr. Doni Monardo acknowledged that the government did not have the capacity to impose a lockdown due to the lack of government resources to meet the basic needs of its 270 million citizens during sustained economic inactivity.[47] Third, a lockdown policy would stop business and working activities, which would bring enormous negative economic consequences.

Derived on those considerations, the most suitable policy to be applied in Indonesia is to maintain physical distance between individuals. The implementation of large-scale social restrictions includes: (i) restrictions on school and work activities (studying and working from home); (ii) restrictions on religious activities (worshiping from home); (iii) restrictions on activities in public places or facilities; (iv) restrictions on social and cultural activities; (v) restrictions on modes of transportation and restrictions on other activities specifically related to defense and security aspects.

This requires a strong community discipline to prevent further transmission of the virus. There are various types of sanctions for the violation of the policy, ranging from social sanctions to imprisonment. Moreover, this policy could also be used by the National Police for prevention measures and law enforcement measures in accordance with the Law so that the PSBB could be implemented effectively.[48]

A month after the announcement, there are 18 regions that implement PSBB with the approval of the Minister of Health of Indonesia. The first province to implement the PSBB is DKI Jakarta, which is from April 10, 2020, followed by other regions surrounding Jakarta.[49]

It should be taken into account that since the implementation of PSBB in several regions, especially in Greater Jakarta, the addition of COVID-19 positive cases remains to continue. In other words, the implementation of PSBB is less effective enough in handling the COVID-19 crisis because Indonesia has not been able to record a downward trend in the number of positive cases in the first two months of the policy implementation.

There are mainly two reasons why PSBB did not bring significant change to cut down COVID-19 positive cases in Indonesia. First, there is a low level of public compliance in practicing physical distancing and in following health protocols established by the government. From March 19–May 19, the police reported that they dismissed 707,578 crowds in a number of areas that violated the provisions of PSBB.[50] Second, there are delays in determining the number of strategic policies by the government. For example, the implementation of PSBB that is not conducted simultaneously had made law enforcement to become more difficult due to the absence of coordinated policy.[51]

Mudik (Homecoming Tradition)

On April 21, President Jokowi announced a regulation that banned citizens from participating in the exodus tradition celebrated during the Islamic holiday Idul-Fitri and banned most commercial travel. The ban would be applied starting from April 24 to May 31 and that the enforcement of sanctions would start on May 7. This decision was in an effort to prevent COVID-19 from spreading further. There are at least three main considerations of why the government finally issued this policy: to prevent the spread of close contact, to isolate the red zone, and to terminate the risk of transmission between humans.

However, this prevention is perceived as premature and too late since millions of people have made their journey going back home. The wave of *mudik* actually started in the first case of the corona pandemic in Indonesia (March 1–5, 2020) and increased sharply when the government issued the PSBB policy on March 16–20, 2020. Jokowi announced that since the end of March, 976 buses had carried approximately 14,000 passengers to many regions: the number has not even taken into account travelers who use private or other public transportation.[52] Based on the data from the Ministry of Health, it is shown that as of May 5, there were already 79 districts/cities that reported cases of local transmission.[53]

Indonesia and the "New Normal"

The COVID-19 pandemic that forces people to stay at home makes the economy slow down. Thus, the government came up with an idea to implement "the new normal." It aims to drive the wheels of the economy that was stagnant during the period of PSBB reflected on the national economic growth in the first quarter of 2020, which only recorded 2.97%. To save the economy, the Coordinating Ministry for Economic Affairs has arranged the opening stages or phases of business and industrial activities in the midst of the COVID-19 pandemic.[54]

On May 27, President Jokowi announced that Indonesia must remain productive but also safe to survive the pandemic. He emphasized in this difficult time, "people should be living coexist with COVID-19." In addition, the new normal socialization program was instructed to be carried out on a large scale.[55] Public is expected to continue to improve discipline in implementing health protocols before entering the new normal lifestyle that is washing hands regularly with soap, wearing a mask when leaving the house, keeping a safe distance, and avoiding crowds.

The following is a preliminary study of economic recovery that will be carried out by Indonesia in stages[56] (Table 8.4).

To maximize the enforcement, TNI and POLRI will be involved in ensuring social discipline. These two agencies will encourage the mechanism of health protocol procedures that could be carried out by communities throughout Indonesia along with cooperation with local governments, community leaders and non-governmental organizations, the central/regional Task Force, and the media.

Table 8.4 Preparation for the New Normal

Phase 1 (June 1, 2020)	Industries and services can start to operate with the COVID-19 health protocol
Phase 2 (June 8, 2020)	Markets and malls are allowed to open following health protocols
Phase 3 (June 15, 2020)	Mall operates like the second phase but will be evaluated for the opening of the salon, spa, and others
Phase 4 (July 6, 2020)	Restaurants, cafes, bars, and others are allowed to open gradually with strict hygiene protocols
Phase 5 (July 20, 2020, and July 27, 2020)	The opening of PSBB with the expectation that by early August, all activities would proceed as usual before the pandemic

Source: Author.

Conclusion

The impact of the COVID-19 pandemic is inevitable in every country, including Indonesia. From the initial cases in March 2020, this pandemic has caused the country to undergo double crises: public health crisis and economic crisis. It hit all sectors of life such as the economic, social, political, and security of the country. However, the rising threat brought by the COVID-19 virus is not proportionally responded to by the government of Indonesia proved by sluggish and uncoordinated policies.

Indonesia's past experiences in dealing with outbreaks do not serve as a solid foundation to deal with the current pandemic. COVID-19 is the first human-to-human transmission that ever happened in the country. The complex interests in domestic politics also contributed to the uncertainty of how the country would deal with the virus.

The pandemic has also resulted in a multidimensional threat to the country. Due to the pandemic, Indonesia is experiencing an economic blowback due to the decline in the tourism sector, loss of many MSME's businesses, and millions of workers getting layoffs. The informal sectors and low-income workers are the most affected by this pandemic. In politics and security, the unpreparedness of the government has caused major uncoordinated policy which could be an opportunity to delegitimize the government.

The responses of the government toward the COVID-19 pandemic can be understood from three periodical categories: defensive response, initial responses, and mixed responses. In the early time of the pandemic, the government seems to downplay the threat of COVID-19 and prioritizes its policy on how to save the country's economy. Furthermore, the government became more alert when Indonesia announced its first cases on March 2, followed by a more responsive policy such as the formation of the COVID-19 Task Force, improvement in public health infrastructure, and economic stimulus to ensure the survival of the country. Entering the second month of the crises, the government appears to issue more agile and compelling policies such as the implementation of large-scale social restrictions (PSBB) and the country's preparation to enter the "new normal."

Indeed, the magnitude of crises of the COVID-19 pandemic has accentuated the need for strong and relevant policy during the time of crises to ensure the survival of the country and importantly its people. In regard to policy formulation, the government should not only focus on using an economic approach but also involve multidisciplinary advice from public health researchers, social scientists, and related parties to create a more comprehensive policy. Further, it should be taken into account the importance of effective crisis communication to support the policy formulation process. This pandemic has shown how poor Indonesia's public health infrastructure is. Therefore, the government should increase its investment in the health sector as well. As the COVID-19 pandemic is recognized as a humanitarian crisis, the government should prioritize using a persuasive approach rather than a coercive approach to prevent the escalation of the crisis into a political crisis.

Notes

1 2020. 'Coronavirus (COVID-19)'. World Health Organization. Retrieved on 6 May 2020 from https://covid19.who.int/.
2 2020. 'COVID-19 Coronavirus Pandemic'. Worldometers. Retrieved on 6 May 2020 from https://www.worldometers.info/coronavirus/?utm_campaign =homeAdvegas1?
3 2020. 'Jumlah Kunjungan Wisatawan Mancanegara per Bulan ke Indonesia Menurut Pintu Masuk, 2017–2020'. Badan Pusat Statistik. Retrieved on 5 May 2020 from https://www.bps.go.id/dynamictable/2018/04/05/1296/jum-lah-kunjungan-wisatawan-mancanegara-per-bulan-ke-indonesia-menurut-pintu -masuk-2017-2020.html.
4 Adrian Wail Akhlas. 2020. 'IMF Projects 0.5% Growth for Indonesia as Global Economy Faces Deep Recession'. The Jakarta Post. Retrieved on 6 May 2020 from https://www.thejakartapost.com/news/2020/04/14/imf-projects-0-5 -growth-for-indonesia-as-global-economy-faces-deep-recession.html.
5 2020. 'COVID-19, MERS & SARS.' National Institute of Allergy and Infectious Diseases. Retrieved on 1 May 2020 from https://www.niaid.nih.gov/diseases -conditions/COVID-19.
6 2003. 'Severe Acute Respiratory Syndrome (SARS)-Multi-Country Outbreak – Update'. World Health Organization. Retrieved on 1 May 2020 from https:// www.who.int/csr/don/2003_03_16/en/.
7 World Health Organization. 2012. H5N1 Avian Influenza: Timeline of Major Events. World Health Organization. Retrieved on 1 May 2020 from https:// www.who.int/influenza/human_animal_interface/H5N1_avian_influenza_ update.pdf.
8 World Health Organization. 2020. Cumulative Number of Confirmed Human Cases for Avian Influenza A (H5N1) Reported to WHO, 2003–2020. World Health Organization. Retrieved on 1 May 2020 from https://www.who.int/ influenza/human_animal_interface/2020_01_20_tableH5N1.pdf?ua=1.

9 Celia Lowe. 2010. 'Preparing Indonesia: H5N1 Influenza through the Lens of Global Health'. Indonesia, (90), 147–170. Retrieved on 5 June 2020, from www .jstor.org/stable/20798236.

10 Purnawan Junadi. 2009. Pandemic Preparedness Operations, Systems and Networks: The Indonesian Case. RSIS Monograph: Pandemic Preparedness in Asia, 16, pp. 27–34.

11 Steven Sanche, Yen Ting Lin, Chonggang Xu, Ethan Romero-Severson, Nick Hengartner, and Ruian Ke. 2020. 'High Contagiousness and Rapid Spread of Severe Acute Respiratory Syndrome Coronavirus 2.' Emerging Infectious Disease, 26 (7). Retrieved on 20 May 2020 from https://pubmed.ncbi.nlm.nih .gov/32255761/.

12 2020. 'Tren Pertumbuhan Kasus Positif Corona di Indonesia Turun, Ini Data Lengkapnya'. Kumparan.com. Retrieved on 12 May 2020 from https://kump-aran.com/kumparannews/tren-pertumbuhan-kasus-positif-corona-di-indonesia -turun-ini-data-lengkapnya-1tK77tXbaiP/full.

13 Steven Sanche, Yen Ting Lin, Chonggang Xu, Ethan Romero-Severson, Nick Hengartner, and Ruian Ke. 2020. 'High Contagiousness and Rapid Spread of Severe Acute Respiratory Syndrome Coronavirus 2.' Emerging Infectious Disease, 26 (7). Retrieved on 20 May 2020 from https://pubmed.ncbi.nlm.nih .gov/32255761/.

14 Margareth S. Aritonang. 2020. 'In COVID-19 Response, Can Jokowi Avoid Military 'Star Wars'?'. The Jakarta Post. Retrieved on 15 May 2020 from https:// www.thejakartapost.com/news/2020/03/26/in-COVID-19-response-can -jokowi-avoid-military-star-wars.html.

15 Retia Kartika Dewi. 2020. 'Gugus Tugas Luncurkan Covid19.go.id, Apa Saja Isinya?'. Kompas.com. Retrieved on 15 May 2020 from https://www.kompas .com/tren/read/2020/03/18/130530565/gugus-tugas-luncurkan-covid- 19goid-apa-saja-isinya.

16 Riza Roidila Mufti, and Marchio Irfan Gorbiano. 2020. 'Indonesia Offers Big Discounts to Attract Foreign Tourists amid Cancellations'. The Jakarta Post. Retrieved on 15 May 2020 from https://www.thejakartapost.com/news/2020 /02/19/indonesia-offers-big-discounts-to-attract-foreign-tourists-amid-cancel- lations.html.

17 Badan Pusat Statistik. 2020. 'Ekspor April 2020 Mencapai US$12,19 Miliar dan Impor April 2020 sebesar US$12,54 Miliar'. Badan Pusat Statistik. Retrieved on 20 May 2020 from https://www.bps.go.id/pressrelease/2020/05/15/1678/ ekspor-april-2020-mencapai-us-12-19-miliar-dan-impor-april-2020-sebesar-us -12-54-miliar.html.

18 Faidah Umu Sofuroh. 2020. 'Data Kemnaker: Pekerja Terdampak COVID- 19 Capai Sekitar 3 Juta Orang'. detikfinance. Retrieved on 20 May 2020 from https://finance.detik.com/berita-ekonomi-bisnis/d-5009421/data-kemnaker -pekerja-terdampak-COVID-19-capai-sekitar-3-juta-orang.

19 Dwi Hadya Jayani. 2020. 'Wabah PHK Akibat COVID-19. April 18'. Katadata .co.id. Retrieved on 20 May 2020 from https://katadata.co.id/infografik/2020 /04/18/wabah-phk-akibat-COVID-19.

20 Moch. Fiqih Prawira Adjie. 2020. 'Jokowi Declares COVID-19 'National Disaster', Gives Task Force Broader Authority'. The Jakarta Post. Retrieved on 20 May 2020 from https://www.thejakartapost.com/news/2020/04/14/ jokowi-declares-COVID-19-national-disaster-gives-task-force-broader-authority .html.

21 The traditional mass migration of Indonesia's Muslims back to their home villages during the upcoming holy month of Ramadhan.

22 Muhammad Choirul Anwar. 2020. 'Mulai Besok, Semua Moda Transportasi Boleh Operasi Lagi'. CNBC Indonesia. Retrieved on 20 May 2020 from https://www.cnbcindonesia.com/news/20200506102523-4-156619/mulai-besok-semua-moda-transportasi-boleh-operasi-lagi.

23 Yuliawati. 2020. 'Survei KIC: Pemudik Akan Didominasi Kaum Muda Berpendapatan Rendah'. Katadata.co.id. Retrieved on 20 May 2020 from https://katadata.co.id/berita/2020/04/20/survei-kic-pemudik-akan-didominasi-kaum-muda-berpendapatan-rendah.

24 Haryanti Puspa Sari. 2020. 'Upaya-upaya TNI dalam Penanganan Pandemi COVID-19'. KOMPAS.com. Retrieved on 20 May 2020. https://nasional.kompas.com/read/2020/04/16/06102901/upaya-upaya-tni-dalam-penanganan-pandemi-COVID-19.

25 Devina Halim. 2020. 'Tugas Polri dalam Penanganan COVID-19: Imbau Warga Jaga Jarak hingga Tindak Penimbun Sembako'. Kompas.com. Retrieved on 20 May 2020 from https://nasional.kompas.com/read/2020/03/20/23012531/tugas-polri-dalam-penanganan-COVID-19-imbau-warga-jaga-jarak-hingga-tindak.

26 Tangguh Chairil. 2020. 'Indonesia Needs to Change Its Security-Heavy Approach to COVID-19'. The Diplomat. Retrieved on 20 May 2020 from https://thediplomat.com/2020/04/indonesia-needs-to-change-its-security-heavy-approach-to-COVID-19/.

27 Muhamad Haripin. 2020. 'Dampak Politik-Keamanan COVID-19'. Pusat Penelitian Politik LIPI. Retrieved on 20 May 2020 from http://www.politik.lipi.go.id/kolom/kolom-2/politik-nasional/1383-dampak-politik-keamanan-COVID-19.

28 2020. 'Mayoritas Warga Anggap COVID-19 Ancam Penghasilan'. Saiful Mujani Research & Consulting. Retrieved on 20 May 2020 from https://saifulmujani.com/mayoritas-warga-anggap-COVID-19-ancam-penghasilan/.

29 Eve Warburton. 2020. 'Indonesia: Polarization, Democratic Distress, and the Coronavirus'. Carnegie Endowment for International Peace. Retrieved on 20 May 2020 from https://carnegieendowment.org/2020/04/28/indonesia-polarization-democratic-distress-and-coronavirus-pub-81641.

30 2020. 'Virus Corona Makin Ganas, Menkes Bilang: Enjoy Aja!'. Warta Ekonomi.co.id. Retrieved on 25 May 2020 from https://www.wartaekonomi.co.id/read268664/virus-corona-makin-ganas-menkes-bilang-enjoy-aja.

31 2020. 'Menkes Tantang Harvard Buktikan Virus Corona di Indonesia'. CNN Indonesia. Retrieved on 25 May 2020 from https://www.cnnindonesia.com/nasional/20200211195637-20-473740/menkes-tantang-harvard-buktikan-virus-corona-di-indonesia.

32 Reza Gunadha. 2020. '5 Cara Indonesia Selamatkan Warganya dari Ancaman Virus Corona'. Suara.com. Retrieved on 25 May 2020 from https://www.suara.com/news/2020/02/01/163313/5-cara-indonesia-selamatkan-warganya-dari-ancaman-virus-corona.

33 2020. 'Policies by the Indonesian Government Related to the Corona Virus (COVID-19) Pandemic'. Ministry of the Foreign Affairs of the Republic of Indonesia. Retrieved on 25 May 2020 from https://kemlu.go.id/brussels/en/news/6349/policies-by-the-indonesian-government-related-to-the-coronavirus-COVID-19-pandemic.

34 A. Muh. Ibnu Aqil, Apriza Pinandita and Fadli. 2020. 'Indonesia Closes Doors to Travelers from China'. The Jakarta Post. Retrieved on 25 May 2020 from https://www.thejakartapost.com/news/2020/02/03/indonesia-closes-doors-to-travelers-from-china.html.

35 2020. 'Indonesia Unveils Nearly $750 Mln Stimulus Package in Response to Virus Outbreak'. Reuters. Retrieved on 25 May 2020 from https://www.reuters

.com/article/indonesia-economy/indonesia-unveils-nearly-750-mln-stimulus
-package-in-response-to-virus-outbreak-idUSJ9N29001A.

36 Ratna Iskana. 2020. 'Cegah Corona, Kemenlu Larang Pendatang dari Iran, Italia, dan Korsel'. Katadata.co.id. Retrieved on 25 May 2020 from https://katadata .co.id/berita/2020/03/05/cegah-corona-kemenlu-larang-pendatang-dari-iran -italia-dan-korsel.

37 Gemma Holliani Cahya. 2020. 'Indonesia Scrambles to Contain Coronavirus as Most Hospitals not Ready'. The Jakarta Post. Retrieved on 25 May 2020 from https://www.thejakartapost.com/news/2020/03/13/indonesia-scrambles-to -contain-coronavirus-as-most-hospitals-not-ready.html.

38 2020. 'COVID-19: WHO Urges Jokowi to Declare National Emergency'. The Jakarta Post. Retrieved on 27 May 2020 from https://www.thejakartapost.com /news/2020/03/14/COVID-19-who-urges-jokowi-to-declare-national-emer-gency.html.

39 Lenny Tristia Tambun. 2020. 'Ini Tugas Gugus Tugas Percepatan Penanganan COVID-19'. Berita Satu. Retrieved on 17 May 2020 from https://www.beritasatu .com/kesehatan/608687-ini-tugas-gugus-tugas-percepatan-penanganan-covid19.

40 Deti Mega Purnamasari. 2020. 'Laporan Lengkap Gugus Tugas COVID-19 Setelah Sebulan Bekerja'. Kompas.com. Retrieved on 27 May 2020 from https:// nasional.kompas.com/read/2020/04/15/11455191/laporan-lengkap-gugus -tugas-COVID-19-setelah-sebulan-bekerja?page=1.

41 2020. 'Additional Measures of The Indonesian Government in Relation to COVID-19 Response'. Ministry of the Foreign Affairs of the Republic of Indonesia. Retrieved on 27 May 2020 from https://kemlu.go.id/portal/en/ read/1135/siaran_pers/additional-measures-of-the-indonesian-government-in -relation-to-COVID-19-response.

42 Addi M Idhom. 2020. 'Daftar Kebijakan Jokowi Tangani Pandemi Corona dan Isi Perppu Baru'. Tirto.ID. Retrieved on 27 May 2020 from https://tirto.id/ daftar-kebijakan-jokowi-tangani-pandemi-corona-dan-isi-perppu-baru-eJYX.

43 Olisias Gultom. 2020. 'Indonesia in the COVID-19 Vortex'. Indonesia for Global Justice. Retrieved on 27 May 2020 from http://igj.or.id/indonesia-in -the-COVID-19-vortex/?lang=en.

44 Adrian Wail Akhlas. 2020. 'Govt Rolls Out $43b Stimulus in Bid to Rescue Economy'. The Jakarta Post. Retrieved on 27 May 2020 from https://www .thejakartapost.com/news/2020/05/18/govt-rolls-out-43b-stimulus-in-bid-to -rescue-economy.html.

45 Andrian Pratama Taher. 2020. 2020. 'Jokowi Minta Alat PCR, Tes Cepat dan Ventilator Segera Diproduksi'. Tirto.ID. Retrieved on 27 May 2020 from https://tirto.id/jokowi-minta-alat-pcr-tes-cepat-dan-ventilator-segera-diprod-uksi-fqie.

46 Lona Olavia, and Heru Andriyanto. 2020. 'Indonesia Imports $50m Worth of Medical Supplies as Coronavirus Cases Show No Sign of Slowing'. Jakarta Globe. Retrieved on 27 May 2020 from https://jakartaglobe.id/news/indone-sia-imports-50m-worth-of-medical-supplies-as-coronavirus-cases-show-no-sign -of-slowing.

47 Jeffrey Neilson. 2020. 'Without Social Safety Nets, Indonesia Risks Political Instability over COVID-19'. New Mandala. Retrieved on 27 May 2020 from https://www.newmandala.org/indonesia-risks-political-instability-over -COVID-19/.

48 2020. 'PSBB Keluar, Presiden Jokowi Minta Pemerintah Daerah Tak Buat Kebijakan Sendiri'. Kompas TV. Retrieved on 27 May 2020 from https://www .kompas.tv/article/73946/psbb-keluar-presiden-jokowi-minta-pemerintah-dae-rah-tak-buat-kebijakan-sendiri.

49 Sania Mashabi. 2020. 'Daftar 18 Daerah yang Terapkan PSBB, dari Jakarta hingga Makassar'. Kompas.com. Retrieved on 27 May 2020 from https://nasional.kompas.com/read/2020/04/20/05534481/daftar-18-daerah-yang-terapkan-psbb-dari-jakarta-hingga-makassar?page=1.

50 2020. 'Polisi Bubarkan 707.578 Kerumunan Massa yang Langgar PSBB '. CNN Indonesia. Retrieved on 30 May 2020 from https://www.cnnindonesia.com/nasional/20200521002024-12-505523/polisi-bubarkan-707578-kerumunan-massa-yang-langgar-psbb.

51 2020. '2 Bulan Jokowi Lawan Corona dan Kurva yang Belum 'Selaw''. CNN Indonesia. Retrieved on 27 May 2020 from https://www.cnnindonesia.com/nasional/20200502154031-20-499418/2-bulan-jokowi-lawan-corona-dan-kurva-yang-belum-selaw.

52 Yuliawati. 2020. 'Survei KIC: Pemudik Akan Didominasi Kaum Muda Berpendapatan Rendah'. Katadata.co.id. Retrieved on 20 May 2020 from https://katadata.co.id/berita/2020/04/20/survei-kic-pemudik-akan-didominasi-kaum-muda-berpendapatan-rendah.

53 2020. 'Situasi Terkini Perkembangan Coronavirus Disease (COVID-19) 6 Mei 2020'. Ministry of Health of the Republic of Indonesia. Retrieved on 27 May 2020 from https://covid19.kemkes.go.id/situasi-infeksi-emerging/info-corona-virus/situasi-terkini-perkembangan-coronavirus-disease-COVID-19-6-mei-2020/#.XtinOC2B1Z0.

54 2020. 'Mulai 1 Juni, Ini Skenario Tahapan New Normal untuk Pemulihan Ekonomi'. Kompas.com. Retrieved on 30 May 2020 from https://money.kompas.com/read/2020/05/26/073708726/mulai-1-juni-ini-skenario-tahapan-new-normal-untuk-pemulihan-ekonomi?page=all.

55 2020. 'Indonesia Menuju New Normal Corona, Ini Protokol Kesehatan COVID-19 yang Harus Dilakukan'. Kompas.com. Retrieved on 30 May 2020 from https://www.kompas.com/sains/read/2020/05/27/163200923/indonesia-menuju-new-normal-corona-ini-protokol-kesehatan-COVID-19-yang?page=1.

56 Muhammad Ahsan Ridhoi. 2020. 'Riuh Skenario New Normal Ekonomi Indonesia Saat Pandemi Belum Reda'. Katadata.co.id. Retrieved on 30 May 2020 from https://katadata.co.id/telaah/2020/05/28/riuh-skenario-new-normal-ekonomi-indonesia-saat-pandemi-belum-reda.

References

Adjie, Moch. Fiqih Prawira. 2020. 'Jokowi Declares COVID-19 'National Disaster', Gives Task Force Broader Authority'. *The Jakarta Post*. Retrieved on 20 May 2020 from https://www.thejakartapost.com/news/2020/04/14/jokowi-declares-COVID-19-national-disaster-gives-task-force-broader-authority.html.

Akhlas, Adrian Wail. 2020a. 'Govt Rolls Out $43b Stimulus in Bid to Rescue Economy'. *The Jakarta Post*. Retrieved on 27 May 2020 from https://www.thejakartapost.com/news/2020/05/18/govt-rolls-out-43b-stimulus-in-bid-to-rescue-economy.html.

Akhlas, Adrian Wail. 2020b. 'IMF Projects 0.5% Growth for Indonesia as Global Economy Faces Deep Recession'. *The Jakarta Post*. Retrieved on 6 May 2020 from https://www.thejakartapost.com/news/2020/04/14/imf-projects-0-5-growth-for-indonesia-as-global-economy-faces-deep-recession.html.

Anwar, Muhammad Choirul. 2020. 'Mulai Besok, Semua Moda Transportasi Boleh Operasi Lagi'. *CNBC Indonesia*. Retrieved on 20 May 2020 from https://www

.cnbcindonesia.com/news/20200506102523-4-156619/mulai-besok-semua
-moda-transportasi-boleh-operasi-lagi.

Aqil, A. Muh. Ibnu, Apriza Pinandita and Fadli. 2020. 'Indonesia Closes Doors to Travelers from China'. *The Jakarta Post*. Retrieved on 25 May 2020 from https://www.thejakartapost.com/news/2020/02/03/indonesia-closes-doors
-to-travelers-from-china.html.

Aritonang, Margareth S. 2020. 'In COVID-19 Response, Can Jokowi Avoid Military "Star Wars"?' *The Jakarta Post*. Retrieved on 15 May 2020 from https://www
.thejakartapost.com/news/2020/03/26/in-COVID-19-response-can-jokowi
-avoid-military-star-wars.html.

Badan Pusat Statistik. 2020a. 'Ekspor April 2020 Mencapai US$12,19 Miliar dan Impor April 2020 sebesar US$12,54 Miliar'. Badan Pusat Statistik. Retrieved on 20 May 2020 from https://www.bps.go.id/pressrelease/2020/05/15/1678
/ekspor-april-2020-mencapai-us-12-19-miliar-dan-impor-april-2020-sebesar-us
-12-54-miliar.html.

Badan Pusat Statistik. 2020b. 'Jumlah Kunjungan Wisatawan Mancanegara per Bulan ke Indonesia Menurut Pintu Masuk, 2017–2020'. Retrieved on 5 May 2020 from https://www.bps.go.id/dynamictable/2018/04/05/1296/jumlah-kunjungan
-wisatawan-mancanegara-per-bulan-ke-indonesia-menurut-pintu-masuk-2017
-2020.html.

Cahya, Gemma Holliani. 2020. 'Indonesia Scrambles to Contain Coronavirus as Most Hospitals not Ready'. *The Jakarta Post*. Retrieved on 25 May 2020 from https://www.thejakartapost.com/news/2020/03/13/indonesia-scrambles-to
-contain-coronavirus-as-most-hospitals-not-ready.html.

Chairil, Tangguh. 2020. 'Indonesia Needs to Change Its Security-Heavy Approach to COVID-19'. *The Diplomat*. Retrieved on 20 May 2020 from https://thediplomat
.com/2020/04/indonesia-needs-to-change-its-security-heavy-approach-to
-COVID-19/.

CNN Indonesia. 2020a. '2 Bulan Jokowi Lawan Corona dan Kurva yang Belum "Selaw"'. Retrieved on 27 May 2020 from https://www.cnnindonesia.com
/nasional/20200502154031-20-499418/2-bulan-jokowi-lawan-corona-dan
-kurva-yang-belum-selaw.

CNN Indonesia. 2020b. 'Menkes Tantang Harvard Buktikan Virus Corona di Indonesia'. Retrieved on 25 May 2020 from https://www.cnnindonesia.com/
nasional/20200211195637-20-473740/menkes-tantang-harvard-buktikan-virus
-corona-di-indonesia.

CNN Indonesia. 2020c. 'Polisi Bubarkan 707,578 Kerumunan Massa yang Langgar PSBB'. Retrieved on 30 May 2020 from https://www.cnnindonesia.com/
nasional/20200521002024-12-505523/polisi-bubarkan-707578-kerumunan
-massa-yang-langgar-psbb.

Dewi, Retia Kartika. 2020. 'Gugus Tugas Luncurkan Covid19.go.id, Apa Saja Isinya?' *Kompas.com*. Retrieved on 15 May 2020 from https://www.kompas.com/tren/
read/2020/03/18/130530565/gugus-tugas-luncurkan-covid19goid-apa-saja
-isinya.

Gultom, Olisias. 2020. 'Indonesia in the COVID-19 Vortex'. *Indonesia for Global Justice*. Retrieved on 27 May 2020 from http://igj.or.id/indonesia-in-the
-COVID-19-vortex/?lang=en.

Gunadha, Reza. 2020. '5 Cara Indonesia Selamatkan Warganya dari Ancaman Virus Corona'. *Suara.com*. Retrieved on 25 May 2020 from https://www.suara.com

/news/2020/02/01/163313/5-cara-indonesia-selamatkan-warganya-dari
-ancaman-virus-corona.

Halim, Devina. 2020. 'Tugas Polri dalam Penanganan COVID-19: Imbau Warga
Jaga Jarak hingga Tindak Penimbun Sembako'. *Kompas.com*. Retrieved on 20 May
2020 from https://nasional.kompas.com/read/2020/03/20/23012531/tugas
-polri-dalam-penanganan-COVID-19-imbau-warga-jaga-jarak-hingga-tindak.

Haripin, Muhamad. 2020. 'Dampak Politik-Keamanan COVID-19'. *Pusat Penelitian
Politik LIPI*. Retrieved on 20 May 2020 from http://www.politik.lipi.go.id/
kolom/kolom-2/politik-nasional/1383-dampak-politik-keamanan-COVID-19.

Idhom, Addi M. 2020. 'Daftar Kebijakan Jokowi Tangani Pandemi Corona dan Isi
Perppu Baru'. *Tirto.ID*. Retrieved on 27 May 2020 from https://tirto.id/daftar
-kebijakan-jokowi-tangani-pandemi-corona-dan-isi-perppu-baru-eJYX.

Iskana, Ratna. 2020. 'Cegah Corona, Kemenlu Larang Pendatang dari Iran, Italia,
dan Korsel'. *Katadata.co.id*. Retrieved on 25 May 2020 from https://katadata
.co.id/berita/2020/03/05/cegah-corona-kemenlu-larang-pendatang-dari-iran
-italia-dan-korsel.

Jayani, Dwi Hadya. 2020. 'Wabah PHK Akibat COVID-19. April 18'. *Katadata.co
.id*. Retrieved on 20 May 2020 from https://katadata.co.id/infografik/2020/04
/18/wabah-phk-akibat-COVID-19.

Junadi, P. 2009. 'Pandemic Preparedness Operations, Systems and Networks: The
Indonesian Case'. RSIS Monograph: Pandemic Preparedness in Asia, 16, pp.
27–34.

Kompas. 2020. 'Indonesia Menuju New Normal Corona, Ini Protokol Kesehatan
COVID-19 yang Harus Dilakukan'. *Kompas.com*. Retrieved on 30 May 2020 from
https://www.kompas.com/sains/read/2020/05/27/163200923/indonesia
-menuju-new-normal-corona-ini-protokol-kesehatan-COVID-19-yang?page=1.

Kompas TV. 2020. 'PSBB Keluar, Presiden Jokowi Minta Pemerintah Daerah Tak
Buat Kebijakan Sendiri'. Retrieved on 27 May 2020 from https://www.kompas.tv
/article/73946/psbb-keluar-presiden-jokowi-minta-pemerintah-daerah-tak-buat
-kebijakan-sendiri.

Kompas.com. 2020. 'Mulai 1 Juni, Ini Skenario Tahapan New Normal untuk
Pemulihan Ekonomi'. Retrieved on 30 May 2020 from https://money.kompas
.com/read/2020/05/26/073708726/mulai-1-juni-ini-skenario-tahapan-new
-normal-untuk-pemulihan-ekonomi?page=all.

Kumparan.com. 2020. 'Tren Pertumbuhan Kasus Positif Corona di Indonesia Turun,
Ini Data Lengkapnya'. Retrieved on 12 May 2020 from https://kumparan.com
/kumparannews/tren-pertumbuhan-kasus-positif-corona-di-indonesia-turun-ini
-data-lengkapnya-1tK77tXbaiP/full.

Lowe, C. 2010. 'Preparing Indonesia: H5N1 Influenza through the Lens of Global
Health'. *Indonesia*, 90, 147–170. Retrieved on 5 June 2020, from www.jstor.org
/stable/20798236.

Mashabi, Sania. 2020. 'Daftar 18 Daerah yang Terapkan PSBB, dari Jakarta hingga
Makassar'. *Kompas.com*. Retrieved on 27 May 2020 from https://nasional.kompas
.com/read/2020/04/20/05534481/daftar-18-daerah-yang-terapkan-psbb-dari
-jakarta-hingga-makassar?page=1.

Ministry of Health of the Republic of Indonesia. 2020. 'Situasi Terkini Perkembangan
Coronavirus Disease (COVID-19) 6 Mei 2020'. Retrieved on 27 May 2020
from   https://covid19.kemkes.go.id/situasi-infeksi-emerging/info-corona-virus

/situasi-terkini-perkembangan-coronavirus-disease-COVID-19-6-mei-2020/#
.XtinOC2B1Z0.

MOFA. 2020a. 'Additional Measures of The Indonesian Government in Relation to COVID-19 Response'. Ministry of the Foreign Affairs of the Republic of Indonesia. Retrieved on 27 May 2020 from https://kemlu.go.id/portal/en/read/1135/siaran_pers/additional-measures-of-the-indonesian-government-in-relation-to-COVID-19-response.

MOFA. 2020b. 'Policies by the Indonesian Government Related to the Corona Virus (COVID-19) Pandemic'. Ministry of the Foreign Affairs of the Republic of Indonesia. Retrieved on 25 May 2020 from https://kemlu.go.id/brussels/en/news/6349/policies-by-the-indonesian-government-related-to-the-coronavirus-COVID-19-pandemic.

Mufti, Riza Roidila and Marchio Irfan Gorbiano. 2020. 'Indonesia Offers Big Discounts to Attract Foreign Tourists amid Cancellations'. *The Jakarta Post*. Retrieved on 15 May 2020 from https://www.thejakartapost.com/news/2020/02/19/indonesia-offers-big-discounts-to-attract-foreign-tourists-amid-cancellations.html.

National Institute of Allergy and Infectious Diseases. 2020. 'COVID-19, MERS & SARS.' Retrieved on 1 May 2020 from https://www.niaid.nih.gov/diseases-conditions/COVID-19.

Neilson, Jeffrey. 2020. 'Without Social Safety Nets, Indonesia Risks Political Instability over COVID-19'. *New Mandala*. Retrieved on 27 May 2020 from https://www.newmandala.org/indonesia-risks-political-instability-over-COVID-19/.

Olavia, Lona and Heru Andriyanto. 2020. 'Indonesia Imports $50m Worth of Medical Supplies as Coronavirus Cases Show No Sign of Slowing'. *Jakarta Globe*. Retrieved on 27 May 2020 from https://jakartaglobe.id/news/indonesia-imports-50m-worth-of-medical-supplies-as-coronavirus-cases-show-no-sign-of-slowing.

Purnamasari, Deti Mega. 2020. 'Laporan Lengkap Gugus Tugas COVID-19 Setelah Sebulan Bekerja'. *Kompas.com*. Retrieved on 27 May 2020 from https://nasional.kompas.com/read/2020/04/15/11455191/laporan-lengkap-gugus-tugas-COVID-19-setelah-sebulan-bekerja?page=1.

Reuters. 2020. 'Indonesia Unveils Nearly $750 Mln Stimulus Package in Response to Virus Outbreak'. *Reuters*. Retrieved on 25 May 2020 from https://www.reuters.com/article/indonesia-economy/indonesia-unveils-nearly-750-mln-stimulus-package-in-response-to-virus-outbreak-idUSJ9N29001A.

Ridhoi, Muhammad Ahsan. 2020. 'Riuh Skenario New Normal Ekonomi Indonesia Saat Pandemi Belum Reda'. *Katadata.co.id*. Retrieved on 30 May 2020 from https://katadata.co.id/telaah/2020/05/28/riuh-skenario-new-normal-ekonomi-indonesia-saat-pandemi-belum-reda.

Sanche, Steven, Yen Ting Lin, Chonggang Xu, Ethan Romero-Severson, Nick Hengartner, and Ruian Ke. 2020. 'High Contagiousness and Rapid Spread of Severe Acute Respiratory Syndrome Coronavirus 2'. *Emerging Infectious Disease*, 26(7). Retrieved on 20 May 2020 from https://pubmed.ncbi.nlm.nih.gov/32255761/.

Sari, Haryanti Puspa. 2020. 'Upaya-upaya TNI dalam Penanganan Pandemi COVID-19'. *KOMPAS.com*. Retrieved on 20 May 2020. https://nasional.kompas.com/read/2020/04/16/06102901/upaya-upaya-tni-dalam-penanganan-pandemi-COVID-19.

Sofuroh, Faidah Umu. 2020. 'Data Kemnaker: Pekerja Terdampak COVID-19 Capai Sekitar 3 Juta Orang'. *detikfinance*. Retrieved on 20 May 2020 from https://finance.detik.com/berita-ekonomi-bisnis/d-5009421/data-kemnaker-pekerja-terdampak-COVID-19-capai-sekitar-3-juta-orang.

Syakriah, Ardila. 2020. 'Climate, Immunity, Incompetence? Indonesia's Zero Recorded Coronavirus Cases Raise Questions'. *The Jakarta Post*. Retrieved on 1 May 2020 from https://www.thejakartapost.com/news/2020/02/08/climate-immunity-incompetence-indonesias-zero-recorded-coronavirus-cases-raise-questions.html.

Taher, Andrian Pratama. 2020. 'Jokowi Minta Alat PCR, Tes Cepat dan Ventilator Segera Diproduksi'. *Tirto.ID*. Retrieved on 27 May 2020 from https://tirto.id/jokowi-minta-alat-pcr-tes-cepat-dan-ventilator-segera-diproduksi-fqie.

Tambun, Lenny Tristia. 2020. 'Ini Tugas Gugus Tugas Percepatan Penanganan COVID-19'. *Berita Satu*. Retrieved on 17 May 2020 from https://www.beritasatu.com/kesehatan/608687-ini-tugas-gugus-tugas-percepatan-penanganan-covid19.

The Jakarta Post. 2020. 'COVID-19: WHO Urges Jokowi to Declare National Emergency'. Retrieved on 27 May 2020 from https://www.thejakartapost.com/news/2020/03/14/COVID-19-who-urges-jokowi-to-declare-national-emergency.html.

Warburton, Eve. 2020. 'Indonesia: Polarization, Democratic Distress, and the Coronavirus'. Carnegie Endowment for International Peace. Retrieved on 20 May 2020 from https://carnegieendowment.org/2020/04/28/indonesia-polarization-democratic-distress-and-coronavirus-pub-81641.

Warta Ekonomi.co.id. 2020. 'Virus Corona Makin Ganas, Menkes Bilang: Enjoy Aja!'. Retrieved on 25 May 2020 from https://www.wartaekonomi.co.id/read268664/virus-corona-makin-ganas-menkes-bilang-enjoy-aja.

WHO. 2003. 'Severe Acute Respiratory Syndrome (SARS)-Multi-Country Outbreak – Update'. World Health Organization. Retrieved on 1 May 2020 from https://www.who.int/csr/don/2003_03_16/en/.

World Health Organization. 2012. 'H5N1 Avian Influenza: Timeline of Major Events'. World Health Organization. Retrieved on 1 May 2020 from https://www.who.int/influenza/human_animal_interface/H5N1_avian_influenza_update.pdf.

World Health Organization. 2020. 'Cumulative Number of Confirmed Human Cases for Avian Influenza A(H5N1) Reported to WHO, 2003–2020'. World Health Organization. Retrieved on 1 May 2020 from https://www.who.int/influenza/human_animal_interface/2020_01_20_tableH5N1.pdf?ua=1.

Worldometers. 2020. 'COVID-19 Coronavirus Pandemic'. Retrieved on 6 May 2020 from https://www.worldometers.info/coronavirus/?utm_campaign=homeAdvegas1?

Yuliawati. 2020. 'Survei KIC: Pemudik Akan Didominasi Kaum Muda Berpendapatan Rendah'. *Katadata.co.id*. Retrieved on 20 May 2020 from https://katadata.co.id/berita/2020/04/20/survei-kic-pemudik-akan-didominasi-kaum-muda-berpendapatan-rendah.

9 Global Security Challenge of COVID-19

A Sociological Observation of Religious Identity in Brunei Darussalam

Ahmad F. Yousif and
Mohammed Hussain Ahmad

Introduction

The demographic characteristics of the Sultanate of Brunei Darussalam, located on the north-west coast of the island of Borneo, in Southeast Asia, has a small population compared to other neighboring countries. The Department of Economic Planning and Statistics in Brunei Darussalam confirmed that the 2019 national population in the country is estimated to be 459,500 persons.[1] Approximately two-thirds (66%) of Brunei's population consist of ethnic Malays, the absolute majority of which are Sunni Muslims, who follow the Shafi'i school of Islamic thought (Madhhab al-Shafi'i). The ethnic Malay community in the country includes Melayu Brunei, Tutong, Belait, Dusun, Kedayan, Murut, and Bisaya, who speak the Malay language (Bahasa Melayu) and use English as a second language. The Chinese community is comprised of 10% of the ethnic distribution, while the remaining "Others" represents 24% of Brunei's population.[2] Members of the Chinese community speak different Chinese dialects including Hokkien, Mandarin, Hakka, and Cantonese.

In terms of religious distributions, Brunei Darussalam is officially a Muslim nation, as stated in the country's Constitution of 1984. The Sultan and Yang Di-Pertuan (a royal title) has been the head of the Islamic faith since the late 13th century. Although Islam is the official religion of the country, religious minorities have the right to observe their religious values and traditions. In this regard, Article 3(1) of the Constitution of Brunei Darussalam (1984) asserts that, "all other religions may be practiced in peace and harmony by the persons professing them in any part of Brunei Darussalam."[3] As far as the religious statistics of Brunei is concerned, the 2018 census indicated that, out of 442,000 population, approximately 67% identified themselves as Muslims, 13% Buddhists, 10% Christians, and the remaining 10% "Others," which includes other religious groups such as Hindus, Sikhs, and non-affiliates.[4]

Influence of Islam in Brunei

Both in the past and in the present, Islamic values, traditions, and ethics have been incorporated and manifested within Brunei's culture, society, and politics.

DOI: 10.4324/9781003291909-10

Proof of the continuous link between religion and state, past and present, is the continuation of the Melayu Islam Beraja or Malay Islamic Monarchy (MIB) philosophy, which has been in existence since Brunei first declared itself a Malay Muslim Sultanate six centuries ago. MIB is the cornerstone of the socio-political ideology of modern-day Brunei, which stresses the importance of maintaining a monarchy political system, Malay race, language, culture, and Islam as a religion of the nation.

Religious institutions for both Muslims and non-Muslims are spreading out around the country. According to the Mosque Affairs Department, there are 107 Mosques and Suraus (prayer hall) and 11 non-Muslim worship places in Brunei as of 2018,[5] including two major state mosques, Masjid Omar Ali Saifuddien and Jame' Asr Hassanal Bolkiah, both of which are considered major tourist attractions for visitors to Brunei.

The majority of Islamic organizations or departments in Brunei are government or semi-government established and maintained. The Ministry of Religious Affairs, established in 1986, is comprised of six different departments, namely, Administration, Islamic Studies, Hajj (pilgrimage), Mosque Affairs, Shari'ah Affairs (Islamic law), and Islamic Religious Council. In addition, educational institutions such as the Islamic Da'wah Center (propagation center), Seri Begawan Religious Teachers University College, and Sultan Haji Hassanal Bolkiah al-Qur'an Tahfiz Institute (http://itqshhb.blogspot.com) are included. The Ministry has an informative website (http://www.kheu.gov.bn/Theme/Home.aspx), which can be accessed in the Malay language. The website designates a full Malay online page to address issues related to COVID-19.[6]

The Islamic Da'wah Center established in January 1985 is responsible for the dissemination and expansion of Islamic teachings among both Muslims and non-Muslims in Brunei Darussalam. It also undertakes research and studies on Islamic-related subjects, publishes Islamic material such as books, pamphlets, periodicals, and networks with other Muslim countries, by exchanging information and organizing intellectual conferences, seminars, and meetings on various contemporary Islamic issues. The Center's Publication Control and Censor Unit monitors books, periodicals, journals, newspapers, and other materials, which contradict Islamic beliefs and teachings.

Moreover, Sufi groups or tariqahs (mystical orders), particularly al-Ahmadiyyah and al-Naqshabandiyyah, have also established themselves in the country. Some of these tariqahs trace their roots directly to the Middle East, while others entered Brunei via neighboring countries such as Indonesia and Malaysia. Many of these groups engage in a weekly Dhikir, a socio-religious ceremony in which religious poems are read and chanted.

The 20th century witnessed the growth and development of Islamic religious education in Brunei. Islamic educational institutions are promoted under schools and colleges affiliated with the Ministry of Religious Affairs, where traditional Islamic subjects are taught in both Malay and Arabic languages. Some of the more reputable religious institutes in the country are the Sultan Haji Hassanal Bolkiah Tahfiz al-Qur'an Institute, the Brunei College of Islamic

Studies (Ma'had), and the Seri Begawan Religious Teachers University College (KUPU SB).

At the tertiary level, the Sultan Omar Ali Saifuddien Centre for Islamic Studies (SOASCIS) was established in 2010, at the University of Brunei Darussalam, to provide postgraduate degrees, i.e., Master of Arts (MA) and Doctor of Philosophy (PhD), by research, on Islamic civilization and contemporary issues (http://soascis.ubd.edu.bn/programs). In fact, SOASCIS is a substitute for the former Sultan Haji Omar Ali Saifuddien Institute of Islamic Studies (IPISHOAS) at the University, which used to provide three different areas of specialization – Islamic law (Shari'ah), theology and propagation (Usuluddin and Da'wah), and Arabic language.

In 2007, with a declaration from the Sultan, IPISHOAS was upgraded to the current Sultan Sharif Ali Islamic University (UNISSA), and becomes the first Islamic institution of higher learning in the country. Today, UNISSA has five faculties and six centers. According to its website, UNISSA is an authentic Islamic university of an international standard, which "offers a variety of programs across disciplines based on Al-Qur'an and al-Sunnah" (http://www.unissa.edu .bn/about-us/corporate-profile/rectors-message). Currently, UNISSA offers undergraduate and postgraduate degrees in major fields of Islamic studies such as Usuluddin (theology), Shari'ah and Islamic law, business and management, Islamic banking and finance, Arabic language, Islamic civilization and development, and Halal science and laws (http://www.unissa.edu.bn/programmes/ programmes-offered).

After the above introduction to Brunei's history, demography, Islamic institutions, and organizations, the following section will explore the developments of COVID-19 and how the state's mechanism continues to manage and control the spread of the virus.

Developments of COVID-19 in Brunei Darussalam

The term "COVID-19" refers to the infectious disease caused by the most recently discovered coronavirus. This virus is related to diseases that are unknown before the outbreak began in Wuhan, China, in mid-December 2019.[7] COVID-19 has been considered a pandemic affecting many countries globally, including Brunei Darussalam. Up to June 29, 2020, there are more than ten millions of confirmed cases and half a million deaths around the world.[8] According to the World Health Organization (WHO), most people infected with the virus will experience mild to moderate respiratory illness and recover without requiring special treatment. WHO states that "the best way to prevent and slow down transmission is to be well informed about the COVID-19 virus, the disease it causes and how it spreads."[9]

Before the outbreak of COVID-19, Brunei Darussalam was and still is a peaceful country "Darussalam" (an Arabic word for "abode of peace"). While the world, including Brunei Darussalam, has become alerted and infected with COVID-19 cases, public perception was that the new coronavirus is only affecting health conditions of older people. This mythological perception was proven to be scientifically unfounded as the virus has been rapidly spreading.

The chronology order of COVID-19 in Brunei Darussalam started on March 9, 2020, when the Ministry of Health confirmed that preliminary coronavirus tests had confirmed positive for a 53-year-old male. This person had returned from a religious gathering of Tabligh Jamat (a global Muslim propagation group) in Kuala Lumpur, Malaysia, on March 3, 2020.[10] He began to experience symptoms on March 7 and was eventually moved for treatment at the National Isolation Centre (NIC), located in the district of Tutong. The Ministry started to follow up with three friends of whom the patient had traveled with and with his family members. On March 9, the Ministry of Health reported five more cases of COVID-19, bringing the total number to six. These five individuals were in close contact with the first case, and, like the previous case, were isolated for treatment at the NIC. Few days later (March 11), the Ministry reported another five new cases, bringing the total number to 11. Three of these individuals had attended the same Tabligh Jamat gathering in Kuala Lumpur on March 3.

Subsequently, the daily news reports on COVID-19 in Brunei Darussalam began to alert the nation particularly policymakers, religious authorities, and security agents. By March 12, the Ministry of Health had confirmed another 14 new cases, bringing the total number to 25 positive-tested patients. Ten of these cases were linked to the same Tabligh Jamat gathering in Kuala Lumpur that the first confirmed patient had attended. Three of these "new" cases were in close contact with the already confirmed patients, while the last case was a 64-year-old man who had recently visited Kuala Lumpur and Cambodia. Two-day later, specifically on March 14, the Ministry of Health in Brunei reported a total of 40 cases who tested positive for COVID-19.

During the month of March 2020, the world had become a pandemic place to live, where life is suddenly replaced with slow death. Waves of COVID-19 cases have attacked countries in Asia and have quickly penetrated the Middle East (specifically Iran) and Europe (Italy, France, Spain, and the United Kingdom). There were daily reports of thousands of infected and dying individuals.

From March 15, 2020 to March 27, 2020, Brunei reported 115 confirmed positive cases of COVID-19, including five recoveries, while the first case of death took place in the country. At the beginning of April 2020, the reported cases in Brunei started to slowly decline compared to an increase in daily recoveries. State officials, including His Majesty, the Sultan, called upon the nation to follow the specific guidelines and policies on how to control the spread of COVID-19 through Brunei's partial "lockdown" implementation. However, positive-tested cases of the virus continue to steadily increase in Brunei, despite all possible measures to control it. For example, during the month of May 2020, only isolated cases started to be detected, including one new case reported on May 5, 2020, which brought the total active cases in the country to 139 persons. On May 6, two more cases were discovered related to the already confirmed case the previous day. Since the second week of May 2020, it has been rarely any reported case(s) in Brunei.

During the COVID-19 era in Brunei Darussalam, the government along with the private sector took serious steps and formulated specific policies to treat and control the virus. Among the measures taken after the partial "lockdown" announced were total closure of religious worship places, closure of educational institutions and changing the learning system to distance online method, closure of health clinics with exception to emergencies, a shutdown of sports and recreational facilities and related activities, forbid social gatherings such as public weddings, and postponed all national celebrations and others. In addition, the Brunei government closed all national borders and suspended flights in and outside the country, except for specially chartered flights related to medical supplies and/or to bring Bruneian citizens home, particularly overseas students. It also barred international visitors from entering the country, including transiting at the international airport. While the government took drastic measures to control the virus, people in Brunei welcomed the new policies and tried to work together to follow international standards required by WHO and Brunei-specific regulations. The *Diplomat* (international current affairs magazine for the Asia-Pacific region) had stated that Brunei "has earned a much more honorable distinction this time around (for) winning the war on the coronavirus."[11]

Two questions need to be addressed in the context of Brunei's era of COVID-19. Firstly, the high level of religious commitment correlates positively with COVID-19, from an individual, family, community, societal, and international perspective? Secondly, how policies and regulations proposed by the Brunei government, during this pandemic period, lead to reinforce individuals' religiosity and reshape Islamic commitment. Responses to the above and other questions will be demonstrated through the following discussion.

Religiously, the extent to which each individual feels the link with his or her own religious commitment varies from one person to another. For a committed Muslim, ritual religious practice is the most significant activity of Islamic identity. Prayer and recitation of the Qur'an, for some Muslims, are the primary rituals that bring them closer to Allah (SWT). They are not just routines, but the means to the achievement of wholeness. Community rituals and gatherings are another mechanism for maintaining Islamic commitment. During community prayer especially Jumah (Friday prayer), Muslims relate to each other, because they are all re-enacting the same ritual, at the same time and in the same place (i.e., mosque). This particular religious rite is different from other customs in other world religions and other kinds of social commitment. Therefore, all of the participants are sharing something that is uniquely theirs.

Social scientists affirmed that commitment to a religious belief system is one of the strongest values influencing the preservation of religious identity. According to Hans Mol, a Canadian sociologist, commitment is an anchoring of the emotions in a salient system of meaning, social, group, or personal whether abstract or concrete.[12] Generally, Muslims possess strong emotional attachments to their religion and therefore attempt to stay true to it in body, mind, and spirit. This is not to say that all Muslims in or outside of Brunei abide perfectly by the rules of their religion, such as performing every Jumah prayer. Instead, it implies that when commitment is strong, there is a strong consistency between belief and practice, and a resultant strengthening of one's identity. When commitment is not strong, and religious belief is not central to the individual's life, he or she often becomes alienated from his or her religion.

While the personal identity of individual Muslims is strengthened through the practice of particular religious rites, social identity is strengthened when a group of individuals comes together to practice religious rites. Mol connects the personal and the communal experience of ritual in this way: "[Ritual] maximizes order by strengthening the place of him/her in the group, or society, and vis-a-vis by strengthening the bonds of a society vis-a-vis the individual... Ritual, thereby, represents society."[13] Accordingly, Friday's prayer rituals performed by Muslims strengthen their religious identity as a distinct group.

During the COVID-19 in Brunei, religious commitment happens at both personal and social levels. On the personal level, the committed Muslim keeps his or her links with Islamic practice, by enforcing the rules of the belief system in all aspects of his or her life. This year (2020), and for the first time, during the month of Ramadan (fasting), mosques in Brunei were completely closed particularly for the annual Taraweeh prayer, which forced people to perform it at home instead. In psychological terms, this personal commitment motivates an individual's behavior and keeps it relatively predictable. This kind of predictability in turn creates security and stability. Commitment, therefore, reinforces identity and systems of meaning and definitions of reality.[14] For instance, if one never violates Islamic ethics because one is committed to Islamic belief and follows its rules, then avoiding forbidden things becomes a predictable element of one's life and a source of stability, i.e., mass-gathering.[15] In other words, if there is an act that is defined as sacrilegious, a person who thinks of himself or herself as religious will never attempt to do it, such as violating the COVID-19 order. Therefore, a "practicing" Muslim in Brunei, who is strongly committed to Islam on an individual level, will act accordingly.

On the second level, "commitment to a social or group identity strongly contributes to the formation of consensus and this makes a society, or group more viable."[16] Social commitment acts as a support system for individual commitment. If there is a large group with which one shares common beliefs, then one is more apt to express that belief and stay within the group. It is with this principle in mind that Muslims in Brunei have organized themselves around religious institutions. The establishment of religious institutions such as mosques and educational centers has been the first priority of Muslims in the country. Today, mosques are now found in almost every major area in the capital Bandar Seri Begawan, small towns, and villages. These mosques are not only the symbols of the fervency of their faith but also important socializing agents and transmitters of cultural values. As a result, Muslims are able to validate their personal beliefs and customs on a much larger scale. In fact, their social commitment reinforces their personal identity. Muslims who do not feel threatened by global COVID-19 because of their own Islamic commitment have a strong sense of identity. Therefore, the Muslim community in Brunei acts as a central base where values and norms come together. Through a commitment to a social community of Islam, identification is reinforced with one's fundamental roots. In this case, the role played by MIB or "Malay, Islamic and Monarchy" has become a fundamentally important instrument to control the spread of COVID-19.

On the technological level, the government of Brunei has introduced BruHealth application (http://www.moh.gov.bn/SitePages/bruhealth.aspx), a modern tool created to assist the public in navigating their daily activities. Today, every person needs to install BruHealth on their smartphone (or print out) with an active "barcode." Daily life in Brunei is slowly becoming connected to this technological application. Recent data show that the absolute majority of Brunei's population (approximately 90%) have BruHealth accounts on their smartphones. As a result, health monitoring officials can easily detect and locate individuals with possible infection of COVID-19.[17] Another advantage of this application is to record, organize, and permit a fixed number of Bruneians to perform Friday prayer in selected mosques. On May 25, 2020, with only 30% of its Friday prayer space allowed, mosques were opened for Jumah prayer since the partial lockdown of the country. No one was allowed to enter the mosque without the "activation of the Friday prayer feature on the BruHealth (application)" including a daily valid barcode.[18]

In addition to permit performing religious duties at worship places, BruHealth also provides "COVID-19 Self-Assessment Tool," an instrument which can be used to assist both authorities and users "to find out what you (applicant) should do to minimize the risk of cross-infection (with COVID-19)." Applicants need to fill out an online form reporting health conditions and possibly any symptoms that they have developed recently. BruHealth also provides the "Quarantine Monitoring" tool which allows quarantine individuals to complete at least 21 days of daily self-reporting, global epidemic updates, personal assessment code, Friday prayer code, COVID-19 knowledge, FAQs on COVID-19, "Nearby" tool, and "Scan QR Code." The "Scan QR Code" allows users to scan their QR codes at business premises or government offices that have the BruHealth QR Code. Entry to these premises is determined by the event code of the user.[19]

Moreover, Brunei's health authority conducted "Rapid Survey on COVID-19 in Brunei Darussalam" to understand people's perception of the new coronavirus. The survey was adapted from WHO's recommendations and aims to measure the public's awareness, knowledge, and ways to stop the spread of COVID-19 in the country.[20]

Among its publications, Brunei's authority produced an informative booklet on the "Measures Undertaken by Government in Addressing the Impact of COVID-19 in Brunei Darussalam." The booklet includes information on how to maintain the well-being of the public, protect employment, and provide alternative supporting systems for individuals, as well as financial assistance for small businesses.[21] For example, on March 30, 2020, the Ministry of Finance and Economy (MOFE) in Brunei allocated BND250 million "Economic Relief Package" which includes a six-month deferment of principal repayments of financing and loans to "businesses in tourism, hospitality and event management, restaurants and cafes, and air transport sectors" (i.e., "Affected Sectors").[22]

In terms of preventive measures, the Ministry of Health alongside other government ministries, departments, and agencies has been coordinating daily efforts on the new virus developments and issued suitable orders and policies to control it. Since early March 2020, the Minister of Health has been providing daily press conferences on Wabak (Arabic term for pandemic) COVID-19, which includes statistical information on the virus development in Brunei. The Minister revealed a total number of cases, new cases, recoveries, and deaths and responded to questions from the media. For example, on June 16, 2020, the official report stated that out of the total 141 cases, there are zero new cases, 138 recoveries, and three deaths.[23] The report shows only the number of cases and health conditions while names and identities of those infected individuals were kept confidential. The de-escalation stages to "normalize" lifestyle and reopening of business in Brunei have started in early June 2020.

The above discussion has demonstrated how Islamic law, values, traditions, and ethics continue to be incorporated and manifested within Brunei Darussalam's culture, society, and politics, as proven during the pandemic of COVID-19. Although the government has played a significant role in creating and developing religious, educational, and financial institutions, as well as supporting community development programs, public responses to coronavirus have shown a positive correlation between religious commitment and implementation of state policies and measures in Brunei Darussalam.

Since COVID-19 is considered a pandemic that affect humanity, the following section will examine the role of religion and medical sciences during the classical era of Islam and their influences on contemporary Brunei Darussalam.

Islamic Tradition of Medical Sciences

In contrast to the predominant view of secular education, which has tended to separate medical sciences from religion, in the Islamic traditions no such division existed. Accordingly, one finds that both the Qur'an and the traditions of the Prophet Muhammad (hadith) are saturated with references to learning, education, observation, and the use of reason, in all realms of life, medicine, and health care included.

Islam teaches individuals and societies how to live their lives in a physically, mentally, and morally up-right manner. The Islamic legal system which is derived from the Qur'an and sunnah (traditions of the Prophet) aims at creating a healthy environment, which will have a positive effect on an individual's physical, mental, and spiritual development.

At a physical level, the Qur'an and sunnah encourage healthy eating, while at the same time forbidding all substances which cause bodily harm (intoxicants, drugs, and others). Food such as fruit and vegetables, dates, yogurt, camel milk, natural honey, black seeds, and zamzam water are especially emphasized for their nutritious quality and benefits.

Although the Qur'an is not a medical textbook per se, it does speak about various diseases (al-Amrad), especially of the heart which often lead to direct or indirect physical and mental ailments. The Qur'an mentions blindness, deafness, lameness, leprosy, and dumbness, as well as mental disorders (junun) including psychoses and neurotic diseases such as sadness and anxiety.

As far as treatments are concerned, the primary focus of Islam is on moral and ethical diseases, rather than those of a physical nature. A large number of Prophetic sayings in the area of medicine and health led to the development of an entire discipline known as al-Tibb al-Nabawi (medicine of the Prophet). Imam Bukhari (the most authentic collector of Prophetic sayings) narrates 129 hadiths directly related to medicine and devotes two entire books to the subject of medicine Kitab al-Tibb (the book of medicine) and patients Kitab al-Muradha (the book of patients).

Without a doubt, classical Islamic literature guidance had a revolutionary effect on the early Muslims in all aspects of life. Prophetic statements such as "there is no disease that Allah has created, except that He also has created its treatment,"[24] proved a strong impetus for Muslim scholars to undertake investigations in the medical field. During the "Golden Age of Islamic Science," which lasted from the 9th to 13th centuries CE, Muslim scholars such as Jalal al-Din al-Suyuti (1445–1505 CE) made numerous contributions to the field of medicine. Al-Suyuti was not merely a medical practitioner, but he possessed an encyclopedic knowledge of theology, law, and philosophy, as well.

The traditional Islamic medical system can be summarized as a mixture between spiritual and physical elements, and between the use of natural substances and certain Islamic supplications for healing and cures. It included preventive measurements, curative medicine, mental healing, surgical experiments, and most importantly spiritual cures, for both the body and the soul. Both Muslim and non-Muslim scholars have agreed that many of the scientific and medical achievements made during the classical Islamic period, had a significant influence on the formation and development of modern medicine in Europe.

In lieu of Islam's glorious past in the medical and health-related fields and subsequent intellectual stagnation (for reasons which we will not dwell on here), how does the present fare, particularly in the Bruneian context? In Brunei today, one finds a variety of approaches to medicine and health care. There are a very small minority of individuals, who completely reject modern medicine, including issues related to COVID-19. Many of them prefer to rely on a combination of du'a (supplications) and traditional medical treatments. Accordingly, it is quite common to find traditional healers (Bomoh) in the modern period, who continue to rely on a mixture of Qur'anic verses, water, local herbs, ornaments, oil, and honey for their medical treatments. One of the shortcomings of this approach, however, is that it is sometimes practiced by people who have little or no medical training, many of whom become involved in superstitious practices that contradict Islamic norms and values.

At the other end of the spectrum, there are some secularly oriented individuals with little knowledge or regard for Islamic injunctions in the medical sphere, who prefer to rely completely on modern medicine. The vast majority of Bruneians, however, fall somewhere between these two groups. On the one hand, they believe that prayer, tahlil (group reciting Yasin-Qur'an: 36), dua' (supplications), Qur'anic recitation, and dhikr (remembrance of Allah) play an important role in healing and recovery, and on the other hand, recognize the benefits of modern medicine. In fact, the decision to utilize traditional and/ or modern medicine, both in and outside Brunei, is often contingent upon an individual's socio-economic and educational status, as well as the nature of the problem at hand. In order for a successful merger between traditional Islamic and modern medicine, appropriate educational and training programs are essential.

In light of the above traditional and contemporary understandings of Islamic medicine, what significance does Islamic tradition have for Brunei Darussalam? The answer to this question can't be separated from what Islam has to offer to mankind in the medical field. Many of the ailments humans suffer from today are diseases of the soul, which stem from societal and environmental factors, that are difficult for medication to cure without completely transforming society. For example, drugs can never remove the causes of racism, which recently has shaken North Americans – but Islamic tradition can.

Secondly, Islam objects to the reduction of humans' ailments and treatments strictly on the physical and mental dimensions, as secular trained and oriented medical practitioners are prone to do. From the Islamic point of view, humans are multidimensional in nature. Accordingly, treatments must be of holistic nature and not restricted to the physical dimension of the problem alone.

A third way Islamic medicine can influence modern medicine is in terms of its perception of illness and disease as in the case of COVID-19. In contrast to contemporary views, disease does not always have a negative connotation but perhaps a "positive" element. According to the classical Islamic scholar Imam Abu Hamid al-Ghazali (d. 1111), "illness is one of these forms of experience by which man arrives at a knowledge of God."[25] Omar Kasule, a former professor of medicine at the University of Brunei Darussalam, argues that falling ill may be Allah's way of forcing the person to take a desired rest or care for the body before it deteriorates further. Not only is patience in the face of severe illness a reason for entering Paradise, Casual said, but the pain is a reminder of the punishment and suffering that the evildoers will suffer on the Day of Judgment.[26]

Fourthly, both medical practitioners and patients must know the limits of the former's capabilities. From a Muslim point of view, life and death are ultimately from Allah. No human being can give or take it away. As such, medical personnel do not have the privilege to say anything definitive about future prognosis. Instead, they are obliged to assist the patient to the best of their abilities and leave the rest. While Muslim physicians may extrapolate based on available data, they must always have the humility to say "Allah knows best."

Lastly, Islamic medicine can also provide a code of ethics for medical practitioners. Muslim medical personnel are subject to Shari'ah (Islamic law), on both personal and professional levels, especially in terms of their obligations towards patients, community, and society. As such, they are obliged to be sincere, humble, and constantly strive to seek the pleasure of Allah, with the consciousness that He is the All-Knowing.

The above discussion represents a general analysis of how Islamic medicine can contribute to modern medicine, particularly at the time when the whole world is trying to control the spread of COVID-19, Brunei Darussalam included.

In conclusion, there is a long list of "negative" impacts of COVID-19 on the individual, community, society, and global levels; however, a "positive" list can also be found, particularly in the context of this pandemic in Brunei Darussalam. A further investigation on the topic will uncover the specific advantages and disadvantages of COVID-19 and their impacts on Brunei.

Notes

1 Cited from http://www.deps.gov.bn/SitePages/Population.aspx, on June 24, 2020.
2 Cited from http://www.deps.gov.bn/SitePages/Population.aspx, on June 24, 2020.
3 Laws of Brunei, Revised Edition 1984, Constitutional Matters I, *The Constitution of Brunei Darussalam.* Cited from https://www.worldstatesmen.org/Brunei1984.PDF, 16, on June 20, 2020.
4 *Brunei Darussalam Statistical Yearbook 2018.* Brunei Darussalam: Department of Statistics, 200.
5 *Brunei Darussalam Statistical Yearbook 2018.* Brunei Darussalam: Department of Statistics, 201.
6 Cited from http://www.kheu.gov.bn/SitePages/Isu-Isu%20Khas%20Mengenai%20Covid19.aspx, on June 6, 2020.
7 World Health Organization (WHO). Cited from https://www.who.int/health-topics/coronavirus#tab=tab_1, on June 21, 2020. "CO" stands for corona, "VI" for virus, and "'D" for disease. Formerly, this disease was referred to as "2019 novel coronavirus" or "2019-nCoV." It was later renamed to "the COVID-19 virus," then commonly referred to "COVID-19."
8 Cited from https://www.who.int/emergencies/diseases/novel-coronavirus-2019, on June 30, 2020.
9 Cited from https://www.who.int/health-topics/coronavirus#tab=tab_1, on June 7, 2020.
10 Report on the "Detection of the First Case of COVID-19 Infection in Brunei Darussalam." Cited from http://www.moh.gov.bn/Lists/Latest%20news/NewDispForm.aspx?ID=366, on June 7, 2020.
11 Austin Bodetti, "How Brunei Beat COVID-19." Cited from https://thediplomat.com/2020/06/how-brunei-beat-COVID-19, on June 24, 2020.
12 Hans Mol. *Identity and the Sacred: A Sketch for a New Socio-Scientific Theory of Religion.* Agincourt, ON: The Book Society of Canada Limited, 1976, 216; See also Hans Mol. *Meaning and Place.* New York: The Pilgrim Press, 1983.
13 Hans Mol. *Identity and the Sacred: A Sketch for a New Socio-Scientific Theory of Religion.* Agincourt, ON: The Book Society of Canada Limited, 1976, 233-4.
14 Hans Mol. *Identity and the Sacred: A Sketch for a New Socio-Scientific Theory of Religion.* Agincourt, ON: The Book Society of Canada Limited, 1976, 218.
15 Siti Mazidah Mohamad (2020), "Creative Production of 'COVID-19 Social Distancing' Narratives on Social Media." *Royal Dutch Geographical Society.* 4. It can be accessed online at https://onlinelibrary.wiley.com/doi/full/10.1111/tesg.12430, June 7, 2020. See also https://www.who.int/emergencies/diseases

/novel-coronavirus-2019/question-and-answers-hub/q-a-detail/q-a-coronaviruses, cited on June 20, 2020.
16　Hans Mol. *Identity and the Sacred: A Sketch for a New Socio-Scientific Theory of Religion*. Agincourt, ON: The Book Society of Canada Limited, 1976, 218.
17　*BruHealth* Application, "Media Statement of the Current Situation of the COVID-19 Infection in Brunei Darussalam." Ministry of Health, Brunei Darussalam, Press Release, June 14, 2020.
18　*BruHealth* Application, "Media Statement of the Current Situation of the COVID-19 Infection in Brunei Darussalam." Ministry of Health, Brunei Darussalam, Press Release, June 14, 2020.
19　Ministry of Health, Brunei Darussalam. Cited from http://www.moh.gov.bn/ SitePages/bruhealth.aspx, on June 23, 2020.
20　"Rapid Survey on COVID-19 in Brunei Darussalam" Cited from https://docs .google.com/forms/d/e/1FAIpQLSe_5GBg7i4lAiXW9ftlXr7feiroxDnOiAv XeM3FtDYLf7ijvQ/viewform, on June 25, 2020.
21　Cited from http://www.moe.gov.bn/Articles/Measures%20Undertaken %20by%20the%20Government%20in%20Handling%20the%20Impact%20of %20COVID-19%20%20issued%2027.04.2020%20v7.pdf, on June 26, 2020.
22　Cited from https://home.kpmg/xx/en/home/insights/2020/04/brunei -darussalam-government-and-institution-measures-in-response-to-covid.html, on June 26, 2020.
23　*BruHealth* Application, "Media Statement of the Current Situation of the COVID-19 Infection in Brunei Darussalam." Ministry of Health, Brunei Darussalam, Press Release, Accessed on June 16, 2020.
24　*Sahih al-Bukhari*, reported by Abu Hurairah, Vol 7, # 582.
25　Imam Abu Hamid al-Ghazali (d. 1111). *The Alchemy of Happiness*. Pennsylvania, USA: General Press, n.pg.
26　Omar Kasule, "Disease (Al-Maradh)." Article was published under "Lectures on Islamic Medicine," p. 4. Cited from http://www.iiu.edu.my/medic/islmed, on May 20, 2002.

References

Al-Suyuti, 2000. *Jalau'd-Din Abdu'ur-Rahman* [d. 911]. Medicine of the Prophet. (ed. Ahmed Thomson). Kuala Lumpur: SAM Publishing Sdn. Bhd.
Amod, Farouk, 1996. *Formation of the Islamic Medical Association of South Africa.* Durban: Islamic Medical Association of South Africa.
Athar, Shahid, ed., 1993. *Islamic Perspective in Medicine: A Survey of Islamic Medicine: Achievements and Contemporary Issues.* Indianapolis: American Trust Publications.
Athar, Shahid, 1995. *Health Concerns for Believers.* Chicago: Kazi Publication.
Badri, Malik, 1997. *The AIDS Crisis: An Islamic Socio-Cultural Perspective.* Kuala Lumpur: International Institute of Islamic Thought and Civilization.
Bakar, Osman, 1996. *Philosophy of Islamic Medicine and Its Relevance to the Modern World.* Penang: Secretariat for Islamic Philosophy and Science.
Brown, Edward G., 2001. *Islamic Medicine* (Fitzpatrick Lectures delivered at the Royal College of Physicians in 1919–1920). New Delhi: Goodword Press.
BruHealth Application, 2020. *Media Statement of the Current Situation of the COVID-19 Infection in Brunei Darussalam.* Brunei Darussalam: Ministry of Health, Press Release. Accessed June 16, 2020.
Department of Economic Planning and Development, 2015. *Brunei Darussalam Millennium Development Goals and Beyond: Towards the Post-2015 Development Agenda.* Brunei Darussalam: Department of Economic Planning and Development.

Department of Economic Planning and Development of Brunei Darussalam, 2016. "Population." Accessed October 19, 2016, from http://www.depd.gov.bn/SitePages/Population.aspx.

Department of Statistics, 2015. *Brunei Darussalam Statistical Yearbook 2015.* Brunei Darussalam: Department of Economic Planning and Development.

Department of Statistics, 2018. *Brunei Darussalam Statistical Yearbook 2018.* Brunei Darussalam: Department of Economic Planning and Development.

Ebrahim, Abul Fadl Mohsin, 1988. *Biomedical Issues: Islamic Perspective.* Mobeni: Islamic Medical Association of South Africa.

Ibn al-Qayim, al-Jawziyah (d. 751), 1993. *Natural healing with the Medicine of the Prophet* (Trans. Shaykh Muhammad Al-Akili, 1993). Philadelphia: Pearl Publishing House.

International Organization of Islamic Medicine, 1982. *Islamic Code of Medical Ethics.* Kuwait: International Organization of Islamic Medicine.

Kasule, Omar Hasan, 1996. "Islamic Medicine: Concepts and Misunderstandings." *Journal of the Federation of Islamic Medical Associations*, 1.

Laws of Brunei, Revised Edition, 1984. "Constitutional Matters I, The Constitution of Brunei Darussalam." Accessed June 26, 2020, from http://www.worldstatesmen.org/Brunei1984.PDF.

Mohamad, Siti Mazidah, 2020. "Creative Production of 'COVID-19 Social Distancing' Narratives on Social Media." *Royal Dutch Geographical Society.* Accessed June 7, 2020, from https://onlinelibrary.wiley.com/doi/full/10.1111/tesg.12430.

Mol, Hans, 1976. *Identity and the Sacred: A Sketch for a New Socio-Scientific Theory of Religion.* Agincourt: The Book Society of Canada Limited.

Mol, Hans, 1983. *Meaning and Place.* New York: The Pilgrim Press.

Nasr, Seyyed Hossein, 1968, also published in 1987. *Science and Civilization in Islam* (2nd ed.). The Islamic Texts Society. Cambridge: Harvard University Press.

Schottmann, Sven Alexander, 2006. "Melayu Islam Beraja: The Politics of Legitimization in a Malay Islamic Monarchy." *Review of Indonesian and Malaysian Affairs*, 40(2), 111–139.

Taha, Ahmad, 1993. *Medicine in the Light of the Qur'an and Sunna.* London: Ta-Ha Publishers Ltd.

Ullmann, Manfred, 1997. *Islamic Medicine.* Edinburgh: Edinburgh University Press.

World Health Organization, 2020. Accessed June 21, 2020, from https://www.who.int/health-topics/coronavirus#tab=tab_1.

Yousif, Ahmad, 2010. "Brunei." In *Religions of the World: A Comprehensive Encyclopedia of Beliefs and Practices*, 2nd edition. Gordon J. Melton and Marin Baumann (eds.). Santa Barbara: ABC-Clio. e-Book: http://www.abc-clio.com/product.aspx?id=52831.

Yousif, Ahmad, 2010. "Islam in Brunei." In *Religions of the World: A Comprehensive Encyclopedia of Beliefs and Practices*, 2nd edition. Gordon J. Melton and Marin Baumann (eds.). Santa Barbara: ABC-Clio. e-Book: http://www.abc-clio.com/product.aspx?id=52831.

Yousif, Ahmad, 2011. *Islam and Science: A Southeast Asian Perspective* (2nd ed.). Kuala Lumpur: IIUM Press, International Islamic University Malaysia.

10 Implication of COVID-19

Response to Islamic Economics in ASEAN

Tulus Suryanto and Mohd Mizan Aslam

Introduction

Coronavirus disease (COVID-19) has an impact on economic activity globally. Previous studies have revealed that there have been 13,000 policy announcements worldwide to respond to COVID-19. This is the first step taken by more than 195 countries in response to this unexpected event (Cheng, Barceló, Hartnett, Kubinec, & Messerschmidt, 2020). Actions taken by the Association of Southeast Asian Nations (ASEAN) countries in response to COVID-19 include the types of government policies implemented with a focus on investment and financing of Islamic financial products, levels of government initiating action, geographic targets of policy actions, human or material targets from policy actions, policy action directions, and travel mechanisms to targets for policy action.

Countries around the world are experiencing economic downturns, including ASEAN. In particular, ASEAN countries with a market for halal products such as Indonesia, Malaysia, Singapore, and Brunei Darussalam have also experienced a decline in purchasing power since the implementation of social distancing and restrictions on international flights. This incident gave birth to major changes in individuals' behavior and lifestyle, government, and private society. The findings suggest that social distancing as a government measure to contain COVID-19 is likely to increase mobility changes as a behavioral response (Warren & Skillman, 2020). But on the other hand, it also encourages feelings of social support between community groups.

The perspective of the community, government, and artificial intelligence technology in responding to COVID-19 has become a topic that has appeared in many studies. Mackworth-Young et al. (2021) investigated the public and health workers' perspectives on COVID-19 and found that society needs moral and material support to survive. Effective government policies support handling the spread of COVID-19 and accelerating economic recovery (Cheng et al., 2020). Another study found a positive relationship between the government's response and the implications of COVID-19. A poor response to the implications of COVID-19 can lead to possible mental and economic stress. Other consequences include increases in prices for necessities, obstruction of formal education, and the possibility of severe socio-economic and health crises, disasters due to climate

DOI: 10.4324/9781003291909-11

change, and infectious diseases during the COVID-19 situation (Bodrud-Doza, Shammi, Bahlman, Islam, & Rahman, 2020; Ciancio et al., 2020). The findings reveal that artificial intelligence (AI) plays a major supporting role in fighting COVID-19. The use of AI is increasing and implementing social distancing policies and other data analyses in many sectors (Sipior, 2020).

Researchers have not found previous studies focusing on Islamic economic sectors' responses, especially in ASEAN countries. Previous studies have focused on Indonesia, Singapore, Brunei, and Malaysia's response by presenting five recommendations towards a more rapid, effective, and comprehensive response. Among them are the response of the national government, the response of the wider community, and recommendations for the resilience of the economic system (Djalante et al., 2020; Kim, Koh, & Xuan, 2020; Haqqi & Hidayati, 2020; Wong, Koh, Alikhan, Abdul Aziz, & Naing, 2020; Arif & Zaim, 2020). From several literature reviews, it is essential to know how the response of ASEAN countries included in the Top Indicator category of Islamic economic scores in responding to the conditions of COVID-19. As one of the regions that are the center of the Islamic economy industry globally, the activities of the halal market share in ASEAN are certainly transforming and playing an important role in the midst of the COVID-19 pandemic situation. The literature states that COVID-19 could be a momentum for the revival of Islamic economics and ASEAN's finance.

Based on the report of the State of the Global Islamic Economy 2019/2020, five ASEAN countries, namely Indonesia, Malaysia, Brunei Darussalam, Thailand, and Singapore, are in the top ten positions in several categories of the world's Islamic economic industry (Dinar Standard, 2020). This shows the results of the performance of the Islamic economy, which is quite encouraging. As a country with a large potential share of the Islamic market amid a pandemic situation, Islamic economic sectors are expected to survive and develop. A projection has predicted that the Top 15 Global Islamic Economic Indicator Score countries' economic growth, including ASEAN in the worst-case scenario, could reach –0.4%. In other words, the decline in economic activity as a whole experiences the worst possibility if it fails to implement the right policies and support from the Islamic economy in particular.

This study seeks to collect and provide brief reporting, analysis, and evaluation of the Islamic economy's rapid response to the COVID-19 events in ASEAN. This research can be seen as an empirical evaluation of some of the most influential Islamic economic dimensions and provides insights for stakeholders. There are at least three objectives of this study. The first is to highlight the implications of COVID-19 and look at the Islamic economic response in Indonesia. The second is to analyze the opportunities in the response. The third is to put forward the recommendations towards developing sectors of the Islamic economy in the short term and sustainability. Several countries that are considered the most prepared and have a large capacity to respond to the outbreak have failed to effectively respond to the pandemic (Kavanagh & Singh, 2020; Sharma, Talan, & Jain, 2020; Karamouzian & Madani, 2020). Of the many countries globally, the country with the most success in responding quickly to COVID-19 is Australia. But during its development, social inequality hampered economic recovery (O'Sullivan, Rahamathulla, & Pawar, 2020). Therefore, stakeholders need to ensure this, considering that the development of the world's Islamic economy has contributed to overcoming the pandemic crisis. If this is so, then the Islamic economy needs full support from the government to spread its wings and ensure that Islamic economic actions taken as a response to COVID-19 are good for effective long-term sustainability and avoid the same failure.

Response

The response is commonly used in psychology to name an emotional reaction or reply to a received stimulus. The answer can be in the form of behavior that appears after stimulation (Subandi, 1982). Behaviorism theory explains that responses are behaviors that arise due to stimuli from the surrounding environment. The response has a significant role or influence in determining whether or not communication is good. If the answer has been conditioned, it will form new behavior towards the conditioned stimuli (Chaplin, 2004). The response is an impression of what has been observed and recognized. There are two types of reactions, namely latent response and actual response. A latent reaction is a response in the subconsciousness, while the precise answer is a response in awareness (Sabri, 2004).

According to Chaffe and Roser (1986), the response occurs because of a symptom of the event that preceded it. In this case, the answer has three criteria: (1) cognitive as a form of response that is closely related to the knowledge of skills and information possessed by individuals that arise due to changes in people's perspective; (2) useful as a form of response that is directly related to emotions, attitudes, and individual assessments of something; and (3) behavioral as a form of response related to daily behavior. McQuail (1987) developed the communication theory that humans have components of attitude, opinion, behavior, cognition, affection, and conation. This theory's main elements are the message or stimulus, the recipient, and the effect received. Stimulus–response results are specific reactions to certain stimuli. The literature reveals that this effect allows individuals to predict the conformity between the message and the communicant's expected reactions (McQuail & Windahl, 2015). The positive effects and adverse effects of the originality of the response model development are carriers over into individuals' or societies' attitudes and behavioral intentions (Yang, Teran, Battocchio, Bertellotti, & Wrzesinski, 2021). Some previous literature mentions the effect of response on social media support (Pöyry, Pelkonen, Naumanen, & Laaksonen, 2019), the effect of strategic communication responses (Tkalac Verčič, Verčič, & Coombs, 2019), and reactions to the initiation of a global event (Schuchat, 2020).

The stimulus given to the communicant has the possibility of being accepted or rejected. In the process of obtaining information, the attention and ability of the communicant to provide meaning to the contents of the message are capable of changing individual attitudes (Petty et al., 2014). The information message received contains a specific stimulus that interacts differently depending on the characteristics of each individual. Thus, it is understood that the response is reciprocal to what is communicated to the community. Without communication elements, the communication process cannot run effectively and efficiently (Petty, Fazio, & Briñol, 2008).

In an organization, social interaction is significant to understand how one individual gets responses from others. The reason is to determine whether the individual is responsible for generating a response with the goal of response mobilization (Stivers & Rossano, 2010). The answer has two factors that influence it – first, internal factors, namely factors that are within (spiritual and physical). A physical element is a physical form that humans can see, while the spiritual or psychological feature includes existence, feeling, mind, fantasy, mental, mental, and motivation. Second, external factors, namely factors that exist in the surrounding environment. The intensity of the stimulus factor occurs due to physical characteristics. Physical aspects relate to objects that can cause stimuli and ignore sense organs (Walgito, 1996). The three kinds of responses are generally known. First, the reaction according to the senses that observe consists of auditive answers (what is heard, both sounds, and beats), visual response (to something seen), and taste responses (to something that is experiencing him). Second, the reaction according to the occurrence consists of a memory response (to something he remembers), a fantasy response (to something imagined), and thought answers (for something to think about). Third, the reaction according to the environment consists of object responses (to objects that approach them) and the response of the words (to the stories he heard) (Greenwald, 1968).

Islamic Economics

Islamic economics is a normative economy that provides a basis for norms in the Al-Quran and As-Sunnah (Haneef, 2009). The models that underlie the Islamic economy are found in Maqasid as Sharia (the highest objective stated in Islamic law) for economic actors about how to behave in fulfilling the needs of life and increasing welfare. This includes maintaining religion, life, reason, family, and property. Islamic economics's main characteristics are the ethical, moral, and socio-economic principles of justice and the balance between spiritual and material needs. Ethical and moral values include everything that is allowed and prohibited in Islam, especially the prohibition of all transactions that have elements of usury, speculation, and obscurity (Harahap, 2014; Iqbal & Mirakhor, 2015; Jumaa, 2016).

Islamic economics has a broad scope, namely the financial sector and the real sector. The financial industry is divided into Islamic commercial finance (profit-oriented) and Islamic social finance (Gabbani, 2011; Salman & Nawaz, 2018), also, halal food and beverage sector, halal cosmetics, halal medicines, Muslim-friendly travel, halal clothing, and Islamic media and tourism (Dinar Standard, 2020). Islamic financial transactions offer a system of cooperation or *mudarabah*.

The principle of this cooperation is based on profit and loss sharing. Islamic economics practice requires an attachment between the financial sector and the real sector so that a potential economic crisis can be avoided. Social finance is based on the obligation of Muslims to help fellow humans. This category consists of three types: zakat, waqf, and infaq, known as ZISWAF (Syafira, Ratnasari, & Ismail, 2020). Zakat is mandatory for the wealthy with the terms and conditions set out in the text, while waqf and infaq are voluntary (Adzrin, Ahmad, Marzuki, Othman, & Sufiyudin, 2015; BAZNAS, 2020).

Method

The research design used was a literature study. In this section, the authors first use social science and behavioral theory to support the implications of the COVID-19 pandemic. The response is aimed at seven sectors of the Islamic economy: (1) Islamic finance, (2) Muslim-friendly travel, (3) halal food, (4) modest fashion, (5) halal pharmaceuticals, (6) halal cosmetics, and (7) halal media and recreation. The research focuses on five ASEAN countries included in the top ten market shares of the world's Islamic economy industry in 2020, namely Indonesia, Malaysia, Brunei Darussalam, Thailand, and Singapore. Next explains the themes provided and how the Islamic economy is organized. Each document obtained includes the implications of COVID-19 for the Islamic economy and the extent of the Islamic economic response to COVID-19. All information mentioned is presented descriptively.

Result and Discussion

The accelerated phase of this pandemic requires an Islamic economic response that is quick to adapt. From early January to late February, the number of COVID-19 cases in ASEAN continued to increase. This causes the country's economy to become unstable. Moreover, the financial industry and private companies are experiencing an economic downturn. The findings in this study have at least three limitations. First, various Islamic economic responses focus on the seven main sectors experiencing the most likely implications for ASEAN. This statement is based on the documentation of the 2020 report from the State of the Global Islamic Economy. Second, an example of a contributing factor to this research is government policies' role during the COVID-19 situation. Third, the response presented is likely to be influenced by limited literature studies, especially estimating the Islamic economic response in the Top 10 Global Islamic Economic Sector category.

Islamic Finance Sector Response

The researcher examines the Islamic financial sector's response with a focus on Islamic banking, Takaful Insurance, and Islamic social finance. Two ASEAN countries were included in the Top 10 Global Islamic Finance in 2020. Malaysia is in the first place in the Top 10 of Islamic Finance and is followed by Indonesia in the fifth position. Malaysia is the country with the highest score on Islamic financial products globally, reaching 111 points. Malaysia achieved momentum and a strengthening of the Islamic economy after the Islamic Finance Services Act (IFSA) 2013 and Financial Services Act 2013. The country has successfully developed a market share of up to 24% for 30 years. In the midst of the COVID-19 conditions, Islamic Bank is trying to provide support in the form of financing for micro, small, and medium enterprises (MSMEs) in the first half of 2020, which reached RM120. Assistance and superior business capital assistance for the MSME sector with a total of more than 50,000 participants. Islamic banks quickly channeled this financing. This effort is carried out because it is often difficult for MSMEs to survive amid limited capital and a pandemic. Also, business capital is followed by *qardhul hasan* loans (loans that do not take profit). The Takaful and Insurance Industry also facilitate certificates and policyholders, namely around 1.1 million certificates. Facilities are provided for those affected by COVID-19 by offering temporary suspension and premiums to increase Takaful protection (Ghaffour, 2020). While COVID-19 peaked in several ASEAN countries, Malaysia is heading for a period of economic recovery.

The 2019 Sharia Economic and Financial Report in Indonesia shows that the Islamic economy's performance, in general, has increased by 5.72% compared to the National Gross Domestic Product (GDP). Bank Indonesia revealed that the Islamic economy is resilient throughout 2020 with great potential for rapid development in the future, including supporting efforts to deal with the impact of the COVID-19 pandemic. The findings explain that the large share of the Islamic market is the main capital for the Islamic economy's sustainability. The biggest step taken by the government to strengthen Islamic financial institutions locally is by merging three Islamic banks, namely Bank Syariah Mandiri (BSM), Bank Rakyat Indonesia (BRI) Syariah, and Bank Nasional Indonesia (BNI) Syariah, where BRI Syariah is surviving. The entity is the merger of the three Islamic banks. The results of Moody's Investors Service survey stated that the three Islamic banks' total melted assets reached 2% of the total assets of all banks in Indonesia, thus placing this Islamic bank at number 7 in terms of assets. The merger was completed in February 2021 and received a warm welcome from the Indonesian people. The merger of these three Islamic banks is a major step towards strengthening Indonesia's Islamic economy in terms of capital, assets, products, and services to customers.

Islamic economic and social finance solutions are also no less competitive in responding to the implications of COVID-19. Distribution of direct cash assistance originating from zakat, infaq, and alms is both from zakat collection units and the community. Especially for cash zakat, the distribution is focused on the poor (the *mustahik* group/those who are entitled to receive zakat according to Islamic provisions) who are directly affected by COVID-19. This response is one of the Islamic economic, philanthropic schemes because of the potential for large zakat, *infaq*, and alms (ZISWAF) collection as the five countries with the largest Islamic economy market share in ASEAN. In the midst of a pandemic situation, the strengthening of zakat, infaq, and alms campaigns continues to be intensified, especially digital payments to facilitate acceptance transactions. Recently, ASEAN countries with ZISWAF institutions formed a mixed financing program oriented towards micro-entrepreneurs in low-income groups. This program is to provide working capital and training programs. Malaysia even managed to collect ZISWAF of US$9.72 million or the equivalent of RM40 million. Another Islamic social finance sector that has responded to the implications of COVID-19 is waqf institutions. The Waqf Board is collaborating with Islamic financial institutions in promoting the waqf scheme so that it can be used for the construction of various waqf-based infrastructures such as the Waqf Hospital (RSW) specifically for COVID-19 patients who are undergoing intensive care and quarantine, waqf masks, waqf clinic, and ventilator procurement waqf.

In economic recovery with the implications of COVID-19, Islamic financial schemes have shown relatively good resilience compared to collapsing domestic and global institutions. The reasons are (1) Islamic finance based on the value-based Intermediation (VBI) agenda applying the principles of justice and transparency; (2) Islamic finance helps in financing nanotechnology where funds come from several sources, both the general public, private companies, and business entities; (3) Islamic finance provides direct loans that the company channels to its employees where the funds can come from and Corporate Social Responsibility (CSR) or other posts; (4) Islamic finance quickly responds to the crisis experienced by society by continuously trying to improve product and service offerings in response to customer needs; and (5) Islamic finance cooperate to form a unity to strengthen the national economy and accelerate economic recovery.

Muslim-Friendly Travel Sector Response

The Muslim-friendly travel sector is the Islamic economic sector that has been hardest hit by COVID-19. Especially for the three countries included in the Top 10 Muslim-Friendly Travel in 2020, namely Malaysia in the first place, Indonesia in the fourth place, and Thailand in the tenth place. Since the enactment of the rules for restricting international flights until the specified time, the government temporarily closes foreign nationals' entry from all countries with a few exceptions. In Indonesia, this policy refers to Standard Operation Procedures (SOP) of the COVID-19 Task Force Number 7 and Number 8 of 2021 in overcoming the COVID-19 pandemic. As a result of this policy, tourist arrivals until March 2021 have decreased. The lack of preparedness for the Muslim-friendly travel business has made most businessmen who have closed their operations for quite a long time unable to survive. Also, the role of certification in convincing tourists and the lack of standardization of halal certification are of particular concern. This inhibiting factor occurs because not all businesses in this sector have halal certificates. This happens because of the low literacy of halal certification among entrepreneurs, especially MSMEs. Previous surveys have stated a relationship between Muslim-friendly travel, travel attitudes towards destinations, images, and intentions of halal tourism trips (Liu, Li, Yen, & Sher, 2018; Henderson, 2016; Abror, Patrisia, Trinanda, Omar, & Wardi, 2020). Various surveys estimate that Muslim-friendly travel can recover in 2023. This sees the demand and supply of the Muslim-friendly travel sector experiencing an increase in Muslim volume and the trend of world halal tourism (Abror, Patrisia, Trinanda, Omar, & Wardi, 2020; Liu et al., 2018; Henderson, 2016).

The Association of Indonesian Hotels and Restaurants (PHRI) suffered losses of more than US $1.5 billion due to COVID-19. In response to this impact, this sector carried out several plans and limited business continuity management (BCPM). One of the government's quick responses is through the Ministry of Tourism and Creative Economics, namely by carrying out promotions targeting travelers who tend to spend more. Although not significant, quality tourism and the reduction of domestic residents' tourism restrictions have made Islamic hotels begin to experience an increase in occupancy, and regional tourism such as Yogyakarta and Lombok are starting to return to their activities. Also, a series of activities in the Indonesia Halal Tourism Summit (IHTS) 2020 were held.

Various stakeholders in this sector have tried their best to work together to survive the crisis. One of them is the Indonesia Sharia Economic Festival (ISEF) and Bank Indonesia. It is an online platform for Muslim-friendly travel entrepreneurs, sharing businesses, discussion forums, and friendly meetings with tourism stakeholders. The literature states that the main concern of halal tourism is the role of certification in convincing tourists and a clear standardization of halal certification (Faiza & Michelle, 2017; Bazazo, Elyas, Awawdeh, Faroun, & Qawasmeh, 2017; Nassar, Mostafa, & Reisinger, 2015; Gabdrakhmanov, Biktimirov, Rozhko, & Khafizova, 2016). The final response that the researcher reviewed from previous findings was to hold an international conference and reaffirm the spirit of reviving the Muslim-friendly travel sector in ASEAN countries.

Other Sector Responses (Halal Food, Modest Fashion, Halal Pharmaceuticals, Halal Cosmetics, Halal Media, and Recreation)

The halal sector is a new type. This sector is diverse, complex, yet integrated with a global reach that crosses geographic, cultural, and religious boundaries. The halal market's potential in ASEAN is huge because most people are Muslim and are starting to realize the importance of a halal lifestyle. Even non-Muslims are starting to be interested in following the halal lifestyle. The State of the Global Islamic Economics notes that there are four ASEAN countries included in the Top 10 category of other halal sectors. There are two countries in the Top 10 halal food: Malaysia is in the second place, and Brunei is in the eighth place. There are three countries in the Top 10 Modest Fashion: Indonesia at the third, Malaysia at fourth, and Singapore at fifth place. With regard to Top 10 Media and Recreation, there are three countries: Malaysia is in the second, Brunei the sixth, and Singapore the seventh place. The last one is Top 10 Pharma and Cosmetics; there are three countries: Malaysia in the second, Singapore in fourth, and Brunei in eighth place. Out of a total of five sectors, only Malaysia ranks in all of the Top 10 categories. This is an outstanding achievement. Malaysia can be one of the trendsetting countries in the Islamic economy sector in ASEAN.

Despite the shock of the COVID-19 condition and the drastic drop in world oil prices, Brunei is still actively responding to the risk of a pandemic. In the Islamic economic sector, namely halal food, media, and recreation, as well as pharma and cosmetics, Brunei through the Brunei Darussalam Authority (AMBD), the central bank, the Ministry of Finance and Economy (MOFE), and the Brunei Bank Association (BAB) agreed to support the economy including the leading sector of Islamic Economics (Wong et al., 2020). Among them are (1) a six-month delay in financing payments to the tourism, hospitality, halal food, pharma, and cosmetics sectors; (2) the suspension extends to importers of food and medical supplies; and (3) all bank fees and fees except third-party fees related to trading transactions and payments for this sector are waived for a period of six months (Haqqi & Hidayati, 2020).

It is imperative to stimulate and map the halal market's rise by looking at the evidence from the field and looking to future progress. Indonesia, Malaysia, Singapore, Brunei, and Thailand respond quickly to the halal market's potential by providing products and services with values that comply with Sharia. Its main values are recommended products (mandub) and products that are not considered disgraceful (makruh) (Kamali, 2010). As stated in the Halal Industry Development Strategy, support for the halal market improves the quality of creative micro, small, and medium enterprises (MSMEs). This is a form of response from these countries, which has lasted until the COVID-19 pandemic occurred. And until now, it is still being encouraged and has even penetrated the digital halal market or e-commerce supported by the Sharia Supervisory Board and government policies. This is done to adjust to the pandemic. The existence of restrictions on economic activity outside the home requires the halal sector to carry out digital transformation and remain productive at home.

Of the five other Islamic economy sectors, namely halal food, modest fashion, halal pharmaceuticals, halal cosmetics, halal media, and recreation, two of them are experiencing an economic downturn, namely fashion and halal cosmetic models. To encourage people's purchasing power, the digital sector has become an enabler in post-pandemic cluster development. Fashion products display e-commerce platforms to virtual fashion shows as a form of response to limitations due to the pandemic.

The halal food, halal pharmaceuticals, and halal media and recreation sectors can survive and become an alternative to meet the domestic community's needs by using e-commerce as a supporting factor. Halal food received a good response in the minority Muslim consumer market and the majority of non-Muslim consumers (Wibowo & Ahmad, 2016). Halal food's potential will increase as Muslim spending on food and beverages is projected to grow by 6.3% compound annual growth rate (CAGR) to $2.0 trillion in 2024 (Dinar Standard, 2020). The literature explains that globally consumer satisfaction and intention towards halal products are increasing every year (Olya & Al-ansi, 2018). The halal logo gets special attention from the public, especially during a pandemic. Even though the crisis period is ongoing, people still pay attention to whether their food products are halal or not. What is clear is that the Islamic economic caravan is gaining momentum thanks to its halal products, which spread vertically and horizontally globally (Wilson, 2014). Increasing public awareness of food quality and health problems has positioned halal products as an attribute of credence. The halal logo's credibility can be a big opportunity in the future (Samori, Ishak, & Kassan, 2014).

Unfortunately, it is predicted that if social distancing restrictions continue, especially in the capital and big cities, this industry is threatened with bankruptcy. Previous studies have revealed that the halal sector's challenges are gaps in knowledge, differences of opinion, and the main concerns that look to the future need to be addressed through continuous progress (Wilson, 2012). Furthermore, issues of Islamic legislation and jurisprudence are debated in global articles. Therefore, there needs to be special attention to the halal sector, especially in the dimensions of halal branding, halal certification, supply chain, and Islamic marketing. This can support the response of the halal sector in encouraging economic recovery in ASEAN countries.

It is commendable that the Islamic economy has played a good role in supporting economic recovery and its ability to survive the COVID-19 situation. The findings revealed that of the seven Islamic economic sectors in five ASEAN countries, Islamic finance accounts for the largest response compared to the other six sectors. Reflecting on the neighboring countries outside ASEAN, namely Australia, it is essential to promote an approach based on justice and transparency based on Sharia for community resilience and preparedness. This aims to avoid social inequalities that can trigger conflict and hinder economic recovery. The government needs to ensure that Islamic finance and other sectors of the Islamic economy can boost the national economy.

Conclusion

Based on the literature study that has been conducted, the implications of COVID-19 have been quickly responded to by various sectors of the Islamic economy in the five ASEAN countries. The seven Islamic economic sectors published by the State of the Global Islamic Economy Report 2020 are (1) Islamic finance, (2) Muslim-friendly travel, (3) halal food, (4) modest fashion, (5) halal pharmaceuticals, (6) halal cosmetics, and (7) halal media and recreation. The biggest response was shown by Islamic finance and halal products. One of the policies that have been taken in the financial sector is a financial investment. Next is to provide financing, restructuring, and Islamic bank mergers. The six other sectors of the Islamic economy have shown a fairly good response to survive the pandemic.

The expected implication is that the Islamic economy can support the economic recovery affected by COVID-19. However, currently, only three ASEAN countries are included in the Top 15 Global Islamic Economy Indicator Score category in 2020, namely Malaysia, Indonesia, and Brunei. However, other ASEAN countries can provide the best response to increasing the halal market share. This is because several ASEAN countries such as

Thailand and Singapore have been included in the Top 10 Categories of other Islamic Economic Sectors. The government needs to develop infrastructure and capital support for Islamic finance and Islamic social finance, especially Islamic banks, which are still very young. Acceleration is needed for the development of innovations in Islamic economy products. Further research can be developed by analyzing the seven sectors of the Islamic economy with more complete and accurate data. This study encourages practitioners and academics to examine further the implications of COVID-19 for the Islamic economic response in various worlds. This study is included in the Top 15 Global Islamic Economy Indicator Score category. So that in the future, the Islamic economy will be able to make a greater contribution to the economy, especially in a situation of economic crisis like today.

References

Abror, A., Patrisia, D., Trinanda, O., Omar, M. W., & Wardi, Y., 2020. Antecedents of word of mouth in Muslim-friendly tourism marketing: The role of religiosity. *Journal of Islamic Marketing.* https://doi.org/10.1108/JIMA-01-2020-0006

Adzrin, R., Ahmad, R., Marzuki, A., Othman, A., & Sufiyudin, M., 2015. Assessing the satisfaction level of zakat recipients towards zakat assessing the satisfaction level of zakat recipients towards zakat management. *Procedia Economics and Finance,* *31*(May 2016), 140–151. https://doi.org/10.1016/S2212-5671(15)01141-7

Arif, A. A., & Zaim, M. A., 2020. The role of zakat institution in facing COVID-19: A case study of the federal territory islamic council (MAIWP) of Malaysia, (January).

BASNAZ, P. K. S.-B. A. Z. N., 2020. *OUTLOOK.* Jakarta Pusat: BAZNAS.

Bazazo, I., Elyas, T., Awawdeh, L., Faroun, M., & Qawasmeh, S., 2017. The impact of Islamic attributes of destination on destination loyalty via the mediating effect of tourist satisfaction. *International Journal of Business Administration,* *8*(4), 65. https://doi.org/10.5430/ijba.v8n4p65

Bodrud-Doza, M., Shammi, M., Bahlman, L., Islam, A. R. M. T., & Rahman, M. M., 2020. Psychosocial and socio-economic crisis in Bangladesh due to COVID-19 pandemic: A perception-based assessment. *Frontiers in Public Health,* *8*(June). https://doi.org/10.3389/fpubh.2020.00341

Chaffe, S. H., & Roser, C., 1986. Involvement and the consistency of knowledge, attitudes, and behaviors. *Communication Research,* *13*(3), 373–399. https://doi.org/10.1177/009365086013003006

Chaplin, J. P., 2004. *Kamus Lengkap Psikologi.* Jakarta: Raja Grafindo Persada.

Cheng, C., Barceló, J., Hartnett, A. S., Kubinec, R., & Messerschmidt, L., 2020. COVID-19 government response event dataset (CoronaNet v.1.0). *Nature Human Behaviour,* *4*(7), 756–768. https://doi.org/10.1038/s41562-020-0909-7

Ciancio, A., Bennett, D., Kapteyn, A., Kämpfen, F., Kohler, I. V., de Bruin, W. B., & Kohler, H. P., 2020. Know your epidemic, know your response: COVID-19 in the United States. *MedRxiv.* https://doi.org/10.1101/2020.04.09.20049288

Dinar Standard, 2020. *State of the global Islamic economy report 2019/20.* Dubai International Financial Centre, 1–174. Retrieved from https://cdn.salaamgateway .com/special-coverage/sgie19-20/full-report.pdf

Djalante, R., Lassa, J., Setiamarga, D., Sudjatma, A., Indrawan, M., Haryanto, B., & Warsilah, H., 2020. Review and analysis of current responses to COVID-19 in Indonesia: Period of January to March 2020. *Progress in Disaster Science, 6,* 100091. https://doi.org/10.1016/j.pdisas.2020.100091

Gabdrakhmanov, N. K., Biktimirov, N. M., Rozhko, M. V., & Khafizova, L. V., 2016. Problems of development of halal tourism in Russia. *Journal of Organizational Culture, Communications and Conflict, 20*(Special Issue 2), 88–93.

Ghaffour, A. R., 2020. Maximising Islamic finance for inclusive growth - from crisis to opportunity. *World Bank Islamic Finance Reports,* (October), 1–4. Retrieved from https://www.bis.org/review/r201007c.pdf

Greenwald, A. G., 1968. Cognitive learning, cognitive response to persuasion, and attitude change. *Psychological Foundations of Attitudes.* https://doi.org/10.1016 /b978-1-4832-3071-9.50012-x

Haneef, M. A., 2009. Developing the ethical foundations of Islamic economics: Benefitting from Toshihiko Izutsu, (July 2015).

Haqqi, A. R. A., & Hidayati, N., 2020. Brunei Darussalam's response to mitigate COVID-19 economic fallouts. Retrieved February 24, 2021, from https:// salaamgateway.com/story/brunei-darussalams-response-to-mitigate-COVID-19 -economic-fallouts

Harahap, Z. A. A., 2014. Konsep Maqasid Al-Syariah Sebagai Dasar Penetapan Dan Penerapannya Dalam Hukum Islam Menurut 'Izzuddin Bin 'Abd Al-Salam (W.660 H). *Tazkir, 9,* 171–190.

Henderson, J. C., 2016. Muslim travellers, tourism industry responses and the case of Japan. *Tourism Recreation Research, 41*(3), 339–347. https://doi.org/10.1080 /02508281.2016.1215090

Iqbal, Z., & Mirakhor, A., 2015. Key virtues of business ethics in Islam. *Ethical Dimensions of Islamic Finance,* 61–80. https://doi.org/10.1007/978-3-319 -66390-6

Jumaa, M. A. A. M. S., 2016. Islamic finance in theory and practice. *Chinese Business Review, 15*(7), 334–355.

Kamali, M. H., 2010. The Halal industry from Shariah perspective. *Islam and Civilisational Renewal, 1*(4), 595–612.

Karamouzian, M., & Madani, N., 2020. COVID-19 response in the Middle East and North Africa: Challenges and paths forward. *The Lancet Global Health, 8*(7), e886–e887. https://doi.org/10.1016/S2214-109X(20)30233-3

Kavanagh, M. M., & Singh, R., 2020. Democracy, capacity, and coercion in pandemic response: COVID-19 in comparative political perspective. *Journal of Health Politics, Policy and Law, 45*(6), 997–1012. https://doi.org/10.1215/03616878 -8641530

Kim, S., Koh, K., & Xuan, Z., 2020. Short-term impacts of COVID-19 on consumption and labor market outcomes: Evidence from Singapore, 1–45. Available at SSRN 3612738. Retrieved from https://www.econstor.eu/bitstream/10419/223796 /1/dp13354.pdf

Liu, Y.-C., Li, I.-J., Yen, S.-Y., & Sher, P. J., 2018. What makes Muslim friendly tourism? An empirical study on destination image, tourist attitude and travel intention. *Advances in Management & Applied Economics, 8*(5), 27–43.

Mackworth-Young, C. R. S., Chingono, R., Mavodza, C., McHugh, G., Tembo, M., Chikwari, C. D., & Ferrand, R. A., 2021. Community perspectives on the COVID-19 response, Zimbabwe. *Bulletin of the World Health Organization*, 99(2), 85–91. https://doi.org/10.2471/BLT.20.260224

McQuail, D., 1987. *Mass communication theory: An introduction.* New York: Sage Publications, Inc.

McQuail, D., & Windahl, S., 2015. *Communication models for the study of mass communications.* New York: Taylor & Francis.

Nassar, M. A., Mostafa, M. M., & Reisinger, Y., 2015. Factors influencing travel to Islamic destinations: An empirical analysis of Kuwaiti nationals. *International Journal of Culture, Tourism, and Hospitality Research*, 9(1), 36–53. https://doi .org/10.1108/IJCTHR-10-2014-0088

O'Sullivan, D., Rahamathulla, M., & Pawar, M., 2020. The impact and implications of COVID-19: An Australian perspective. *The International Journal of Community and Social Development*, 2(2), 134–151. https://doi.org/10.1177 /2516602620937922

Olya, H. G. T., & Al-ansi, A., 2018. Risk assessment of halal products and services: Implication for tourism industry. *Tourism Management*, 65, 279–291. https:// doi.org/10.1016/j.tourman.2017.10.015

Pöyry, E., Pelkonen, M., Naumanen, E., & Laaksonen, S. M., 2019. A call for authenticity: Audience responses to social media influencer endorsements in strategic communication. *International Journal of Strategic Communication*, 13(4), 336–351. https://doi.org/10.1080/1553118X.2019.1609965

Sabri, A., 2004. *Psikologi Umum dan Perkembangan.* Jakarta: Pedoman Jaya.

Salman, A., & Nawaz, H., 2018. Islamic financial system and conventional banking: A comparison. *Arab Economic and Business Journal*, 13(2), 155–167. https://doi .org/10.1016/j.aebj.2018.09.003

Samori, Z., Ishak, A. H., & Kassan, N. H., 2014. Understanding the development of Halal food standard: Suggestion for future research. *International Journal of Social Science and Humanity*, 4(6), 482–486. https://doi.org/10.7763/ijssh .2014.v4.403

Schuchat, A., 2020. Public health response to the initiation and spread of pandemic COVID-19 in the United States, February 24–April 21, 2020. *The COVID-19 Reader*, 69(18), 142–151. https://doi.org/10.4324/9781003141402-16

Sharma, G. D., Talan, G., & Jain, M., 2020. Policy response to the economic challenge from COVID-19 in India: A qualitative enquiry. *Journal of Public Affairs*, 20(4). https://doi.org/10.1002/pa.2206

Sipior, J. C., 2020. Considerations for development and use of AI in response to COVID-19. *International Journal of Information Management*, 55, 102170. https://doi.org/10.1016/j.ijinfomgt.2020.102170

Stivers, T., & Rossano, F., 2010. Mobilizing response. *Research on Language and Social Interaction*, 43(1), 3–31. https://doi.org/10.1080/08351810903471258

Subandi, A., 1982. *Psikologi Sosial.* Jakarta: Bulan Bintang.

Syafira, F. N., Ratnasari, R. T., & Ismail, S., 2020. The effect of religiosity and trust on intention to pay in Ziswaf collection through digital payments. *Jurnal Ekonomi Dan Bisnis Islam (Journal of Islamic Economics and Business)*, 6(1), 98. https:// doi.org/10.20473/jebis.v6i1.17293

Tkalac Verčič, A., Verčič, D., & Coombs, W. T., 2019. Convergence of crisis response strategy and source credibility: Who can you trust? *Journal of Contingencies and Crisis Management*, *27*(1), 28–37. https://doi.org/10.1111/1468-5973.12229

Walgito, B., 1996. *Pengantar Psikologi Umum*. Yogyakarta: Universitas Gadjah Mada Press.

Warren, M. S., & Skillman, S. W., 2020. *Mobility Changes in Response to COVID-19*. ArXiv.

Wibowo, M. W., & Ahmad, F. S., 2016. Non-Muslim consumers' Halal food product acceptance model. *Procedia Economics and Finance*, *37*(16), 276–283. https://doi.org/10.1016/s2212-5671(16)30125-3

Wilson, J. A., 2012. Charting the rise of the Halal market – tales from the field and looking forward Citation. *Journal of Islamic Marketing*, *3*(3), 57–77. https://doi.org/10.1108/jima.2012.43203caa.001

Wilson, J. A. J., 2014. Islamic economics 2.0 - creating a Halal wealth and knowledge economy. *Zawya*, 1–7. Retrieved from http://gala.gre.ac.uk/id/eprint/11418

Wong, J., Koh, W. C., Alikhan, M. F., Abdul Aziz, A. B. Z., & Naing, L., 2020. Responding to COVID-19 in Brunei Darussalam: Lessons for small countries. *Journal of Global Health*, *10*(1), 1–4. https://doi.org/10.7189/JOGH.10.010363

Yang, J., Teran, C., Battocchio, A. F., Bertellotti, E., & Wrzesinski, S., 2021. Building brand authenticity on social media: The impact of Instagram ad model genuineness and trustworthiness on perceived brand authenticity and consumer response. *Journal of Interactive Advertising*, *2021*. https://doi.org/10.1080/15252019.2020.1860168

11 Malaysia Border Security and Pandemic COVID-19

Ainuddin Iskandar Lee Abdullah

Introduction

In early December 2019, the first pneumonia cases of unknown origin were identified in Wuhan, the capital city of Hubei Province. The pathogen has been identified as a novel enveloped RNA beta coronavirus that has currently been named severe acute respiratory syndrome coronavirus 2 (SARS-CoV-2), which has a phylogenetic similarity to SARS-CoV. Patients with the infection have been documented both in hospitals and in family settings. The World Health Organization (WHO) has recently declared coronavirus disease 2019 (COVID-19) a public health emergency of international concern. As of February 25, 2020, a total of 81,109 laboratory-confirmed cases had been documented globally. In recent studies, the severity of some cases of COVID-19 mimicked that of SARS-CoV (W. Guan et al., 2020).

A new coronavirus disease, now known as COVID-19, was first identified in Wuhan, People's Republic of China (PRC), in early January 2020. From the information known at this point, several facts are pertinent. First, it belongs to the same family of coronaviruses that caused the severe acute respiratory syndrome (SARS) outbreak in 2003 and the middle east respiratory syndrome (MERS) outbreak in 2012.

Second, the mortality rate (number of deaths relative to the number of cases), which is as yet imprecisely estimated, is probably in the range of 1–3.4% – significantly lower than 10% for SARS and 34% for MERS, but substantially higher than the mortality rate for seasonal flu, which is less than 0.1%. Third, even though it emerged from animal hosts, it now spreads through human-to-human contact. The infection rate of COVID-19 appears to be higher than that for the seasonal flu and MERS, with the range of possible estimates encompassing the infection rates of SARS and Ebola (The Economic Impact of the COVID-19 Outbreak on Developing Asia, ADB Briefs. No. 128 March 2020).

Coronavirus disease 2019 (COVID-19) is a global pandemic. As of April 28, 2020, infected patients were present in 185 countries and there were more than 3,000,000 cases reported worldwide, with more than 210,000 fatalities. The outbreak began in China, but the number of cases outside of China exceeded those in China by March 15, 2020, and rose at an exponential rate (Kevin J. Clerkin, 2020).

DOI: 10.4324/9781003291909-12

The study of human mobility is one of the main factors that contribute to the worldwide dissemination of microorganisms. The spread of coronavirus disease 2019 (COVID-19) was recently reported to transmit to neighbouring countries with relocation diffusion. With most of the studies focusing on China, Western Europe and the USA, little is known about its evolution and genome variability in Southeast Asian (SEA) countries. SEA is home to more than half a billion or 9% of the world's population.

As the region grapples with a surge in infection cases since March 2020, it is important to investigate purported mutations and the role of geographical proximity in shaping the genetic structure of the SARS-CoV-2 in SEA countries. On March 4, 2020, the World Health Organization (WHO) outlined that only nine of the 11 countries have the capacity to test for COVID-19, suggesting that the lack of testing facilities could hinder the preparedness and response planning of these countries towards COVID-19. Among the SEA countries, Malaysia, Thailand and Singapore employ a large number of migrant workers, with Malaysia being the top importer with approximately 2.23 million people.

Concurrently, there has been a mass exodus of Malaysians seeking greater economic security in Singapore, with approximately 450,000 people crossing the Malaysia–Singapore border daily. The Indonesian authorities reported that more than 64,000 Indonesian migrant workers had returned from Malaysia amid the country's ongoing lockdown.

Another type of human mobility is refugees. The political instability which holds sway in Myanmar has forced 10% of the population to emigrate in search of refugees. More boats carrying Rohingya refugees were spotted off the coasts of Malaysia and southern Thailand, adding to the challenges faced by these countries fighting the pandemic outbreak. This trend of massive internal mobility is expected to continue as the countries ease the lockdown in the foreseeable future, continuously shifting the genetic drift of the viral population. Studies have shown that human migration (gene flow) is a remarkable factor to consider in virus evolution (Polly Soo Xi Yap et al., 2020).

With regard to the impact of border closures, almost all countries have responded to the spread of COVID-19 by closing borders and tightening immigration regimes. As options for cross-border movements dwindle, incoming migrants and travellers are pushed back or quarantined at borders and forced to stay in informal, overcrowded, and underserved transit sites, where they face threats to their health, dignity and survival. Border closures have made it virtually impossible for incoming asylum seekers to apply for international protection. International refugee resettlement operations have largely come to a halt due to increasing travel restrictions, despite some limited initiatives for the resettlement/ relocation of unaccompanied minors. Refusal of relevant countries to grant a safe port to rescue vessels and quarantines imposed on both migrants rescued at sea and the ships' crews of rescue vessels have further hindered rescue missions in the Central Mediterranean, increasing the risks that migrants face in what was already the most dangerous crossing in the world. People travelling abroad, or already in transit through a third country when travel bans were adopted, have found themselves unable to reach their destination – as was the case for over 25,000 Filipino outbound workers.

These disruptions might have far-reaching consequences for migrants and families who have borrowed money to pay recruiters and travel agents, only to find themselves unable to start a job and repay their debt. More generally, closed borders might push an increased number of people towards informal, more risky migration channels. Conversely, thousands of migrants and travellers worldwide have been stranded in countries that closed their borders. Prolonged travel bans might result in many of them having to overstay their visa. Migrants who were on home leave or travelling out of their host country (including for visa renewal) when the bans came into place might be unable to return to their job, their studies, their homes and families.

All over the world, lockdowns and border closures have sparked the return of migrants who have lost support and networks, employment options and ultimately the possibility of dignified living in places of destination due to the pandemic. Such movements create significant health risks both in migrants' home countries and communities and in locations in host and transit countries through which they travel. Few countries have managed to avoid the complete limitation of internal and international movements by investing in testing, contact tracing and isolation measures. Self-quarantine systems for incoming migrants, and quarantine facilities that comply with basic standards and protection principles, can in any case help avoid border closure and guarantee the application of the non-refoulement principle (Lorenzo Guadagno, 2020).

The first confirmed case of COVID-19 in Malaysia was detected on 25 January 2020. While the pandemic first spread slowly in Malaysia, there was a rapid rise in the number of confirmed cases in March, from 29 cases on 1 March to 2,766 by the end of the month. Following the enactment of the Movement Control Order (MCO) on 18 March, the number of new cases began to decline by mid-April and shrunk to double digits in most of May, suggesting that Malaysia had begun to flatten its epidemic curve. As of 1 June, Malaysia recorded a total of 7,857 confirmed cases of COVID-19. Initially, the Ministry of Health (MOH) released data on new cases by citizenship only intermittently.

On 25 April, it was announced that out of the total 14,187 foreign workers who tested for the virus, 676 tested positive. Compared with the country's tally of 5,742 then, this means foreign workers made up 11.8% of the total number of confirmed cases in Malaysia, proportionate to the size of non-citizens who make up a little over 10% of the population. Infections can only be confirmed through testing, which is key to tackling the pandemic. As of 25 April, the total number of tests carried out in Malaysia was 3.9 per 1,000 people. Compared with countries known for their mass testing such as Singapore (17.1) and South Korea (11.6), Malaysia still has much room for improvement in detecting the spread of COVID-19 in the country. The Singapore data was for 27 April, the closest date for the corresponding data for Malaysia. Testing foreign workers in Malaysia may be especially difficult as non-citizens are dispersed all over the country, with most being in Sabah (where 35.3% of non-citizens are located), Selangor (20.2%),

Johor (10.2%) and Kuala Lumpur (7.5%). COVID-19 cases may be particularly difficult to detect amongst undocumented foreign workers, as they fear making their presence known due to the possible legal ramifications.

Since May, there seems to be a rise in new cases among foreign workers in Malaysia. On 1 June, the MOH announced that out of the total 35,811 non-citizens tested for the virus, 2,014 were tested positive, constituting 25.6% of total cases. Though the data did not confirm that they were all foreign workers, this is likely the case given MOH's increased effort in targeted testing among foreign workers after learning from Singapore's experience. In general, the Malaysian government has provided limited assistance for the care of the country's foreign worker population. Senior Minister Datuk Seri Ismail Sabri Yaakob has made clear that the welfare of foreigners is the immediate responsibility of their respective embassies.

Based on his comments, the Malaysian government will offer support in terms of coordinating and purchasing supplies, if necessary. So far, one of the most prominent government initiatives related to foreign workers is the 25% cut for foreign worker levy introduced as part of the Prihatin Plus Economic Stimulus Package. This is extended to employers for payments due between April and December 2020, introduced mainly to alleviate the financial burden on hard-hit small- and medium-sized enterprises (SMEs). There are various estimations of the number of undocumented foreign workers, ranging from 1.2 million to 5 million. Non-citizens form the majority of cases in active clusters throughout May, including a factory cluster in Maran and Pedas, security guards cluster in Cheras, construction site clusters in two Kuala Lumpur areas and Setia Alam, a cleaning company cluster in Kuala Langat and Seremban, a plantation cluster in Bera, and clusters involving markets in Chow Kit, Pudu and Selayang. Furthermore, more than 400 cases were recorded in Bukit Jalil, Semenyih and Sepang immigration detention centres which are likely to house undocumented foreign workers.

By 1 June, the total number of tests carried out in Malaysia was 17.3 per 1,000 people. Several foreign institutions have stepped in to provide labour protection for foreign workers in Malaysia, given reports of unpaid wages and unfair terminations which have surfaced since the MCO. For example, the Bangladesh High Commission in Malaysia has been working with employers on salary issues, while the International Labour Organization (ILO) has been documenting labour and contractual violations committed by employers. As for access to COVID-19 testing and treatment for foreign workers, there has been somewhat conflicting messaging given by the Malaysian government throughout the pandemic.

In January, the MOH released a circular announcing that foreign workers who are suspected of being infected with the coronavirus or are close contacts of COVID-19 patients are exempted from COVID-19-related outpatient fees. However, on 23 March, the Prime Minister stated that foreign workers must pay for testing and treatment of COVID-19, in contradiction to MOH's policy, although the statement was quickly refuted.

Another measure related to testing among foreign workers is the introduction of a subsidy of RM150 to employers for each COVID-19 screening undertaken by foreign workers who are Social Security Organisation (SOCSO) contributors. The Malaysian government has also changed its stance on detaining undocumented migrants. In March, Datuk Seri Ismail Sabri Yaakob announced that undocumented migrants would not be arrested during this crisis; however, the immigration raids that have taken place since May indicate otherwise. Indeed, on 31 May, Datuk Seri Ismail Sabri Yaakob confirmed that amnesty for undocumented immigrants to get tested without legal repercussions had ended, meaning that the government would continue detaining undocumented migrants.

These migrants would be tested in detention centres, and if found positive, they will be moved to the quarantine centre at the Malaysia Agro Exposition Park Serdang (MAEPS) for treatment. For those not infected, they will be deported back to their home countries with the governments of Indonesia, Nepal and Bangladesh agreeing to receive them. As of mid-April, the Malaysian Trades Union Congress (MTUC) had reported several violations of migrant workers' labour rights, which include unfair termination, unpaid wages, poor living conditions, requiring workers to continue working in jobs that are non-essential, and uncertainty about employment status due to limited contact with employers. The MTUC has been following up on specific cases and filed complaints to the Labour Department for investigation.

Overall, help available to foreign workers in Malaysia has come in a fairly fragmented form, with the embassies, civil society organisations (CSOs), Malaysian Trades Union Congress (MTUC) and international organisations chipping in wherever the government has left out. This is not surprising given the assisting role the government has intentionally taken from the start when it comes to the welfare of foreigners. As such, despite the existing efforts taken by multiple parties, it is believed that without a systematic approach, aid is far from sufficient, and a large number of foreign workers, including those in hiding for fear of arrest as well as those in remote areas such as the plantation, manufacturing and domestic work, are bound to be left behind (Tan Theng Theng, Nazihah Muhamad Noor and Jarud Romadan Khalidi, 2020).

Although Malaysia has experienced vast economic development since independence, some of the neighbouring states' regions at the periphery of her borders are still lacking in terms of socioeconomic development. This has resulted in a flourishing black market economy in these areas that thrive on the smuggling of controlled items (in Malaysia) such as cigarettes, rice, fuel, small arms, illegal immigrants, human trafficking, and other criminal activities. The Northern borders of Peninsula Malaysia, the Straits of Malacca, the East Coast of Sabah (East Malaysia) and small portions in border areas of Sarawak (East Malaysia) with West Kalimantan (Indonesia) are critical entry points for such smuggling activities. Human trafficking and illegal entry of foreigners are mostly concentrated in the Northern borders of Peninsular Malaysia, East Coast of Sabah (East Malaysia) and the Straits of Malacca (Mohd Zaini Saleh, Adam Leong Kok Way, 2018).

Though the implementation of the Movement Control Order (MCO) has succeeded in controlling the spread of the disease within the country, the pandemic has brought about an influx of illegal foreign workers and immigrants, representing a significant challenge for Malaysia.

Two scenarios have led the Malaysian government to focus on border security enforcement amid the pandemic. First, rapid socioeconomic development has made Malaysia a major focus for foreign workers. With rising labour needs in various sectors such as manufacturing, construction and agriculture, the influx of illegal foreign workers has increased. However, due to their limited access to healthcare and sanitation systems, the possibility of these workers being infected with the new coronavirus now threatens the livelihood of the local population.

Second, Malaysia is a preferred destination for Rohingya immigrants; the country is an attractive location for the persecuted community from Myanmar as it is a Muslim-majority nation and has been a major recipient of Rohingyas for humanitarian reasons. It was estimated that 2,000 Rohingya individuals were screened for COVID-19 in Malaysia after participating in the mosque gathering in February 2020. The presence of this cluster has been more visible during the pandemic and the MCO period, with a number of boats carrying Rohingyas arriving at Malaysian shores. As a result, Malaysia has faced challenges in drawing a clear line between humanitarian assistance and national security (https://thediplomat.com/2020/06/COVID-19-is-reshaping-border-security-enforcement-in-malaysia/).

Strict border control is a necessary key to ensure that there is no COVID-19 import case, even though the government of Malaysia introduced the Conditional Movement Control Order (PKPB) to increase control at all border checkpoints.

Officers and security personnel also remain vigilant in monitoring any party attempting to smuggle into the country through various rat routes and illegal roads through forests and farms, which are also used for smuggling activities.

The task of controlling and guarding the entire country's borders is not an easy task, with about 3,000 km of land and sea borders over 4,600 km shared by Malaysia with neighbouring Thailand, Singapore, Brunei Darussalam, Indonesia, the Philippines and Vietnam. But that task needs to be done. It is reported that security personnel are now conducting inspections everywhere, in an effort to ensure that the border area is under control.

On the Perlis and Kedah border with Thailand, mostly the police force will conduct intelligence periodically to obtain information on the possible entry of foreigners into the country. Only individuals who have gone through the screening process conducted by the Ministry of Health can go to the Immigration counter. The operations at the Immigration, Customs, Quarantine and Security (ICQS) Complex in Bukit Kayu Hitam, including the Heavy Vehicle Complex and Light Vehicle Complex, went on as usual screening. More patrols are carried out in 'hotspot' areas such as Wang Kelian, Kuala Sanglang, Padang Besar and Chuping, especially in rat routes favoured by foreigners and smugglers. There was an increase in the smuggling of ketum leaves, with 8.4 tonnes worth RM472,000

seized in April 2020 (https://www.bharian.com.my/berita/nasional/2020/05
/684214/COVID-19-kawalan sempadan-kunci-elak-kes-import).

Tighter controls on the Malaysia–Thailand border in Kelantan by various
security agencies have helped to check the entry of foreigners and reduce the
smuggling of goods at the border. The Border Control Agency (AKSEM) has
always worked closely, especially since the Movement Control Order (PKP) came
into force on March 18. The cases of smuggling involving goods decrease within
three phases of PKP from March 18 to April 28. Patrols intensified in Pengkalan
Hulu, Perak, which is the Malaysia–Thailand border with Betong in the southern
Yala Province of Thailand. The security forces did strict monitoring on rat routes
used by foreigners and smugglers, especially in Ops Pagar 3 which covers the
Felda Lepang Nenering area, Ayer Panas. The stricter inspections were also carried out at the Immigration, Customs, Quarantine and Security Complex (ICQS)
in Bukit Berapat, Pengkalan Hulu, and apart from adding roadblocks at the com-
plex. The border operation was carried out jointly with the Criminal Investigation
Department, the Drug Crime Investigation Department and the Pengkalan Hulu
District Police together with the Border Control Agency (AKSEM).

In an effort to effectively enforce the PKP, the Sabah Marine Police has implemented an operational action plan looking at the establishment of 14 checkpoints
at sea, to tighten border controls on the entry of foreigners, smuggling, illegal
fishing by foreign fishermen, kidnapping and cross-border crime.

The Sabah Region Marine Police monitoring the maritime security has mobi-
lised border control operations in Indonesia via Sungai Tawau recently. Tawau has
become a stopover centre for crabs that are trusted by the international market.
Sarawak also increases assets to further enhance border control in the Kalimantan
area, Indonesia, during the PKP to prevent the entry of illegal immigrants into
Sarawak. Additional focus on Long Singut, Kapit Division, which has the closest
settlement to the Sarawak–Kalimantan border in the interior of the state.

With tighter border controls, health authorities can be confident that no one
will smuggle into Malaysia carrying COVID-19 and start a new cluster in the
country. The Malaysian Armed Forces (ATM) is constantly strengthening the
country's maritime, land and airspace borders, making it a priority to ensure the
peace and sovereignty of the country is always preserved.

Although the country was facing a contagious COVID-19 epidemic situation, the border control operation was further tightened following the instructions of the government. The order was issued to prevent illegal immigrants from
crossing the country's borders through 'rat lanes,' thus preventing them from
bringing in the COVID-19 epidemic. The integrated operation was also named
Operation Fortress which involved ATM personnel and assets in addition to
security agencies and other enforcement officers including the Royal Malaysian
Police (PDRM), the Malaysian Maritime Enforcement Agency, the Ministry of
Health, the Malaysian Civil Defense Force, the Immigration Department and the
Malaysian Volunteer Department (RELA). The operation also involved the assis-
tance and operations of other agencies, namely the Malaysian Fire and Rescue
Department, the Malaysian Border Control Agency, the Malaysian Marine

Department and the Customs Department and the National Anti-Drug Agency (AADK) (https://www.hmetro.com.my/mutakhir/2020/05/578656/per-ketat-kawalan-sempadan-elak-kluster-baharu-COVID-19-metrotv).

The matter proves that the government is able to overcome and restrict the entry of illegal immigrants through rat lanes and national borders. In addition, the government has identified rat lanes, among others on the West Coast of the Peninsula, the East Coast of Sabah such as Semporna and Lahad Datu as well as in Sarawak.

The International Law Enforcement Agency and the Anti-Tobacco Action Team, the Australian Border Team praised Malaysia's efforts to strengthen border control as the COVID-19 pandemic was raging. The directive was not only an initiative to control the spread of viruses across countries but also had the potential to stop or reduce illegal trade. The agency's consultant, Rohan Pike, mentioned that the Malaysia's government was taking serious strategies to combat the spread of the COVID-19 pandemic at the international border. As law enforcement, the easy-going borders not only threatened the security of a country and the health of the people but also damaged the economy through the proliferation of illegal trade. The Malaysian border was filled with so many rat lanes that allowed illegal or undocumented visitors from foreign countries to invade Malaysia and potentially carry the COVID-19 virus. With the implementation of the Movement Control Order (PKP), it is the right time to refocus on efforts to tighten the Malaysian border to prevent unwanted visitors and products from entering the country.

The International Chamber of Commerce (ICC) in 2017 found that global trade in counterfeit and pirated goods was estimated to generate between AUD 923 billion (RM4 trillion) and AUD 1.13 trillion (RM4.9 trillion) a year covering cross-border trade, domestic trade and print digital robbery. Recently, the Brand Advocacy and Retail Trade (RTBA) report showed that the continued illegal tobacco trade resulted in significant revenue losses to governments and legitimate businesses in the Asia-Pacific region (https://www.hmetro.com.my/mutakhir/2020/04/567344/perketat-sempadan-mampu-kawal-penularan-COVID-19-perdagangan-haram).

The border between Singapore and Malaysia, before COVID-19 restrictions were in place, more than 300,000 people, many of them Malaysians working in Singapore, crossed the land checkpoints between the two countries daily. While some Malaysian workers have remained in Singapore since the Movement Control Order came into force on March 18 – resulting in families being separated – others are stuck in Malaysia, which has affected Singapore businesses that rely on Malaysian manpower. Both countries take into account the required health protocols and available medical resources in both countries to ensure the safety of citizens of both sides well executed the pandemic of COVID-19 (https://www.thestar.com.my/aseanplus/aseanplus-news/2020/07/26/COVID-19 singapore-malaysia-travel-arrangements-for-permit-holders-business-travellers-finalised).

The government formed the National Task Force (NTF) to manage illegal entry to Malaysia. The Malaysian Armed Forces (MAF) was given the mandate to coordinate an integrated operation with other security enforcement agencies within the NTF. The main elements that drive this task force are the MAF, the Royal Malaysian Police (RMP) and the Malaysian Maritime Enforcement Agency (MMEA). Aside from the main three main security enforcement agencies, close cooperation and strong collaboration with other government agencies, such as the Malaysian Immigration Department, Royal Malaysian Customs, the Civil Defense Agency, the Ministry of Health and the Malaysian Border Security Agency, have been implemented (https://thediplomat.com/2020/06/COVID -19-is-reshaping-border-security-enforcement-in-malaysia/).

The NTF was formed as an integrated operation to carry out tasks assigned by the government. It is responsible for developing a plan by gathering all the information, coordinating security measures, and monitoring the illegal encroachment of immigrants and undocumented foreign workers at all entrances and border areas of the country both by land and by sea. The operation identified corridors in the West Coast of Peninsular Malaysia, the East Coast of Sabah and along the inland border of Sarawak. Managing and executing remedial actions immediately and effectively during the COVID-19 pandemic is crucial. With the newly established task force, it is clear that Malaysia seeks to implement new mechanisms to deal with illegal border crossings as part of its disease control response. Sharing information and domain awareness is a step in the right direction in addressing pandemic border security in Malaysia (https://thediplomat.com/2020/06/COVID-19-is-reshaping-border-security-enforcement-in-malaysia/).

The RTBA report entitled Illegal Tobacco in the Asia-Pacific region: causes and conclusions found that in terms of turnover alone, the total tax loss in all 19 markets in the region monitored was over USD 5.8 billion (RM25.3 billion) in 2017. Almost 50% of it happens in only two markets namely Australia and Malaysia. The impact of the illegal tobacco trade alone has resulted in huge losses to the economy, and the prevalence of this problem stems from border security which is less effective in the region. More than 50% of smuggled cigarettes in Malaysia entered ports and rat lanes while ironically in Australia more than 40% of the products were imported from or unloaded ships through Malaysia.

In fact, the latest news reports showed that smugglers used food delivery services or e-hailing to distribute contraband cigarettes during PKP because legitimate cigarette manufacturers were not allowed to distribute cigarettes. Most of these smuggled cigarettes come from outside the Malaysian border. If border security is not tightened, the increase in smuggled cigarettes will be so robust, making it almost impossible to eradicate it. It will damage the country socioeconomically. As a result, the government's loss in terms of tax revenue was not collected due to smuggled cigarettes, which is currently at the level of RM5 billion a year.

Early in September 2020, Malaysia National Task Force (NTF) made 28 arrests in Operation Fortress after detaining 83 illegal immigrants. The operation involved various enforcement agencies of the country to control the country's borders in an integrated manner from being booed by illegal immigrants to curb cross-border crime, besides blocking the spread of COVID-19. The operations under NTF involved the Malaysian Armed Forces (ATM), the Royal Malaysian Police (PDRM), the Malaysian Maritime Enforcement Agency (APMM) and the Malaysian Border Control Agency. The 171st Rehabilitation Control Order (PKP) and the 87th day of the Rehabilitation Movement Control Order (PKPP) have been implemented (https://www.hmetro.com.my/mutakhir/2020/09/617146/kawalan-sempadan-diperketat-elak-penularan-COVID-19).

In the position of combating the matter, government instructions to all relevant enforcement agencies such as the Royal Malaysian Police (PDRM), the Malaysian Armed Forces (ATM), the Royal Malaysian Customs Department (JKDM) and the Malaysian Immigration Department (JIM) to tighten border security were appropriate. The attention to border security increased not only to control the COVID-19 pandemic to save lives but also to business.

In addition to mobilising relevant agencies, the Malaysian government also looks at aspects of enhancing cross-border intelligence sharing and monitoring to identify and close the rat route with advanced technology such as drones, scanners and the latest CCTV can also be used in areas that are suspected to be such illegal routes. It aims to prevent illegal immigrants from crossing the rat lane at the country's borders, thus giving space to bring COVID-19 into the country. Along the country's borders, there are rat lanes used by foreigners to get out and enter our country. All agencies involved were responsible to tighten control along the country's borders. Strict border control by the Malaysian government has given the community confidence that in such a way, it can curb the spread of COVID-19 in border areas and at the same time creates a safe environment for re-energising economic and social activities in the country.

References

Kevin J. Clerkin, Justin A. Fried, Jayant Raikhelkar, Gabriel Sayer, Jan M. Griffin, Amirali Masoumi, Sneha S. Jain, Daniel Burkhoff, Deepa Kumaraiah, LeRoy Rabbani, Allan Schwartz, Nir Uriel, 2020. In Depth COVID-19 and Cardiovascular Disease. https://www.ahajournals.org/doi/pdf/10.1161/CIRCULATIONAHA.120.046941.

Lorenzo Guadagno, 2020. Migrants and the COVID-19 Pandemic: An Initial Analysis. *International Organization for Migration*. Migration Research Series, No 60. https://publications.iom.int/system/files/pdf/mrs-60.pdf

Mohd Zaini Salleha, Adam Leong Kok Wey, 2018. Shut the Door! Military Cooperation at the Borders: Malaysian Initiatives and Capabilities. *ZULFAQAR International Journal of Defence Management, Social Science & Humanities*, 1(1): 1–10. National Defence University of Malaysia, Kuala Lumpur.

Polly Soo Xi Yap, Tse Siang Tan, Yoke Fun Chan, Kok Keng Tee, Adeeba Kamarulzaman, Cindy Shuan Ju Teh, 2020. An Overview of the Genetic Variations of the SARS-CoV-2 Genomes Isolated in Southeast Asian Countries. *Journal of Microbiology and Biotechnology*, 30(7): 962–966. https://doi.org/10.4014/jmb.2006.06009

Tan Theng Theng, Nazihah Muhamad Noor, Jarud Romadan Khalidi, 2020. June. Discussion Paper 8/20. COVID-19: We Must Protect Foreign Workers.

Khazanah Research Institute. International Organization for Migration, Route des Morillons. Geneva.

W. Guan, Z. Ni, Yu Hu, W. Liang, C. Ou, J. He, L. Liu, H. Shan, C. Lei, D.S.C. Hui, B. Du, L. Li, G. Zeng, K.-Y. Yuen, R. Chen, C. Tang, T. Wang, P. Chen, J. Xiang, S. Li, Jin-lin Wang, Z. Liang, Y. Peng, L. Wei, Y. Liu, Ya-hua Hu, P. Peng, Jian-ming Wang, J. Liu, Z. Chen, G. Li, Z. Zheng, S. Qiu, J. Luo, C. Ye, S. Zhu, N. Zhong, 2020. Clinical Characteristics of Coronavirus Disease 2019 in China. *The New England Journal of Medicine.* Massachusetts Medical Society. https://www.nejm.org/doi/pdf/10.1056/nejmoa2002032

12 The Securitization of the Coronavirus Crisis in Jordan

Saud Al-Sharafat

Introduction

The coronavirus spread to Jordan on March 2, 2020, when the Prime Minister of Jordan Omar Razzaz reported the first case of coronavirus in Jordan.[1] The Government responded immediately; the Ministry of Health launched an official website to provide reliable information about COVID-19 from a standardized source. The website aims to disseminate awareness and care within all groups of society by providing information about the virus, how it is spread, its signs and symptoms, and methods of prevention, as well as the procedures in cases of suspected COVID-19 infection and reducing its risk, and hotline: 111.[2] And there is a portal for all government platforms related to dealing with COVID-19: http://one.gov.jo.

On 6 March, the Jordanian government made an agreement with Facebook to launch an awareness campaign regarding COVID-19. Facebook will present all site visitors from within the Kingdom with links to the Ministry of Health website promoting its content intended to increase awareness of the outbreak, preventative measures and tips to reduce the spread, and the dedicated facilities for testing and treatment.[3]

On March 17, Jordan's King Abdullah II issued, A "Royal Decree" approving the cabinet's decision to announce the implementation of the National Defence Law No. 13 of 1992 in Jordan, as of Wednesday, 17 March. Article 2 of the Defense Law explains its objectives. It stipulates that

> upon a decision and a Royal Decree, a National Defence Law shall be passed in case of emergency that would threaten the "national security" or public safety in all parts of the Kingdom or in a region due to war, disturbances, armed internal strife, public disasters or the spread of a pest or epidemic.

To implement the "National Defence Law No. 13 of 1992," King Abdullah sent a letter to Prime Minister Omar Razzaz. Following is the English translation:

[In the name of God, the Compassionate, the Merciful,

Your Excellency Dr Omar Razzaz,

The Prime Minister,

DOI: 10.4324/9781003291909-13

Peace, God's mercy and blessings be upon you,

I convey to you and your colleagues my greetings and deep thanks and appreciation for your efforts, in coordination with the various state institutions, to address these exceptional conditions facing our dear nation.

As the challenges arising from the global conditions caused by the spread of the novel coronavirus obligate us to protect the health and wellbeing of our fellow Jordanians and ensure their safety; and as part of our commitment to this responsibility; we have decreed the approval of the Cabinet's recommendation to proclaim the activation of the Defence Law number 13 for the year 1992, out of our keenness to ensure the continuation of exerted efforts and remove any obstacles that may arise while countering this plight.

I hereby direct the Government to ensure that the implementation of the Defence Law and the orders issued under it will be within the most limited scope possible, without infringing on Jordanians' political and civil rights, but, rather, safeguarding them and protecting public liberties and the right to self-expression enshrined in the Constitution and in accordance with regular laws currently in effect, and guaranteeing the respect of private property, be it real estate, or movable and immovable funds.

For the goal of promulgating this exceptional law is to provide an additional tool to safeguard public health, protect the wellbeing of citizens, enhance performance, and increase coordination among all to counter this epidemic.

Your Excellency,

Since the start of this pandemic, I have been closely following the minutest of details regarding its spread and means to counter it, and I have directed the Government to take pre-emptive measures, set plans, and implement procedures to safeguard our nation and our citizens as the top priority. These measures, with God's grace, have proven effective.

My faith in the awareness of Jordanians is unwavering. They have proven, time and again, to be up to that trust, and I fully believe, from what I have observed, that they are the main pillar in addressing the current exceptional circumstances and countering this epidemic and preventing its spread by following instructions and adhering to regulations that all serve the sole purpose of safeguarding their health and wellbeing.

It would be remiss not to commend the efforts of all those working in the Government and our civil, military, and security agencies, which have had a tangible effect on citizens' trust. And I reaffirm my pride in the level of public awareness in dismissing rumours that serve no purpose beyond undermining the effectiveness of these efforts.

Your Excellency,

The measures taken to alleviate the impact on citizens and meet their needs for healthcare, education, and basic commodities are effective and necessary. The Government must step up and continue efforts to mitigate burdens on citizens, and take the necessary measures to safeguard and maintain their health, wellbeing, and living requirements, through effective coordination among the various relevant state institutions.

The Government must also take all the measures needed to sustain the private sector and its institutions, while maintaining the operation of public facilities, particularly those that serve citizens.

I would like to express my pride in the personnel of the Jordan Armed Forces-Arab Army and security agencies, as well as every doctor, nurse, and technical and administrative staff member working in our medical institutions, for their great efforts amidst these conditions.

Once again, I reaffirm that the health of Jordanians is a sacred matter, and their wellbeing is above all else. They are at the top of my priorities, and we must all work diligently to counter this plight, which we will overcome, with God's support, and with the awareness of our dependable people.

May God protect Jordan and Jordanians, and grant us success in serving our dear people.

Peace, God's mercy and blessings be upon you.

Abdullah II ibn Al Hussein

Amman, 22 Rajab 1441 Hijri

17 March 2020].[4]

The Prime Minister Omar Razzaz pledged to carry it out to the "narrowest extent" and stated that it would not impinge on political rights, freedom of expression, or private property, and the Jordanian government announced several precautionary measures.

On March 20, 2020, the Jordanian government declared a state of emergency as part of a series of measures to limit the spread of COVID-19, the Prime Minister imposed a mandatory curfew pursuant to the law. Violation of the curfew is punishable by up to one year in prison. The Public Security Directorate said it had arrested 693 individuals for violating the curfew on March 21.[5]

The king's Royal Decree – was the turning point and the milestone in Jordan's march towards the implementation of securitization. That's why I prefer to cite it as it is because I think it is the basis on which Jordan today applies its own securitization model.

On May 11, 2020, King Abdullah, chairing a National Policies Council (NPC) meeting attended by Crown Prince Al Hussein bin Abdullah II, the King called for stricter health measures on all border crossings to prevent the spread of coronavirus disease (COVID-19) in Jordan and called for plans to ensure private sector institutions retain their employees and stressed the importance of devising a comprehensive plan for distance learning for schools and universities, as well as a plan for holding exams for secondary school and university students during the current exceptional circumstances.[6]

Importantly, the King delivered the speech in military uniform so the Crown Prince.

Securitization Theory

Securitization in international relations theory can be conceptualized as a particular kind of speech act that elevates issues of concern above normal politics. "Securitization," relay deeply on the "Copenhagen School of security studies" (CS), which places particular emphasis on the non-military aspects of security, representing a shift away from traditional security studies.[7]

Within the analysis of securitization, one must ask: first, "who" securitizes; then, what is the referent of the securitization act (i.e., the state, people, the environment, the civilization); and then, what is the threat. The social constructivist framework of securitization analysis, then, also rests on the idea of an inter-subjective space. Thus, how audiences understand and give consent to securitization speech acts is at least as important as "who" speaks security; the act of securitization is negotiated between securitizer and audience." Theorists associated with the school include Barry Buzan, Ole Waever, and Jaap de Wilde.[8]

Essentially, securitization means

> the process of state actors transforming subjects into matters of "security": an extreme version of politicization that enables extraordinary means to be used in the name of security. Issues that become securitized do not necessarily represent issues that are essential to the objective survival of a state, but rather represent issues where someone was successful in constructing an issue into an existential problem. Securitization is a "rule-governed practice, the success of which does not necessarily depend on the existence of a real threat, (i.e. Coronavirus pandemic) but on the discursive ability to effectively endow a development with such a specific complexion.[9]

Therefore, "Ole Waever" emphasized that security is a speech act with distinct consequences in the context over international politics. By making use of speech act, a (state) actor tries to move a topic away from politics into an area of security concerns, thereby legitimating extraordinary means against the socially constructed threat.[10]

Over the past decades, the securitization of health had been claimed to be a permanent feature of public health governance in the 21st century.[11] So it is worth to emphasize that threat posed by infectious diseases has been increasingly framed as a security issue.[12] The UN Security Council's Resolution 1308, which designated HIV/AIDS as a threat to international security, evidenced the securitization process. The World Health Organization (WHO) has tended to securitize infectious diseases since 2000.[13]

At the same time, previous academic studies have "explored the securitization of past pandemics. Many of these focus on the failures to securitize the pandemic or on the normative implications of securitization."[14] However, despite this existing engagement with securitization theory, existing literature has paid less attention to global health issues as security threats in Jordan and the Middle East.[15]

Securitization Processes in Jordan

Macrosecuritization

The idea of macrosecuritization as a higher-level securitization, which provides an overarching context through which to interpret and prioritize different perceived threats.[16] Without any exaggeration, the virus crisis was "globally politicized" and become a matter of countries image, and political competition after its spread. WHO itself did not respond to questions about whether it has in some cases provided political cover for authoritarian governments concerned about negative media coverage on the coronavirus.[17]

I believe that "Macrosecuritization" buds grow and flourish up in the womb of globalization. In an increasingly globalized world, health challenges (like coronavirus) can "no longer afford being solved by the health sector alone. Coronavirus Shown that contagions have an innate ability to transcend national borders and alter life faster than any other menace known to humankind."[18]

Jordan is a deeply globalized country with the de facto rank (38) for 2019 in the world,[19] but unfortunately this led to one negative effect of globalization processes, which made the political system structure fragile in the face of the effects of globalization.

So in the milieu of macrosecuritization, Jordan has sought to improve his image in front of citizens and the world through extensive media campaigns and publicity (speech acts) about the effectiveness and accuracy of the actions it has taken quickly to contain and address the virus crisis.

In consequence, "as an exceptional condition facing the nation," Jordan introduced and implemented some of the toughest anti-coronavirus measures in the world. These measures included an indefinite curfew, a one-year prison sentence for those who violated it and the closing of all businesses in Jordan, in addition to the direct supervision of the return of Jordanians and students through airports to Jordan, and the preparation of quarantine places for them in hotels and caravans at a quarantine center in the Dead Sea.

But despite these exceptional conditions, there have also been positive social changes as the country has sought to respond to the crisis. Increasing social solidarity and cooperation between neighbors and citizens, especially in relation to Jordan's distinct Arab communities such as Iraqis and Egyptians, is all visible in the wake of the crisis. Moreover, there has been a strong adherence to Jordanian regulations and laws, along with many going above and beyond by donating to Jordanian sovereign funds. These trends have the potential of remaining even after the end of the crisis if they are cultivated and encouraged.[20]

The Securitization Dilemma

The "securitization dilemma" describes the situation when "securitizing an issue in one sector negatively impacts upon another sector. This creates a dilemma for the securitizer as to whether they should securitize the issue or not?"[21]

Healthcare has long been treated

> as a less important political priority. Despite widely available literature, and the precedent of global health catastrophes, healthcare continues to be treated as a mere "soft" issue in the framework of international and domestic politics alike. International relations have long been defined by numerical variables, where national interests are attached to economical values and reinforced with multilateral agreements to protect an economic interest. This restricted perspective frequently prioritized issues it viewed as being big enough over issues it deemed to be secondary.[22]

I believe that the securitization dilemma in the Jordanian experience lies in the process of trade-off between public healthcare and the economy, where Jordan (the securitizer) has chosen – as I will explain – to securitize the public healthcare. Therefore, since the beginning of the coronavirus spread to Jordan on March 2, 2020, the government has resorted to securitize the response to the coronavirus and turning the "public health" into a securitized sector, by a securitizer actor through reliance on speech acts (i.e., the utterances that label something as a security issue) to frame a threat (coronavirus) as a security issue.[23]

In his March 23 address to the nation, King Abdullah II applied the "act of speech" as a "securitising actor" in this vein during his remarks:

> My brothers and sisters, my family, my people, and my source of fortitude Over the past weeks, we have all seen our dear Jordanian brothers and sisters, each in their own capacities, rise to the challenge, working day and night to counter this threat. They stand united with their brothers and sisters in our armed forces, for the dignity (karamah) of Jordanians, the dignity all Jordanians have fought and sacrificed for, led by the martyrs and Nashama of the Arab Army and security agencies, to whom we proudly pay tribute on the anniversary of Karamah Battle, each and every one of you is a soldier of this nation, each in your own post.[24]

In discussing the posed by the virus, King Abdullah used the acts of speech

> the metaphor of war by invoking the *Battle of Karamah*,[25] which was marked in Jordan two days before, on March 21. 31 By invoking the Battle of Karamah, King Abdullah called on Jordanians to show the same spirit of bravery, honor, and sacrifice as the Jordanian soldiers had done fifty years earlier. The King said that today, each and every Jordanian "is a soldier" in Jordan's campaign against the virus. Importantly, the King delivered the speech in military uniform.[26]

All of these measures are implemented by the force of the Jordanian Armed Forces-Arab Army (JAF), Civil Defence Department (CDD), and security agencies according to the instructions issued by the "coronavirus crisis cell" at National Center for Security and Crisis Management,[27] further emphasizing the securitization of the threat."[28]

In coordination, Jordan

> employed (JAF), along with other security forces to deliver supplies such as food, water, oil, and other necessities to the various communities, especially Jordan's refugee camps. The (JAF) has proven instrumental not only in controlling and checking the movement of the population during this crisis but also in offering services.[29]

For Jordanians, the sight of JAF, along with police and security agencies deployment in the streets – including check points in all 12 Jordanian provinces – has solidified the image of coronavirus as a war military with police and security agencies' supervision of social distancing in the streets, and commercial movement has included in-person and drone monitoring of citizens' compliance with defense laws and ensure there are no violations of the curfew. Sirens call for a full curfew every day at 6 p.m.[30]

These clear securitization manifestations are notably unprecedented for many younger Jordanians. The appearance of army patrols as they roam the streets, on checkpoints, along with the isolation of Amman from the rest of the provinces and the closing of other provinces has not occurred since the 1970s. These previous measures were last implemented during the events of "the Black September, 1970"[31] and in the aftermath of the expulsion of Palestinian guerillas from Jordan.[32]

The sirens are reminiscent of the Second Gulf War, when Saddam Hussein fired Scud missiles against Israel in early 1991. As such, the current measures against coronavirus resemble the state's response to major security events in Jordanian history, further solidifying a sense of securitization.[33]

Even so, the state is also enacting other measures to counter the secondary effects of the lockdown, focusing particularly on its economic implications. Special fundraising efforts have solicited funds from institutions and individuals alike, establishing three specialized funds to support the Ministry of Health and affected sectors.[34]

The "Central Bank of Jordan" creates a package of precautionary measures in order to contain the negative repercussions of the pandemic on the performance of the local economy. Banks are now allowed to restructure the loans of individuals and companies, especially small and medium-sized loans, which have been affected by the repercussions of this virus. The Central Bank has also decided to inject additional liquidity to the national economy of 500 million dinars through reducing mandatory cash reserves, reducing the cost of financing, and increasing the time limits for existing and future facilities for economic sectors. This is all in addition to support for the Jordanian Loan Guarantee Company's procedures by reducing the commissions of the company's programs and raising the percentage of insurance coverage for the local sales guarantee program.[35]

Notably, the process of securitization and concurrent economic efforts are being met with public approval; the state's response to the crisis has increased the popularity of King Abdullah II. A number of popular heroes within the state have also emerged, including the Minister of Health and Minister of State for Media Affairs and Government.[36]

Limits to Securitization

After reviewing all the measures taken by the Jordanian government to deal with the coronavirus, it is clear now that the virus has changed the "behavior" of the state and society in a broad and profound way. The securitization process was one of the most important manifestations of this change in the conduct of the state, especially in the short term. It also became clear today that Jordan, through securitization, avoided a "Pyrrhic victory"[37] over the virus, with many losses of life and property.

This may explain why Jordanian government passed 12 defense orders, during the period (March 2, 2020–May 3, 2020) to deal with the virus, all of which are subject to the application of the armed forces and security agencies. In all these "defense orders," the government has dealt with institutions in the public and private sectors and citizens of all types of life as soldiers in the war with the virus.

Securitization deepened in Jordan as a result of "functional actors" like the media, academia, non-governmental agencies, and think tanks. Jordanian individuals themselves helps to frame storylines about the existentially threatening nature of the virus add to that the failure of relevant ministries such as industry and trade, labor, social development, and transportation to deal with the virus crisis (i.e., failure to distribute bread to homes in Jordan),[38] so the armed forces and security agencies intervened clearly and explicitly to fill the vacuum and perform the task instead.

The coronavirus in Jordan has gone beyond identifying the disease a "critical public health crisis" due to concerns that a medical emergency would not provide the speed and agility necessary for dealing with the virus and to prevent its spread. Jordan's "securitization model" has in many ways proven itself as an effective, quick, and strict way to mobilize all needed resources available in the face of the pandemic to preserve lives and property before the disease was able to infect a large proportion of the population.[39]

There are many signs that Jordan's securitization strategy has been a relative success in the face of a major threat. However, the state's decision to approach the challenge through a securitized lens should not be interpreted as the response of a strong state able to quickly mobilize its army and security forces, impose lockdowns, and maintain domestic stability in the face of a global crisis. Rather, a quick and decisive response to the crisis was seen as a necessity to prevent a mass outbreak because of the government's awareness of the lack of the necessary resources to deal with the COVID-19 crisis.

Similarly, as Jordan looks to maintain its successes, it will be faced with a new challenge of how and when to reopen to the outside world. The pandemic is global, and no one state can eliminate the threat without a concerted and international effort. This may explain the call in a joint article in the *Financial Times* by King Abdullah II and leaders of four other countries, led by Germany, for a new global alliance to accelerate scientific research and enhance its funding to access the new coronavirus vaccines.[40]

Moreover, the lasting effects of this crisis are still in the process of emerging. Like most countries, Jordan's political, economic, social, and security will certainly suffer from the crisis. There will be significant challenges in all sectors, from bankruptcies to high unemployment rates, disruption of the tourism sector Jordan has worked so hard to build, and reduced remittances from workers abroad.

There are also drawbacks specific to securitization. Securitization runs the risk of stunting human development, democratic transformations, and the evolution of political, parliamentary and civil society institutions, especially when emergency laws are extended. In the medium turn, a sense of decreased freedoms may lead to the emergence of serious societal challenges, such as high crime, robbery, theft, widespread drug use, increased mental illness, and possibly suicide.[41]

Social unrest in the midst of a crisis can become a self-fulfilling cycle. Domestic unrest is likely to increase the burden of the various security agencies, especially the General Intelligence Department (GID) making them more vulnerable to threats from different terrorist groups like ISIS "the spread of the pandemic and its impact on governments and militaries around the world, represents an opportunity for ISIS to emphasize the weakness of its enemies to renew its attacks."[42]

Political activists, opposition movements, and many intellectuals in Jordan are wary of the political consequences of securitization, as the extraordinary means employed to deal with the security threat could lead to an erosion of democratic norms.[43] There is a particular fear that the continuation of these measures will lead to a tightening of public freedoms, freedom of the press, and hinder the difficult democratic process in the country. Although it is not clear how Jordanian intellectuals abroad view the "securitization model," there is certainly a wealth of information being shared between those abroad and those who remain at home, and scenes in Jordan are featured on social media.[44]

I have noted that these legitimate wary have prompted Michael Page, deputy Middle East director at Human Rights Watch, to comment on the Jordanian actions, saying

> Jordanian authorities should stick by their commitment not to abridge basic rights under the state of emergency and to ensure that all measures taken are

necessary and proportional to the threat posed by the pandemic, The test of every nation is how it treats its citizens in times of crisis.[45]

Yet despite what may be valid concerns, available polling (16 April) – although many Jordanians question the accuracy of these polling – suggests that a large majority of Jordanians (77.9%) are satisfied with the government's performance during the crisis, and 74.1% believe very much that government decisions are for the interest of the citizen.[46] This suggests that most Jordanians, at least for now, see the trade-offs as warranted and a variation of the difficult calculations most countries have made. That said, the question still whether this support will last if these restrictions continue remains to be seen in the long term.

Jordan's early response and implementation of several laws and containment policies

> can be justified given the many challenges facing the country even before the pandemic. Yet the current measures must be understood as merely a short-term palliative. The country will soon need to rethink its longer-term situation in the wake of the pandemic. For a country with such social, economic, and environmental stresses, the coronavirus could serve as a wake-up call, triggering the switch from its existing crisis adjustment policy to a robust crisis management and alleviation policy. Such changes can only be implemented through political will—and the risks either way are unavoidably substantial.[47]

In the meantime, Jordan can build on its successes from short-term securitization by ensuring that this securitization does not become a continuous state of affairs. The government can continue to reassure the public through two strategies. The state must first gradually remove all military manifestations from public streets – especially within cities, communities, workplaces, and shopping places. This move must be communicated publicly through press briefings by the National Center for Security and Crisis Management, the Minister of State for Media Affairs and Government, and the Minister of Health – which has been conducted daily since the beginning of the crisis.[48] The second key factor is the resumption of an official political process. Jordan's general election for parliamentarians is scheduled for September and King Abdullah II confirmed in late February that these elections will take place.

Now, Jordan must ensure that the political process continues with the implementation of appropriate safety standards.[49] On-time elections will send an important political message that Jordan is a strong country that is capable of dealing with a pandemic while continuing its standard political process. Both a withdrawal of the military and removing all aspects of securitization in public life and elections will further confirm that Jordan's securitization strategy was applied only when necessary, and will not permanently hinder the country's societal freedoms in the long term.

Notes

1 Jordan News Agency (Petra) (2020) https://petra.gov.jo/Include/InnerPage .jsp?ID=129088&lang=ar&name=news.
2 The Ministry of Health in the Hashemite Kingdom of Jordan (2020), https:// corona.moh.gov.jo/en/page/1033/Covid%20-%2019.
3 Ibid.
4 The Royal Hashemite Court (2020). Royal Decree approves Cabinet decision to proclaim Defence Law, https://rhc.jo/en/media/news/royal-decree-approves -cabinet-decision-proclaim-defence-law.
5 Human Rights watch (2020). Jordan: State of Emergency Declared, Government Promises to Respect Rights in COVID-19 Response, https://www.hrw.org/ news/2020/03/20/jordan-state-emergency-declared.
6 Royal Hashemite Court (2020). King urges strict health measures on all border crossings to prevent COVID-19 spread, https://kingabdullah.jo/en/news/king -urges-strict-health-measures-all-border-crossings-prevent-COVID-19-spread.
7 Collins, Alan, ed. (2016). *Contemporary Security Studies* (4th ed.). Oxford, United Kingdom: Oxford University Press.
8 Buzan, Barry; Wæver, Ole; de Wilde, Jaap (1998). *Security: A New Framework for Analysis*. Boulder, Colo.: Lynne Rienner Pub. ISBN 978-1-55587-603-6. p26.
9 Balzacq, Thierry (2005). "The Three Faces of Securitization: Political Agency, Audience and Context". *European Journal of International Relations.* **11** (2): 171–201. doi:10.1177/1354066105052960.
10 - Buzan, Barry; Wæver, Ole; de Wilde, Jaap (1998). *Security: A New Framework for Analysis*. Boulder, Colo.: Lynne.
11 Al Bayaa, Ali (2020). Global Health Diplomacy and the Security of Nations Beyond COVID-19, https://www.e-ir.info/2020/05/22/global-health-diplo- macy-and-the-security-of-nations-beyond-COVID-19/?utm_source=MadMimi &utm_medium=email&utm_content=Weekly+Roundup+from+E-International +Relations&utm_campaign=20200517_m158394507_Weekly+Roundup+from +E-International+Relations&utm_term=Global+Health+Diplomacy+and+the +Security+of+Nations+Beyond+COVID-19.
12 Elbe, S. (2010). Haggling Over Viruses: The Downside Risks of Securitizing Infectious Disease, Health Policy and Planning, 25 (6), 476–485.
13 Jin, Jiyong & Karackattu, Joe Thomas (2011). Infectious diseases and securitiza- tion: WHO's dilemma. Biosecurity and bioterrorism: biodefense strategy, prac- tice, and science. 9. 181–7. 10.1089/bsp.2010.0045.
14 Lewis Eves and James Thedham (2020). Applying Securitization's Second Generation to COVID-19, https://www.e-ir.info/2020/05/14/applying-secu- ritizations-second-generation-to-COVID-19/.
15 Adam Hoffman (2020), The Securitization of the Coronavirus Crisis in the Middle East.
16 -Lewis Eves and James Thedham (2020) Applying Securitization's Second Generation to COVID-19, https://www.e-ir.info/2020/05/14/applying-secu- ritizations-second-generation-to-COVID-19/.
17 Mike, Eckel (2020), Counting The Dead: How Do Countries Tally The Toll From COVID-19?, https://www.rferl.org/a/coronavirus-counting-the-dead -different-countries-russia-usa-tajikistan-belgium/30624320.html.
18 Al Bayaa, Ali (2020).
19 Gygli, S., Haelg, F., Potrafke, N. et al. (2019). The KOF Globalisation Index – revisited. Rev Int Organ **14,** 543–574 (2019). https://doi.org/10.1007/ s11558-019-09344-2.
20 Saud, Al-Sharafat (2020) Securitizing the confrontation with the Coronavirus in Jordan, http://www.shorufatcenter.com/4169/%d8%a3%d9%85%d9%86%d9

%91%d9%86%d8%a9-%d8%a7%d9%84%d9%85%d9%88%d8%a7%d8%ac%d9%87
%d8%a9-%d9%85%d8%b9-%d9%81%d9%8a%d8%b1%d9%88%d8%b3-%d9%83
%d9%88%d8%b1%d9%88%d9%86%d8%a7-%d9%81%d9%8a-%d8%a7%d9%84%d8
%a3/.

21 Ibid.

22 Al Bayaa, Ali (2020).

23 Hansen, L. (2000). The Little Mermaid's Silent Security Dilemma and the
    Absence of Gender in the Copenhagen School. Millennium, 29(2), 285–306.
    https://doi.org/10.1177/03058298000290020501.

24 Royal Hashemite Court (2020). Video message by His Majesty King Abdullah II
    (Translated from Arabic). https://kingabdullah.jo/en/speeches/video-message
    -his-majesty-king-abdullah-ii.

25 *Battle of Karamah was a military battle between the Israel Defense Forces and the
    Jordanian Arab Army and Palestinian guerillas in March 21, 1968, in which the
    Jordanian forces forced the Israeli forces to retreat and inflicted heavy casualties on
    the IDF. The battle's legacy in Jordan shattered the myth of the invincibility of the
    Israeli army, and its outcome was embraced by the late King Hussein.*

26 Hoffman, A. (2020). The Securitization of the Coronavirus Crisis in the Middle
    East. POMEPS Study on the COVID-19 Pandemic in the Middle East and North
    Africa.

27 Al-Ghad newspaper(2020). The Armed Forces start implementing the plan to
    evacuate Jordanian students to quarantine areas, https://alghad.com/%D8%A7
    %D9%84%D9%82%D9%88%D8%A7%D8%AA-%D8%A7%D9%84%D9%85%D8
    %B3%D9%84%D8%AD%D8%A9-%D8%AA%D8%A8%D8%AF%D8%A3-%D8%AA
    %D9%86%D9%81%D9%8A%D8%B0-%D8%AE%D8%B7%D8%A9-%D8%A5%D8
    %AE%D9%84%D8%A7%D8%A1-%D8%A7%D9%84/.

28 Saud, Al-Sharafat (2020). Securitization of the Coronavirus Crisis in Jordan:
    Successes and Limitations, https://www.washingtoninstitute.org/fikraforum/
    view/COVID-19-Jordan-Middle-East-Securitization.

29 Manjari, Singh (2020). Jordan after COVID-19: From Crisis Adjustment to
    Crisis Management, https://www.washingtoninstitute.org/fikraforum/view/
    Jordan-response-COVID19-pandemic-Middle-East.

30 Saud, Al-Sharafat (2020).

31 Shlaim, Avi (2008). Lion of Jordan: The Life of King Hussein in War and Peace.
    Vintage Books.

32 *The Black September (Arabic: أيلول الأسود; Aylūl Al-Aswad) was a conflict fought in the
    Hashemite Kingdom of Jordan between the Jordanian Armed Forces (JAF), under
    the leadership of King Hussein, and the Palestine Liberation Organisation (PLO),
    under the leadership of Yasser Arafat, primarily between 16 and 27 September 1970,
    with certain aspects of the conflict continuing until 17 July 1971.*

33 Saud, Al-Sharafat (2020). Securitization of the Coronavirus Crisis in Jordan:
    Successes and Limitations, https://www.washingtoninstitute.org/fikraforum/
    view/COVID-19-Jordan-Middle-East-Securitization.

34 Ibid.

35 Saud, Al-Sharafat (2020). Securitization of the Coronavirus Crisis in Jordan:
    Successes and Limitations, https://www.washingtoninstitute.org/fikraforum/
    view/COVID-19-Jordan-Middle-East-Securitization.

36 Ibid.

37 *"Pyrrhic victory" refers to" Pyrrhus of Epirus" a Greek general from the Hellenic
    period (319 BC-272 BC).*

    *In response to congratulations for winning a costly victory over the Romans, at the
    Battle of Asculum he is reported to have said: "If we are victorious in one more battle
    with the Romans, we shall be utterly ruined". Plutarch. Parallel Lives: Pyrrhus, 21.9,*

The Parallel Lives by Plutarch published in Vol. IX of the Loeb Classical Library edition, 1920, http://penelope.uchicago.edu/Thayer/e/roman/texts/plutarch/lives/pyrrhus*.html.

38 Zaid Al-Dabisi (2020). Failure to distribute bread to homes in Jordan, https://www.alaraby.co.uk/economy/2020/3/24/%D9%81%D8%B4%D9%84-%D8%A2%D9%84%D9%8A%D8%A9-%D8%AA%D9%88%D8%B2%D9%8A%D8%B9-%D8%A7%D9%84%D8%AE%D8%A8%D8%B2-%D8%B9%D9%84%D9%89-%D8%A7%D9%84%D9%85%D9%86%D8%A7%D8%B2%D9%84-%D9%81%D9%8A-%D8%A7%D9%84%D8%A3%D8%B1%D8%AF%D9%86.

39 Saud, Al-Sharafat (2020). Securitizing the confrontation with the Coronavirus in Jordan, http://www.shorufatcenter.com/4169/%d8%a3%d9%85%d9%86%d9%91%d9%86%d8%a9-%d8%a7%d9%84%d9%85%d9%88%d8%a7%d8%ac%d9%87%d8%a9-%d9%85%d8%b9-%d9%81%d9%8a%d8%b1%d9%88%d8%b3-%d9%83%d9%88%d8%b1%d9%88%d9%86%d8%a7-%d9%81%d9%8a-%d8%a7%d9%84%d8%a3/.

40 Royal Hashemite Court (2020). King co-authors Financial Times op-ed with presidents of Germany, Singapore, Ethiopia, and Ecuador, https://kingabdullah.jo/en/news/king-co-authors-financial-times-op-ed-presidents-germany-singapore-ethiopia-and-ecuador.

41 Saud, Al-Sharafat (2020). Securitization of the Coronavirus Crisis in Jordan: Successes and Limitations, https://www.washingtoninstitute.org/fikraforum/view/COVID-19-Jordan-Middle-East-Securitization.

42 Sigalit Maor-Hirsh)2020(. ISIS in the Age of Coronavirus: From Islamizing the Pandemic to Implementing the Jihadist Strategy, https://irintheageofcorona.com/isis-in-the-age-of-coronavirus-from-islamizing-the-pandemic-to-implementing-the-jihadist-strategy/.

43 Saud, Al-Sharafat (2020). Securitization of the Coronavirus Crisis in Jordan: Successes and Limitations, https://www.washingtoninstitute.org/fikraforum/view/COVID-19-Jordan-Middle-East-Securitization.

44 Ibid.

45 Human Rights watch (2020). Jordan: State of Emergency Declared, Government Promises to Respect Rights in COVID-19 Response, https://www.hrw.org/news/2020/03/20/jordan-state-emergency-declared.

46 Ibid.

47 Manjari, Singh (2020), Jordan after COVID-19: From Crisis Adjustment to Crisis Management, https://www.washingtoninstitute.org/fikraforum/view/Jordan-response-COVID19-pandemic-Middle-East.
   Saud, Al-Sharafat (2020).

48 Ibid.

49 Ibid.

References

Al Bayaa, Ali, 2020. Global health diplomacy and the security of nations beyond COVID-19, https://www.e-ir.info/2020/05/22/global-health-diplomacy-and-the-security-of-nations-beyond-COVID-19/?utm_source=MadMimi&utm_medium=email&utm_content=Weekly+Roundup+from+E-International+Relations&utm_campaign=20200517_m158394507_Weekly+Roundup+from+E-International+Relations&utm_term=Global+Health+Diplomacy+and+the+Security+of+Nations+Beyond+COVID-19.

Al-Ghad Newspaper, 2020. The armed forces start implementing the plan to evacuate Jordanian students to quarantine areas, https://alghad.com/%D8%A7%D9%84

%D9%82%D9%88%D8%A7%D8%AA-%D8%A7%D9%84%D9%85%D8%B3%D9
%84%D8%AD%D8%A9-%D8%AA%D8%A8%D8%AF%D8%A3-%D8%AA%D9%86
%D9%81%D9%8A%D8%B0-%D8%AE%D8%B7%D8%A9-%D8%A5%D8%AE%D9
%84%D8%A7%D8%A1-%D8%A7%D9%84/.

Al-Sharafat, Saud, 2020a. Securitizing the confrontation with the coronavirus in Jordan, http://www.shorufatcenter.com/4169/%d8%a3%d9%85%d9%86%d9%91%d9%86%d8%a9-%d8%a7%d9%84%d9%85%d9%88%d8%a7%d8%ac%d9%87%d8%a9-%d9%85%d8%b9-%d9%81%d9%8a%d8%b1%d9%88%d8%b3-%d9%83%d9%88%d8%b1%d9%88%d9%86%d8%a7-%d9%81%d9%8a-%d8%a7%d9%84%d8%a3/.

Al-Sharafat, Saud, 2020b. Securitization of the coronavirus crisis in Jordan: Successes and limitations, https://www.washingtoninstitute.org/fikraforum/view/COVID-19-Jordan-Middle-East-Securitization.

Balzacq, Thierry, 2005. The three faces of securitization: Political agency, audience and context, *European Journal of International Relations*, 11(2): 171–201. https://doi.org/10.1177/1354066105052960.

Buzan, Barry, Waever, Ole, & de Wilde, Jaap, 1998. *Security: A New Framework for Analysis.* Boulder, CO: Lynne Rienner Pub.

Clara, Eroukhmanoff, 2018. Securitization theory: An introduction, https://www.e-ir.info/2018/01/14/securitisation-theory-an-introduction/

Collins, Alan, ed., 2016. *Contemporary security studies* (4th ed.). Oxford: Oxford University Press.

Elbe, S., 2010. Haggling over viruses: The downside risks of securitizing infectious disease, *Health Policy and Planning*, 25(6): 476–485.

Eves, Lewis & Thedham, James, 2020. Applying securitization's second generation to COVID-19, https://www.e-ir.info/2020/05/14/applying-securitizations-second-generation-to-COVID-19/.

Gygli, S., Haelg, F., Potrafke, N. et al., 2019. The KOF globalisation index – revisited. *Review of International Organizations*, 14, 543–574. https://doi.org/10.1007/s11558-019-09344-2.

Hansen, L., 2000. The little mermaid's silent security dilemma and the absence of gender in the Copenhagen school. *Millennium*, 29(2): 285–306.

Hoffman, A., 2020. The securitization of the coronavirus crisis in the Middle East: POMEPS study on the COVID-19 pandemic in the Middle East and North Africa. https://doi.org/10.1177/03058298000290020501.

Human Rights Watch, 2020. Jordan: State of emergency declared, government promises to respect rights in COVID-19 response, https://www.hrw.org/news/2020/03/20/jordan-state-emergency-declared.

Jin, Jiyong & Karackattu, Joe Thomas, 2011. Infectious diseases and securitization: WHO's dilemma. *Biosecurity and Bioterrorism: Biodefense Strategy, Practice, and Science*, 9: 181–187. https://doi.org/10.1089/bsp.2010.0045.

Manjari, Singh, 2020. Jordan after COVID-19: From crisis adjustment to crisis management, https://www.washingtoninstitute.org/fikraforum/view/Jordan-response-COVID19-pandemic-Middle-East.

Mike, Eckel, 2020. Counting the dead: How do countries tally the toll from COVID-19?, https://www.rferl.org/a/coronavirus-counting-the-dead-different-countries-russia-usa-tajikistan-belgium/30624320.html.

Royal Hashemite Court, 2020a. King co-authors financial times op-ed with presidents of Germany, Singapore, Ethiopia, and Ecuador, https://kingabdullah.jo/en

/news/king-co-authors-financial-times-op-ed-presidents-germany-singapore
-ethiopia-and-ecuador.

Royal Hashemite Court, 2020b. King urges strict health measures on all border
crossings to prevent COVID-19 spread, https://kingabdullah.jo/en/news/king
-urges-strict-health-measures-all-border-crossings-prevent-COVID-19-spread.

Royal Hashemite Court, 2020. Video message by his majesty king Abdullah II,
(Translated from Arabic). https://kingabdullah.jo/en/speeches/video-message
-his-majesty-king-abdullah-ii.

Shlaim, Avi, 2008. *Lion of Jordan: The life of king Hussein in war and peace*. London:
Vintage Books.

Sigalit Maor-Hirsh, 2020. ISIS in the age of coronavirus: From Islamizing the
pandemic to implementing the Jihadist strategy, https://irintheageofcorona.com
/isis-in-the-age-of-coronavirus-from-islamizing-the-pandemic-to-implementing
-the-jihadist-strategy/.

The Ministry of Health in the Hashemite Kingdom of Jordan, 2020. https://corona
.moh.gov.jo/en/page/1033/Covid%20-%2019.

The Royal Hashemite Court, 2020. Royal decree approves cabinet decision to
proclaim defence law, https://rhc.jo/en/media/news/royal-decree-approves
-cabinet-decision-proclaim-defence-law.

13 The COVID-19 Pandemic and Its Impact on Violent Extremist Movement in the Philippines

Joshua Snider

Introduction

The Indo-Pacific region has been particularly hard-hit by the coronavirus disease (COVID-19) pandemic. The Philippines in particular has been disproportionately impacted by pandemic conditions. In addition to already grinding levels of economic inequality, the pandemic brings new and unwelcome challenges to an already fragile state. The country faces economic vulnerability at the best of times, born from a mix of over-reliance on Overseas Filipino Workers (OFW) and remittances, elite capture of the economy, subsistence employment, corruption, and frequent natural disasters. These factors and more make the Philippines uniquely vulnerable and generally lacking in society-level resilience mechanisms to cope with long-term pandemic conditions. Beyond the country's general economic precariousness, the impact of the pandemic on the simmering ethnoreligious conflict in the south of the country remains a point of concern. Despite a peace agreement with the mainstream insurgent elements, in recent years the conflict has been driven by recalcitrant violent extremist movements that challenge the state and pose a threat to communities. The Philippines Violent Extremist Organization (VEO) space has undergone a transformation in recent years. While legacy movements such as Abu Sayyaf have always maintained linkages with regional and international Jihadist movements, post-Arab spring conflicts have further radicalized and internationalized the local VEO space. In 2017, two new Islamic State of Iraq and Leven (Syria) (ISIL)-linked VEOs – Bangsamoro Islamic Freedom Front and the Maute Group (BIFF) – occupied the Marawi region and waged against the Armed Forces of the Philippines in a brutal months-long confrontation. The synergistic effects of the ferocity of this iteration of violent extremism and the state's response to it have diminished prospects for either a swift military victory or a negotiated settlement. Moreover, there is concern that the state is over-reaching and in particular that the Duterte's government's new suite of anti-terror laws could further alienate Muslim Malays in the South without addressing any of the root causes (Abuza, 2002).

The pandemic's impact on the extremist threat environment remains an open question. While there is literature looking at how Jihadist movements have used pandemic conditions to exploit anti-state narratives, this has not been fleshed out in the context of VEOs in the Philippines. Anecdotally, there is evidence to

DOI: 10.4324/9781003291909-14

suggest that pandemic conditions have disrupted VEO activity – i.e., stemming the flow of foreign militants into the south with air and sea routes being cut off. At the same time, there is evidence that VEOs use pandemic conditions as a recruitment tool to further radicalize vulnerable constituencies. While the drivers of radicalization amongst Jihadist VEOs vary from location to location and group to group, these dynamics in the Philippines have traditionally been fed by an opaque mixture of ethnocultural and religious grievance and economic dispossession. There is concern that the pandemic has exacerbated both sources of tension and will thus result in a net increase in extremist activism.

This chapter will address several key areas in relation to the pandemic, including (1) anti-state narratives adopted by Jihadist VEOs during the pandemic; (2) trajectories of recruitment and radicalization amongst leading VEO and the extent of pandemic-related recruitment disruption; (3) the extent to which the pandemic has changed of violent and non-violent activism amongst Jihadist VEOs; and (4) the pandemic's impact on Preventing and Countering Violent Extremism (PCVE) activities. All of this will be argued in an attempt to show that the pandemic is challenging all states; the government of the Philippines is making decisions that will exacerbate tension in the south and possibly feed a new generation of conflict and extremist violence.

The COVID-19 Pandemic in the Philippines

According to the World Health Organization (WHO), the Philippines has over 400,000 confirmed COVID-19 cases and over 8,000 deaths, as of November 2020. New cases of the virus climbed steadily through the spring, peaked in August, and have been slowly declining since late September (WHO 2020). In addition to the issues nearly all countries have faced with community transmission, the Philippines has had the added complication of repatriating 320,000 overseas foreign workers, many from COVID-19 global hotspots (Government of the Philippines 2020). This large influx placed greater stress on the health infrastructure of Manila, where returnees were required to undergo quarantine and any medical care before returning to the provinces. Regions of the Philippines with higher Muslim populations, such as Northern Mindanao and Cagayan Valley, have had relatively few COVID-19 deaths (119 and 41, respectively) compared to the major metro areas of the Philippines (Outbreak News Today 2020). However, while the highest numbers of cases have been in Manila and the surrounding region, there has been a recent increase in cases in Mindanao, where Davao recorded the highest number of new cases in the country in October 2020 (Outbreak News Today 2020). The increase in new cases in the area of the Philippines with the highest Muslim population could increase the impact of COVID-19 on Islamic extremism. Like elsewhere in the Global South, there are issues with both the reliability of testing and data in the Philippines. Thus, while the government is reporting infection and fatalities rates, given resource constraints and issues with the overall governance of the Philippines COVID-19 response, it is likely that the numbers being reported represent more of an estimate than a true representation of the scale of the pandemic.

Violent Extremism in the Philippines

The rise of Islamist-inspired religio-political activism in the Philippines is a byproduct of the longstanding ethnoreligious struggle between the Moros (Muslim community in Mindanao) and the Catholic-dominated central government. The Islamization of the "Southern struggle" in the 1980s and 1990s resulted in the creation of religiously motivated insurgency movements and terror organizations, notably the Moro Islamic Liberation Front and the Abu Seyyef Group (ASG). While the roots of extremist narratives have been (a) local and (b) grievance oriented, there has always been a distinctly transnational element to extremist activism and discourse. Operationally and ideologically the founding of local Jihadist movements such as the Abu Seyyef Group (ASG) drew heavily from the wider Salafi-Jihadist milieu. ASG was founded with assistance from the Al-Qaeda (AQ) core and in the 1990s' AQ operatives including Ramzi Yousef, lived and trained with ASG fighters and used the Philippines as a sort of Asian hub. In the early 2000s, following a large-scale intervention from the Armed Forces of the Philippines aided by US advisors, ASG was weakened and devolved into a rent-seeking and organized crime syndicate. The Mindanao Islamic Liberation Front's (MILF) peace agreement with Manila resulted in further fragmentation of the Islamist space to include the Bangsamoro Islamic Freedom Fighters (BIFF). Over the past five years, there has been an uptick in Islamist-inspired extremism driven by a mix of old grievances and ISIL's inroads in the region, which saw the BIFF and ASG pledge loyalty to ISIL. This upsurge in activity culminated in the 2017 siege at Marawi where a coalition of various Jihadist actors occupied the region for several months.

COVID-19 and Violent Mobilization

Push and Pull Factors

A number of analysts including Tova Norlen (2020), have argued that Salafi-Jihadist groups across the world have been "emboldened" by COVID-19 and have increased their activities in other areas in the Middle East, Asia, and Africa. While Norlen doesn't discuss the Philippines directly, her analysis is relevant. In the Philippines content, the COVID-19 pandemic may have a chilling effect on factors that fuel their operations, such as funding sources, recruitment, and retention of group members, and the ability to take violent actions such as bombings, during a time of travel restrictions (Norlen 2020).

In the Philippines, vulnerable populations, such as those in Mindanao, are under increased economic stress from the measures taken by the government to control the pandemic. Several non-governmental organizations (NGOs) focused on counter-extremism have expressed concern that the local media and social media's focus on the pandemic and how the government response is exacerbating social divisions creates fear and anxiety that could lead to violence and public unrest. In addition, others in the civil society sector have raised issues with corruption in the local governments as a factor leading to radicalization and potential violence. Thus, there is limited evidence that VEOs use COVID-19 dynamics (depicting the state as weak, feeble, and corrupt) to tap into deep anti-state feelings.

The causal linkage between poverty, under-development, and extremism is complicated. While there might be a linkage between the appeal of extremist discourses and these issues, it is difficult to trace them precisely. In any case, the government lockdowns limit the actualization of violence by domestic actors carrying out attacks in the individuals' local area. Instead, they push lone actor attacks, which are less appealing to radicalized individuals in a Philippines context, further lowering the volume of attacks. Consequently, the actualization of violent intent is likely reduced during COVID-19.

Several analysts have argued that Muslims' spiritual, cultural, and religious practices have been disrupted as a result of pandemic-related movement restrictions, which exacerbated their feeling of "otherness" in the context of being a minority group in the Philippines (Jones 2020). During Ramadan, there were food shortages due to supply chain issues and travel restrictions in Marawi, restrictions on prayers at mosques, and limits to the hours that citizens could leave their houses to run errands and visit family that did not consider suhoor or iftar, even in areas with a large Muslim population (BenarNews 2020). While Eid'l Fitr fell on a Monday in 2020, the Philippine government also placed the public holiday on the following Tuesday, which resulted in Muslims in areas like Cotabato City, being unable to leave their homes on the holiday, as Sunday was declared a "no movement day" (CNN 2020).

Mindanao has 370,000 internally displaced people (IDPs) from violence and natural disasters and combined with the COVID-19 pandemic, this creates a situation that disproportionately burdens women and girls (Abo and Ayo 2020). Given the socio-cultural and gender dynamics in Muslim Filipino culture, women shoulder a majority of the burden for child-rearing. There is also evidence that strict COVID-19 closures and quarantine measures enforced by large security force presence have caused further harm and spread fear in local communities as armed groups tend to target areas where there is a large military presence (Banlaoi 2020). Thus, when military forces set up camp near evacuation centers or villages, residents fear they will be collateral damage when the inevitable firefight erupts (Banlaoi 2020).

In spite of these factors that would tend to increase radicalization, COVID-19 has produced conditions that limit the actualization of violence by these groups in different parts of the world. Salafi-Jihadi rhetoric has focused on issues such as the virus as "divine punishment" or justifications for individual actors to engage in violent activity against local Western targets or political authorities rather than fighting the virus (Norlen 2020). Banlaoi (2020) and Jones (2020) have both argued that COVID-19 restrictions have limited the ability of foreign actors to enter and exit the country (significant as a majority of suicide bombings in particular have been carried out by foreigners), and violent extremism activity has been further limited by the frequent restrictions on movement into and out of Metro Manila and between provinces (Jones 2020). They also argue that extremist groups are also discouraged from bombing population centers because the closure of streets and regulations on social distancing makes these areas less crowded.

Given the extent to which Islamist VEO agendas are inspired by a mix of local and transnational issues, extremists (particularly those engaged in state-seeking national liberation struggles) have to walk a fine-line in their target selection process. This point is supported by Tobias Ide who argues that: "Starting or intensifying attacks during the COVID-19 crisis is likely to decrease the local (and international) legitimacy of armed groups, especially if health infrastructure is affected" (Ide 2020). Thus, in light of the highly local-ized conflict that drives extremist grievance, it is possible that actors located in Muslim-majority areas in the south of the Philippines may be disincentivized to attack structures that provide for their own communities. While they may not have the same affinity for preserving structures, including healthcare structures, in largely Christian cities in the Philippines such as Manila, the inter-province travel restrictions may limit their ability to carry out attacks outside of their own communities.

Additionally, extremist groups are facing more difficulty obtaining fund-ing during COVID-19. Government of the Philippines report noted that the Sawadjaan group (concentrated in Sulu) that conducts attacks in Sulu and kidnap-pings in Sabah is experiencing resource scarcity due to the pandemic. Moreover, the global economic downturn has impacted international financing available, and that the reduction of tourism in Sabah had directly impacted their ability to secure financing, food, and ammunition. Additionally, "because civilian support is being blocked by rapid military operations and local government policies on COVID19 limit the mobility of civilian population there are less supplies and foreign assistance."

Recruitment

Many of the violent extremist attacks in the Philippines in recent years have been carried out by foreigners who come to the Philippines, largely from Malaysia and Indonesia (Jones 2020). Travel restrictions have largely reduced these movements from the majority who enter through formal immigration channels, although there are very porous borders between the interconnected islands of Malaysia, Indonesia, and the Philippines, particularly Mindanao and Sabah pro-viding another possible vector for entry. These foreign actors bring funding and weapons and train the local fighters (Banlaoi 2020). The flow appears currently to have been reduced.

Various sources also affirm that local recruits are interested in fighting against government forces rather than engaging in suicide bombings, which is why sui-cide bombings in the past have been largely committed by foreigners. This state-ment reflects a key tension within VEO activist space in the southern Philippines whereby local Islamists are fighting for autonomy and national liberation and need the support of local people, while foreign volunteers lack local connections and are often more willing to engage in unrestrained violence. Moreover, with COVID-19, there is likely to be a disconnect between the types of extremist activities local recruits want to engage in, and those that are available due to government restrictions. It has been noted by several NGO officials' via media reporting that COVID-19 has not had an effect on recruitment and radicalization itself, which they argue has stayed constant (Jones 2020).

Individual pathways towards radicalization are complex and often involve a mixture of ideological indoctrination combined with social exposure, which occurs at the family level. This view was confirmed by a report from a Philippines-based conflict NGO which argues: "when the father in ASG, the rest of the family become members," including wives and children of the family patriarch. This has been demonstrated recently through suicide bombings conducted by close family members of slain or martyred fighters. In the context of COVID-19 and reduced mobility, there is some concern that extremists who might not otherwise be home will attempt to indoctrinate family members, exacerbating this family phenomenon.

Given the grievance narrative that drives the southern autonomy struggle, there is every reason to believe the state's handling of the crisis and the comparatively high infection rates in the south will play into existing anti-state feelings. According to Abo and Ayao (2020), the failure on the part of the Philippine government to consult with the local population on issues that directly affect them and to address grievances such as "injustices against the Bangsamoro people, socio-economic disparities, discrimination, and disenfranchisement from political processes play a key role in the continuation of the conflict." Thus, the failure to respond to COVID-19 effectively and the disproportionate impact on the south will no doubt be added to the list of injustices that inspire Islamist VE as a justification for the autonomy struggle.

Narrative and Rhetoric

Doctrinally, Salafist-Jihadist movements across the world have been consistent in advancing the position that COVID-19 was sent by Allah to attack infidels, and ISIL has taken the step further and called for its members to use this time of relative weakness in Western powers to conduct attacks (Norlen 2020). However, this rhetoric can become problematic as the pandemic affects Muslim populations. Worldwide, the closure of mosques in many places has meant Jihadi clerics are able to offer more extremist views in sermons online than they could issue in government-monitored mosques (Norlen 2020).

It should be noted that while Salafi-Jihadi ideology has had the most penetration amongst VEOs in the Philippines context, like elsewhere adherents to this movement often don't have a great understanding of their own ideology. For example, Singh and Haziq (2020) argue that members of local extremist groups are often not well-educated on religious doctrine, and "these youths received religious education in informal, poorly funded schools staffed by radical preachers who were educated in informal extremist circles overseas." For example, a widely circulated video (during the pandemic) from an ISIS-affiliated group includes a misquote of a hadith.

Pandemic-driven mosque closures have been a particular source of concern in countering extremist narratives. Local mosques are seen as a moderating influence and there is concern that their closure leads to a bifurcation of the Muslim community whereby more moderate less radicalized would not attend mosques and therefore become less radicalized (Jones 2020). Conversely, those already more radicalized would follow extremists online in the absence of more mainstream narratives proffered by state-sanctioned mosques (Jones). Essentially, mosque closures have a disproportionate impact on moderates who rely more on in-person religious interactions than their radical peers.

Beyond ideology, VEOs in conflict environments often justify their agendas and attract members by capitalizing on the grievance, injustice narratives, and the ineptness of the state (Kenlan 2020). There is some limited data on the exact means by which the Philippines-based groups have incorporated COVID-19 narratives and the extent to which they have integrated it into their messaging. In response to the previously discussed restrictions on mosques on movement during Eid'l Fitr, "BIFF claimed that virus containment measures prohibiting mosque services were attempts by the state to 'destroy Islam' and called for attacks to be carried out in retaliation" (Howe 2020). Based on the past behavior of VEO, it is reasonable to assume that VEOs have capitalized on pandemic conditions to justify anti-state narratives. Given that pathways towards radicalization are driven by a mix of material and ideological factors, it is reasonable to argue that heightened economic vulnerability and the perception that the state has exacerbated this vulnerability would fit their agenda (USAID 2013). For example, VEOs have a long tradition of highlighting corruption and the general ineptness of the governments of the day. This view was reinforced by a former VEO member who said that: "the most pressing factors for radicalization in the Philippines have been the local conditions, perceptions of inequality and ethnic and religious disenfranchisement, rather than the global rhetoric of the Salafi-Jihadi movement" (USAID 2013).

VEOs have also used new terrorism law (signed July 2020) to attract new followers. This new legislation is a powerful recruitment tool to the extent that it is both draconian and plays into neo-colonial northern domination narratives. After the new terrorism law was introduced in the midst of the COVID-19 pandemic, Filipino extremists on social media have threatened "to kill and bomb Christians in the Philippines and strengthen jihadism in Mindanao" (Singh and Haziq 2020).

Attacks and Plots

The Philippines had an increase in the number of battles and explosions per month in the initial month of the pandemic, while it also had a rapid increase in COVID infections and strict implementation of COVID restrictions (Ide 2020). However, the rise was mostly driven by the Communist New People's Army (NPA), and therefore unrelated to Islamic extremist violence. The NPA and the

Philippine government both agreed to unilateral ceasefires in late March, but ended them in late April (Ide 2020).

The following attacks in the Philippines have taken place during the COVID pandemic according to The Armed Conflict Location & Event Data Project (ACLED) data and are either attributed to Islamic violent extremist groups or are not specifically attributed to a group, but given the location and methods can reasonably be assumed to have been committed by Islamic extremist groups. While the volume of attacks overall seems down, the pattern of activity reflects a consistency with earlier attacks, with some more recent shifts – for example, the growing use of women by ASG to launch suicide attacks. There is little clarity around whether these strategic decisions are linked to COVID-19 and its fall-out.

Suicide Bombings

On 24 August 2020, two suspected Abu Sayyaf suicide bombers – reportedly the wives of previously slain Abu Sayyaf leaders – consecutively set off two bombs near the town police station in Barangay Walled City (Jolo, Sulu, Bangsamoro Autonomous Region in Muslim Mindanao). At least 17 people died: the two suicide bombers, eight soldiers, one police officer, and six civilians. At least 74 others, including soldiers, police officers, and civilians, were also wounded. The military blamed the attack on the Abu Sayyaf, though the Islamic State East Asia Province – which has ties to some Abu Sayyaf factions – also claimed responsibility. The military was also investigating claims that local police with ties to the Abu Sayyaf might have been involved in the bombing, and that the bombing might be related to the 29 June killing of four military intelligence officers by Jolo police officers. The four intelligence officers killed on 29 June were reportedly on the trail of the two suicide bombers who carried out this latest bombing (Raleigh et al. 2020).

An Indonesian woman was arrested in October 2020 on suspicion of planning an additional suicide attack in the same area. She is a widow of a man killed in an attack in Sulu in August and believed to be the daughter of suicide bombers who committed an attack in Jolo in 2019.

These incidents point to an increase in women involved in planning and carrying out suicide bombings, and also suicide bombings conducted by either Filipinos or Indonesians who were related to Filipinos (and presumed to live in the Philippines). In contrast, suicide bombings from 2018 to 2019, which were primarily conducted by foreigners who came to the Philippines for the purpose of planning an attack or otherwise supporting armed groups. The coordination of the attacks ties in to the literature showing that local actors prefer to be involved in group efforts rather than lone actor attacks. The purported close relationship between the suicide bombers and slain leaders demonstrates that additional personal motivation contributes to the actualization of violence during COVID.

Armed Assaults on Military Targets

BIFF attacked three army detachments on May 21 (Singh and Haziq 2020).

Improvise Explosive Devices (IEDs)/Bombs

The following is a list of bombings or IED explosions that have taken place in Mindanao during the COVID pandemic. Key takeaways are that they are primarily targeting the military, with also one attack on civilian government and one religious target. In some cases of buried IEDs, these could potentially have been planted prior to COVID. Most other targeting of individuals in the area (such as shootings) has not been attributed to an armed group or ideological motivation.

- On February 14, 2020, an IED was detonated by unidentified assailants near the Saint Therese of the Child Jesus Parish. No one was hurt in the explosion (Raleigh et al. 2020).
- On March 15, 2020, a government soldier was killed while two other soldiers were wounded after a landmine planted by suspected Abu Sayyaf militants detonated in Barangay Limbubong, Maluso, Basilan (Raleigh et al. 2020).
- On June 22, 2020, the mayor of South Upi, Maguindanao, survived an explosion from a bomb detonated by unidentified assailants as the mayor's vehicle passed by Barangay Romangaob, South Upi, Maguindanao (Raleigh et al. 2020).
- On September 18, 2020, a government soldier was killed while four others were wounded during an explosion of a roadside bomb planted by suspected BIFF militants in Barangay Limpongo (Datu Hoffer Ampatuan, Maguindanao, Bangsamoro Autonomous Region in Muslim Mindanao). The bomb exploded as a military convoy was passing by the area (Raleigh et al. 2020).
- On September 24, 2020, three soldiers were wounded in an explosion of an IED planted by suspected BIFF militants in Barangay Salman (Ampatuan, Maguindanao, Bangsamoro Autonomous Region in Muslim Mindanao). One of the wounded soldiers later died at the hospital (Raleigh et al. 2020).
- On October 23, 2020, two soldiers and two active auxiliaries of the military's Citizen Armed Force Geographical Unit were wounded in an explosion of a roadside IED suspected to have been planted by BIFF militants in Barangay Salman (Ampatuan, Maguindanao, Bangsamoro Autonomous Region in Muslim Mindanao) (Raleigh et al. 2020).
- On September 23, 2020, a farmer was wounded in an explosion of an IED planted by suspected Dawlah Islamiyah militants in Barangay Tonggol (General Salipada K. Pendatun, Maguindanao, Bangsamoro Autonomous Region in Muslim Mindanao). A second IED was found a few meters away but was defused by authorities (Raleigh et al. 2020).

Local Authority Response

Armed groups in many countries, including the Philippines, have announced limited ceasefires in response to the COVID-19 pandemic, though this has been against selected groups (and did not include VEOs relevant to this paper) (Ide 2020). President Duterte announced on March 18 that the government would have a unilateral month-long ceasefire specifically against communist rebels (the NPA), specifying that the declaration of ceasefire did not apply to other armed groups as well (Howe 2020). Notably, the NPA did not make their own unilateral declaration of ceasefire until one week after the government's declaration. Despite the information about a (short-lived) ceasefire during COVID-19 between the Philippines government and the communist terrorist group, there is no publicly available information or evidence of COVID-19-related ceasefires with the Islamic extremist groups in the Philippines.

President Duterte signed the Anti-Terrorism Act of 2020 on July 3, and it took effect by mid-August. It is not known if the time of this legislation is related to the COVID-19 pandemic. This supersedes an existing terrorism law and expands upon the government's powers. The new law is extraterritorial, meaning that non-Filipinos can be charged and individuals can be charged for actions they take against Filipinos outside the territory of the Philippines (Zicolaw.com 2020). This is likely relevant to the foreign members of extremist groups that operate in the Philippines and to cover the acts of terrorism that are committed on the Philippine–Malaysia border. The law also now covers preparation or planning for acts of terrorism, even when no harm has been done (*Arab News* 2020). The sweeping powers allowed under the law, including arrests without warrants, 24-day detention without charges, and surveillance of communications and banking records of alleged terrorists. There have been over 30 petitions charging the law as unconstitutional, with particular concerns citing overly broad definitions of "terrorism" and "terrorist activities" in the law and the expansive powers of the newly established Anti-Terrorism Council (Zicolaw.com 2020). The Indonesian woman arrested for plotting a suicide bombing was the first person charged under the new law.

Conclusion

Based on analysis presented in this chapter, it is clear that more research needs to be done in this area, both in the context of the Philippines and other states in Southeast Asia. In a general sense, research in this area is complicated by a lack of literature and a lack of data-focused research. At this stage, most of the information linking extremism and COVID-19 in the Philippines comes from the media and to a lesser degree think tanks. A vast majority of media reporting focuses on the possible risk of COVID-19-related extremism rather than specific incidents. There has been no systematic research done on any of the key research questions.

There is good reason to believe COVID-19 has impacted the push and pull factors for extremism. Anecdotally, it would appear that COVID-19 pandemic has impacted push and pull factors, but the extent remains unclear. Moreover, the VEOs (ASG, BIFF, and Maute) all draw from distinct constituencies and operate in specific areas. While there has been discussion of VEOs during the pandemic, we do not know if all VEOs have been impacted evenly, or if some have been grown or shrunk due to the pandemic. It seems that while physical meetings have been restricted more activism is taking place online. Given the relationship between Islamist-inspired violent extremism and the overall conflict environment, it is difficult to isolate the run of the mill anti-state grievance that drives extremism with trajectories of extremism driven uniquely by the COVID-19 pandemic. It is reasonable to conclude that "push factors" such as conflict, marginalization, discrimination, and limited access to resources might be exacerbated due to movement restrictions and impact of economic slowdown. For example, the socioeconomic factors resulting from the COVID pandemic (decreased livelihoods, increased economic instability) might increase radicalization. However, the government lockdowns limit actualization of violence to domestic actors carrying out attacks in the individuals' local area and often to lone actor attacks, which are less appealing to radicalized individuals in a Philippines context. Thus, the actualization of violent intent is likely dampened during COVID. There is more conclusive data on "pull factors" such as the appeal of extremist narratives. For example, ISIL-affiliated groups use the government's handling of the pandemic to justify anti-state narratives, though it is unclear if this has been effective in terms of inspiring more and more violent extremism.

It seems that VEOs are using COVID-19 in their rhetoric, but its effect is unclear. As previously mentioned, VEOs around the world, including in the Philippines, are using COVID-19 conditions to justify both ideology and anti-state narratives. It is also clear that VEOs are resilient and despite movement restrictions find ways (online) of spreading messages. It is unclear if this is working in the sense that more people are joining VEO and/or those within VEO are more active.

Finally, at this stage it is unclear how or of COVID-19 has impacted the Philippines government's Counter Terrorism (CT) or Preventing/Countering Violent Extremism (P/CVE) efforts. There is little data or discussion on the impact of the pandemic on CVE activities. Informally, there have been reports that the lockdown has curtailed the delivery of CVE program-related activities. The biggest piece of new policymaking during COVID-19 has been the new CT law, which does not appear to be specifically related to the pandemic. There is currently no publicly available information on the ways in which government-led CT activities have been impacted by the pandemic.

References

Abo, N., & Ayao, A. 2020. Conflict forces Mindanao's displaced to choose: Violence or the virus. *The New Humanitarian*. Retrieved November 19, 2020, from https://www.thenewhumanitarian.org/opinion/2020/06/01/Philippines -Mindanao-coronavirus-violence-women-girls

Abuza, Z. 2002. *Militant Islam in Southeast Asia: Crucible of terror*. New York: Lynne Rienner.

Arab News. 2020. Indonesian woman first to be tried under Philippines' new anti-terror law. Retrieved November 24, 2020, from https://www.arabnews.com/ node/1749001/world

Banlaoi, R. 2020. Philippines: Threats of violent extremism and terrorism amidst COVID-19 pandemic – analysis | Yerepouni Daily News. *Yerepouni-news.com*. Retrieved November 18, 2020, from https://www.yerepouni-news.com/2020/08/10/philippines-threats-of-violent-extremism-and-terrorism-amidst-COVID-19-pandemic-analysis/

BenarNews. 2020. Philippines: COVID-19 brings new challenges to Ramadan in Muslim South. Retrieved November 24, 2020, from https://www.benarnews.org/english/news/philippine/philippines-coronavirus-04242020150213.html

Gov't repatriates nearly 320K OFWs amid health crisis. 2020. *Pna.gov.ph*. Retrieved November 23, 2020, from https://www.pna.gov.ph/articles/1122593

Herbert, S. 2019. *Conflict analysis of the Philippines*. K4D Helpdesk Report 648. Brighton: Institute of Development Studies.

How Filipino Muslims have celebrated Ramadan amid the pandemic. 2020. CNN Philippines. Retrieved November 24, 2020, from https://www.cnn.ph/life/culture/2020/5/23/ramadan-quarantine.html

Howe, J. 2020. *Conflict and coronavirus: How COVID-19 is impacting Southeast Asia's conflicts*. Issues & Insights. Pacific Forum.

Ide, T. 2020. COVID-19 and armed conflict. *SSRN Electronic Journal*. http://doi.org/10.2139/ssrn.3603248

Jones, S. 2020. COVID-19 and extremism in Southeast Asia. *Asia Pacific Journal: Japan Focus*, 18(15): 1–8.

Kenlan, A.K. 2020. COVID-19 is an 'ally' for ISIS in the Philippines, DoD report finds. *Military Times*. August 13, 2020. Retrieved from https://www.militarytimes.com/news/your-military/2020/08/13/COVID-19-is-an-ally-for-isis-in-the-philippines-dod-report-finds/

Mainstreaming pro-ISIS groups 'cooperation and inter- regional ties across clans and ethnic bonds in the Southern Philippines. (n.d.). 2004.

Norlen, T. 2020. The impact of COVID-19 on Salafi-Jihadi. *Connections: The Quarterly Journal*, 19(2): 11–23. http://doi.org/10.11610/connections.19.2.01

Outbreak News Today. 2020. Philippines: Davao City reports most new COVID-19 cases, Measles/Polio vaccination campaign in La Union. *alj Today*. Retrieved November 23, 2020, from http://outbreaknewstoday.com/philippines-davao-city-reports-most-new-COVID-19-cases-measles-polio-vaccination-campaign-in-la-union-58280/

Philippine new anti-terrorism law enacted. 2020. *Zicolaw.com*. Retrieved November 24, 2020, from https://www.zicolaw.com/resources/alerts/philippine-new-anti-terrorism-law-enacted/

Philippines arrests woman suspected of planning suicide attack. 2020. *Aljazeera.com*. Retrieved November 24, 2020, from https://www.aljazeera.com/news/2020/10/10/philippines-arrests-woman-suspected-of-planning-suicide-attack

Philippines: WHO coronavirus disease (COVID-19) dashboard. 2020. *Covid19.who.int*. Retrieved November 23, 2020, from https://covid19.who.int/region/wpro/country/ph

Raleigh, C., Linke, A., Hegre, H., & Karlsen, J. 2020. Introducing ACLED-armed conflict location and event data. *Journal of Peace Research*, 47(5): 651–660.

Singh, J., & Haziq Jani, M. 2020. COVID-19 and terrorism in the Southern Philippines: More trouble ahead. *Thediplomat.com*. Retrieved November 25,

2020, from https://thediplomat.com/2020/08/COVID-19-and-terrorism-in -the-southern-philippines-more-trouble-ahead/

USAID. 2013. Violent extremism and insurgency in the Philippines: A risk assessment. Retrieved from https://msi-inc.com/sites/default/files/additional-resources /2018-12/Violent%20Extremism%20and%20Insurgency%20-%20Philippines.pdf

14 Security Threats and Challenges of Coronavirus Outbreak

General Policy Analysis

Mamdouh Abdelmottlep

Introduction

Emergencies, which affect public health, pose special challenges for security, police, and law enforcement agencies. This threat may be man-made (such as anthrax or biological terrorist attacks) or naturally occurring (such as Flu or Corona epidemics). Security strategies differ as per the threat cause and level, in addition to the potential risk to the security, police, and law enforcement forces.

These strategies deal with infected cases of police officers and their families. Medical emergencies require coordination and rapid response from public health officials in the country and supportive bodies of public emergency states. Security, police, and law enforcement agencies' role may include enforcing public health orders (such as quarantine or travel restrictions), securing surrounding areas where the epidemic outbreaks, securing health care units, controlling the crowded people, investigating suspected biological terrorism scenes, or protecting national vaccines or other drugs stocks. In cases of epidemics outbreak on a wide scale, such as Corona, the security, police, and law enforcement officials will resort to balance their resources and efforts among these new responsibilities and daily service requirements on the security of the community and safety of its individuals.

The ability of the Ministry of Interior and law enforcement agencies to respond effectively to any emergency condition whether related to the public health scale or not mainly depends on the readiness and planning of these agencies with their strategic partners to challenge these emergencies. Learned lessons from the country's response to biological threats and health epidemics state the importance of accurate planning in preparing security, police, and law enforcement agencies and communities towards any kind of risks and the necessity of guaranteeing the safety of security, police, and law enforcement officials and their families.

This is a vital issue to ensure an adequate workforce to execute the urgent response to emergencies about health. Various security, police, and law enforcement agencies should be able to exceed the restrictions of legal jurisdiction to access the resources and essential assistance to face these cases. The cases of epidemics outbreak stated the importance of dealing with the polluted area as soon as possible, obtaining the necessary drugs and vaccines, and providing the proper

DOI: 10.4324/9781003291909-15

personal protective equipment to the first responders. This requires community cooperation on large scale and approval to comply with the quarantine and isolation orders, the necessity of spreading community's awareness of public health threats and taking the necessary measures to avoid an outbreak of infectious diseases.

This policy declares the main issues assigned to security, police, and law enforcement officials to be solved following the health emergency states and preparing for emergency health conditions in the future, including epidemics and biological terrorism incidents. It is hoped that security, police, and law enforcement officials carefully consider the issues that require a solution in the planning operation for all dangers in their departments. Public safety and responded issues discussed here may be considered relatively new in this era of security work. Therefore, it requires more coordination and cooperation between various police and security agencies on one hand and between the other bodies concerned in law enforcement on the other hand. This policy tackles the security challenges, which relate directly to security, police, public security, state security, Ministry of Interior, and its parallel agencies.

Scope of Study

A respiratory disease resulting from a new virus has been discovered for the first time in China. Soon it quickly reached to about 170 international sites. This virus was named "SARS-CoV-2" and the disease due to it was called "Coronavirus Disease 2019" or "COVID-19". On January 30, 2020, the International Health Regulations Emergency Committee of the World Health Organization declared that the disease outbreak is a "Public Health Emergency of International Concern (PHEIC)"; at the beginning of March 2020, it has been declared as an international epidemic (WHO, January 30, 2020).

The World Health Organization defines "Coronavirus Family" as a species that includes viruses, which may cause a group of diseases in humans, ranging from common Flu and Severe acute respiratory syndrome (SARS). The latest discovered "Coronavirus" causes "Coronavirus COVID-19" disease. The viruses belonging to this species also cause several diseases to animals. As this virus is new, the organization collaborates with other countries and partners to get more information about it and test its effects on public health (WHO, March 15, 2020).[1]

The WHO declared on the morning of March 19, 2020, Coronavirus outbreak developments all over the world, indicating that there are 218.709 thousand confirmed infected cases all over the world, 76.003 thousand recovered cases, and 8.936 thousand death cases. China came in the first place in the number of infected cases and deaths, followed by Italy, Iran, Spain, Germany, the United States, France and South Korea, Switzerland, and Britain. In Arab countries, Qatar came in the first place as there was about 340 confirmed infected cases, followed by Bahrain, then Saudi Arabia with a several infected cases reached 238 (Saudi Ministry of Health, March 19, 2020), then Egypt with several cases at 210.[2]

The rapid outbreak of this disease caused a direct effect on the number of sectors, including security, police, and law enforcement sectors. On the morning of March 18, 2020, the British Guardian newspaper published news about suspending police investigations regarding some crimes. It also reported that there was a frequent delay in responding to urgent cases, resulting in an increasing number of infected confirmed cases of Coronavirus in the United Kingdom to become 2,626 confirmed cases and 104 dead cases. The newspaper called for adopting governmental emergency plans to help police forces to overcome the severe Coronavirus outbreak. The British police have warned that nearly a fifth of the workforce may be infected during the potential peak of the epidemic outbreak. Action plan composed of twenty-eight pages warned that a group of measures will be put in place if the virus shifts to "post-Contain Phase" defined currently (The Guardian, March 18, 2020).[3]

These cases refer to a group of challenges and threats that face security, police, and law enforcement agencies in various countries that may face any threats related to health risks. Therefore, problems may appear related to security services' ability to face these threats and its ability to balance between its ordinary works regarding the security of the society and its individual's safety, rapid, and growing outbreak challenges of infected and vulnerable cases, taking into consideration, limited security resources whether at the human level or material potentials.

There were also problems related to protecting members of the security or police community itself (including police officers, individuals, and their families) from any infections or diseases and its consequences on the security agency's ability to provide the security services as required. Finally, the problem of societal gatherings may arise, which security, police, and law enforcement agencies deal with by describing it as effective attempts or not, such as officials in the patrol police, firefighting, rescue, ambulance, employees in airports and border outlets, officials in police stations and centers, or workers in the prison and penal institutions. Then, how can the security and police agencies deal in case of disease outbreak between prisoners, security forces or emergency forces?

Public policies paper will help officials of security, police, and law enforcement agencies to understand the **mechanism of infectious diseases outbreak and its threat to public health and safety**. It summarizes the main assignments charged to the officials of security, police, and law enforcement agencies to deal with it when they are preparing to deal with an epidemic caused by a virus or other public health emergencies. The paper contains three main sections**, the first one is: Related to how to keep the security operation of police and security forces, the second section is: Related to the protection of police and security forces** and their families, and **the third section** is: **Related to social security and safety of its individuals.**

Available Alternative Discussion

Mechanism of Infectious Diseases Outbreak and Its Threat to Public Health and Safety

The World Health Organization and the Centers for Disease Control and Prevention developed a list of six phases for any epidemic outbreak as follows: **First Stage: Per-Epidemic Period:** There is no new subtype of viruses that has been discovered in humans. If these viruses are discovered in animals, the risk of human infection or disease is low. **Second Stage:** There is no new subtypes of viruses that have been discovered in humans: However, the subtype of the viral animal virus represents a major risk to humans. **Third Stage: The Epidemiological Warning Period:** Whereas the infection occurs in humans with a new virus subtype, it only spreads limitedly. **Fourth Stage:** Virus spreading within a small group or groups: with a limited transmission of infection from human to human. This indicates that the virus does not adapt well to humans. **Fifth Stage: Major spread in groups:** This indicates that the virus has become more adapted to humans.

Sixth and Final Stage: Epidemic period: It is characterized by increasing the transmission of the virus infection among people in general. (Edward P. Richards, "The Role of Law Enforcement in Public Health Emergencies," 2006).[4]

The mechanism by which infectious diseases are transmitted can be understood by dividing it into **three categories**.

First Category: Food and Waterborne Diseases

These diseases are spread through bacterial contamination of food or drinking water in general. These diseases represent a threat to security, police, and law enforcement personnel as for the population in general. The risk of catching these diseases may increase in cases where the infrastructure has been severely damaged, as in the case of hurricanes or biological attack. Law enforcement personnel of police and security are considered the first responders to help the public health authorities and municipalities to close shops or areas to prevent spreading of the infection—food and waterborne diseases among people while their assistance in the evacuation, rescue, and recovery.

The spread of food and waterborne diseases can be controlled if the infected individuals and people who were in close contact with them are prevented from preparing food or supplying water until the medical tests reveal that they are not in infection. If the biological terrorists pollute the water supply, eliminating the excess chlorine through the water supply system can lead to eliminating the pollution easily. In case of a bioterrorist attack on the food supply, coordination with the public health authorities can determine the source and pollution extent and work to control it.

Second Category: Bloodborne Diseases

Bloodborne diseases represent a major threat to security, police, and law enforcement personnel, especially if they work in penal institutions or are in close contact with injecting drug users. In addition, minor injuries often occur to both suspects and officers during quarrels, arrests, and during vehicle and traffic accidents. This leads to potential exposure to bloodborne causes, especially hepatitis B, as it is more infected than HIV. Security, police, and law enforcement agencies can protect their employees by providing them with preventive vaccinations, as well as obligating them to use health protection equipment.

Third Category: Respiratory Disease

These respiratory diseases, which are transmitted through breathing including Coronavirus, are considered one of the most dangerous diseases in society. Due to virus ability to spread both humans and animals, because of easily transmit through the air. Hence, the basic principle of protecting the respiratory system is through wearing a protective mask and pre-vaccination for common respiratory diseases. Personnel of security, police, and law enforcement agencies need protective eyeglasses and masks that fit comfortably the nose and mouth. Taking into consideration, that officials who have asthma or other respiratory illnesses may not be able to tolerate the decrease of airflow.

Based on the previous concept about the spread of infectious diseases mechanism and the threat to public health and safety, the insurance and law enforcement plans related to large-scale health emergency cases must apply to all types of public health risks. Therefore, it can be applied regardless of whether a public health emergency was intended, such as biological terrorist actions, or naturally occurred, such as the spread of Coronavirus. More significantly, the plans must guarantee better protection for officers and individuals from the risks of the daily dealings of the security and police services. Several countries have chosen to put their emergency response plans with the help of security, police, and law enforcement sectors. The security, police, and law enforcement personnel must review their planned roles to be aware of the expectations of the government and local agencies in case of a serious epidemic.

Singapore is a successful model; until now, there have been around 313 cases of coronavirus infection without any deaths, and the rates of recovery cases outweigh the infected ones. Singapore's success is a result of several factors that may not easily be repeated in another country. These include the limited population of about 5.6 million, the high level of health care, early preparedness and implement accurate and strict procedures to monitor infection cases. In addition, citizens accepting of the restrictive governmental measures and employing the social media and platforms to promote the importance of hygiene and governmental measures.

Suggested Solutions and Options

There is a difference in terminology between security, police, and law enforcement. The term security refers to everything related to community security and the safety of the individuals residing in this community. Because security is the responsibility of the society, it includes all the roles assigned to the private and public security services. The police term is limited to the role which is played by the state for achieving public security, whether for society or individuals. It concerns the Ministry of the Interior and the National (State) Security. The term "law enforcement" means all the concerned agencies in the country that have been given the authority to enforce its rules by the Law and therefore it includes the police, security, municipalities, government departments, and others.

We believe that the policy recommendations in this regard are represented in **three** main elements, **the first one is: How to keep the sustainability of security works, the second one is:** How to protect police, security, and law enforcement personnel from being infected with the epidemic or minimize its effect after catching the infection, and **the third one is: How to protect the community** whether the internal community of security, police, and law enforcement agencies or local community.

First Element: Keep the Sustainability of Security Operations

The main challenge represents in health emergency plans, to be taken into consideration by police, security, and law enforcement agencies is to ensure operation sustainability. Therefore, it is conceivable, there will be a decrease in security and police workforce because some of them catch the infection and expand the scope of its work to a large extent because of the disease outbreak. Thus, all police, security, and law enforcement agencies shall set plans to include preparing for work with a reduced number of workforces significantly considering potential reductions of workforce ranging from 10 to 40%.

The routine of security and police personnel during performing their daily works such as arresting, requesting a driving license, drawing up a report, inspecting a car, controlling gatherings in mega-events, dealing with a prisoner, or transporting them to prisons may cause them to become infected, especially in diseases transmitted via breathing or touching such as Flu, Corona, measles, and others.

Hence, police, security, and law enforcement personnel shall give special priority to diseases, which spread via accidental contact between individuals. Since the infected cases increase in the community, it is expected that the number of infected ones will also be increased among police, security, and law enforcement agencies personnel as long as there are no special protective measures that have been taken.

The reduction in police workforce results in:

- Give priority to classified high-risk security reports rather than fewer risk reports as per approved security plans in each security sector with determining the top responsibilities and assignments and how to deal with other lower priority assignments.
- Reconsider the types of calls that often required sending patrols or officers to prepare reports about the incident such as the cases of property damage, vehicle accidents, or others and using reports via phone or Internet.

This requires the following:

- Training forces and officials on performing alternative jobs as the patrollers can train on firefighting, rescue, ambulance operations; draw up reports in departments and police stations or doing administrative works as per the jurisdiction. Moreover, the employees who perform assistant jobs such as human resources or training sector may resort to performing the primary response tasks to security reports.
- Coordination between police, security, and law enforcement agencies within each geographical scope to provide services during health emergency periods through interoperability between such agencies.

In addition, business continuity factor requires the following:

- Strict enforce of the legislation regarding the resistance of safeguards and control measures, disturbing the medical practices, attack staffs at the medical facilities, intentional spreading of Coronavirus through an infectious person, exploitation of the epidemic for profiting from the medical consumables, producing or selling faked or crimes of poor quality medical products, disorders crimes by publishing rumors, crimes of using the epidemic as a cause to illegally collect or embezzle the donations or changing the usage of the donated assets without prior permission.
- Notifying the public with legal basis regarding imposing restrictions on public health, while keeping all measures symmetric with the type and the scope of the damage sought to be prevented, avoiding inordinate influence over the citizen's right and the rapporteur system.
- Working on explaining the health measures to encourage social cooperation, considering the public feelings during the epidemic, to avoid public dissatisfaction (Law Enforcement in the Time of the Coronavirus, China's Ministry of Justice, March 7, 2020).[5]
- Dissemination channels to submit complaints and reports concerning law enforcement activities and to prevent and control epidemics. Besides, appointing expert employees to review and respond immediately to any complaints or suggestions.

Second Factor: Protecting Personnel of Police, Security, and Law Enforcement Agencies from Health Risks Related to the Epidemic

The World Health Organization declared six states of emergency in the last twenty years: swine flu epidemic was declared in 2009, poliomyelitis epidemics was declared in 2014, Ebola in 2014, Zika virus in 2016, Ebola again in 2019, and now this is the sixth state that declared an unexpected epidemics known as coronavirus 2020 (WHO website, March 15, 2020).[6]

This repetition of the declaration of emergency state for a short period indicates the necessity of working on set up police, security, and law enforcement agencies upon any kind of emergency state on the public health, whether it was ordinary due to the prevalence of the diseases or an epidemic attack or biological terrorist.

This preparation will be delivered regularly through constituent and training courses, manuals, periodic instructions, and continuous monitoring of mechanisms of publishing the health awareness among the employees. As well as they should do regular checks annually. In the case of epidemic outbreaks, they should be checked monthly.

This preparation shall include the following:

- Implementation of an occupational health and safety program, through short courses and on-the-job courses.
- Basic knowledge about infectious diseases biology, patterns of infection transmission, disease interventions, basic precautionary measures, proper use of personal protective equipment, how to use antimicrobial gloves during close personal communications with the public, and methods of frequent hand washing and sterilization and disinfection strategies.
- Vaccination for common diseases and annual vaccination against influenza, vaccination with Smallpox, yellow fever, cholera, and typhoid fever vaccines, anthrax vaccine for people dealing with animals. Police, security, and law enforcement agencies may impose on the applicant to be vaccinated against infectious diseases (like measles, mumps, rubella, chickenpox, poliomyelitis, and diphtheria) before employment, as this condition is considered one of the important protective measures for the personnel of the police, security, and law enforcement agencies.
- In infectious diseases related to health emergency states, countries usually give priority to some groups that should benefit from vaccinations or obtaining health protective equipment. Medical service providers are often at the top of the list, then personnel in police, security, and law enforcement agencies.
- Force personnel of police, security, and law enforcement agencies to carry protective equipment. This equipment should be in bags or on the waist belt, which personnel wear. Protective equipment includes three main categories: manual contact protective equipment, protective equipment from body liquids, and respiratory system protective equipment.
- Establishing a mechanism for disposing of all personal protective equipment has been used, considering them as hazardous medical waste.
- Pay attention to effective protective measures in the workplace, developing a more flexible policy for having paid sick leave for employees, because a single infectious person, work for few hours, can transmit the disease to many other persons. For example: at the time of SARS, virus outbreak in Toronto, Canada, one infectious employee transferred the virus to forty-nine persons in one day. Consequently, they were unable to perform their job duties for

at least ten days. Similarly, each person infected with coronavirus will pass the infection to nearly five persons according to a medical analysis by the World Health Organization.

- Provide public places with thermal tracking devices whether in airports, Border ports, placing where crowdedness or they may be installed in places where the employees gather at the entry and exit gates.
- Paying special care to families of police, security, and law enforcement agencies for two reasons. The first one is due to direct contact of the personnel with his family, as if he or one of his family was infected; this will affect his job performance. The second one: the sick leave system or vaccination plans usually include employees without their families. Whereas effective control of epidemic diseases requires protective activity systems including all close contacts with the employee.

One of the best global practices in this field is the occupational health and safety program, Toronto Police Services, Canada. As it guarantees to receive all security and police officers and some civilian personnel training in the field of communicable disease risk management, as well as receiving the proper personal protective equipment (personal protective equipment). In addition, according to WHO analyses, each person infected with the Coronavirus will transmit the disease to approximately five people. Every patrol officer and some civilians who are subjected to these risks, like Prosecutorial Security Officers, court, prison officers, and staff who work in the forensic laboratories.

The officers have been obligated to carry protective equipment, which should always be in their bags or on the police's belt. This equipment includes the following: antimicrobial gloves, disinfected towels, salt solution, and unidirectional face mask. Improved, high-level equipment should be stored in officer's patrol boxes such as N95 masks, protective eyeglasses, washing hands without antiseptic, needle container, Tyvek covers or other similar materials, heavy rubber gloves, and storage bags designed for contaminated clothes (Occupational Health and Safety Program, Toronto Police Service, Canada, 2020).[7]

Identification of officers who need personal protective equipment was one of the lessons learned during epidemic times of severe acute respiratory syndrome (SARS) and other events like anthrax. Through the assessment of health risks, Toronto police services decided that there was a need for officers who can respond to natural or synthetic heath emergency states. So, officers have been trained and prepared for this preparation. They have been equipped with (SCBA), full cover and complete isolation, and biological containment crews. Officers have trained to identify, assess, and combat biological risks, reducing effects of biological hazards, which result from the emergency states through appropriate means. Like: (Containment, isolation, and decontamination) then investigation in the event including completing and collecting evidence then drawing up a model, this has been done in all Canada.

Third Factor: Protection of Society

It has been taken over many years, strategies of community policing and problem-solving police in many countries, as an essential component for law enforcement. As they facilitate community involvement and common ownership of initiatives and security programs oriented to society. They also provide opportunities to educate the society about the importance of law compliance (Mamdouh Abdelmottlep, Introduction to Police Sciences, 2019, Page 380).[8]

Adopting these strategies helps police, safety, and law enforcement agencies during cooperating with the population before contagious diseases outbreak. Whereas personnel of law enforcement and local community representatives may meet for an open dialogue to discuss plans and common interests. These strategies also help in motivating community public health officials to work as a team with law enforcement authorities.

It is important for police in societies that lack such strategies to work immediately on building bridges of cooperation with its community. These measures will largely enhance all its efforts of supporting and coordinating the effective response to emergency states of public health. In addition, society is involved in developing plans for combating contagious or epidemic diseases. These plans should include initiatives regarding methods related to guide people with a plan of police services in case of medical emergencies announcement. Particularly, in case of health isolation or medical quarantine cases. Effective and meaningful partnership with local community representatives has led to coordinated planning, exchanging information, and formal memorandum of understanding and mutual assistance agreements. These partnerships help all parties on determining challenges and abilities inside their institutions, developing and testing response plans and alternatives based on collecting knowledge and resources.

China has succeeded in dealing with Coronavirus 2020; it provides its successful experience to South Korea, Iran, and Italy. The Ministry of Justice in China issued a major document on law enforcement at the time of the Coronavirus outbreak. This document shall not only include the security and policing work, but also include maintaining the coordination between these multiagencies concerned for enforcement of the law.

Among the many important steps to facilitate law enforcement, there were three topics that merit attention. The first one: It focused on "courtesy" during law enforcement, noting that the public opinion and emotions may be variable during the epidemic. The second one: Focusing on using technology and online methods as possible. Finally, the necessity of searching in all related to combating the epidemic and the necessity of sustaining the work.

Collaborative work and information sharing ensure a clear understanding of roles and responsibilities and help security departments in meeting the expectation of other local responders. It also can predict effectively where their resources will be needed, potential deficiencies and type of activities that will be required according to the nature and location of the threat.

Therefore, that, partnerships between police, security, and law enforcement agencies and local community representatives in the governmental departments should focus on the following:

- Officials training.
- Educating and sensitizing the community on its role during public health emergencies and the basics of communicable disease prevention.
- Developing new methods of providing updated and consistent information for the public at the time of the emergency.
- A designated plans for the hospital of dealing with the overflow of patients and how to maintain medical and security systems at the same time in these health institutions.
- Setting mechanism of dealing with the numbers of death, particularly with many them.
- Emergency measures for schools, universities, hospitals, medical centers, and shopping centers.
- Setting mechanism of dealing with the expected violence cases when forcing isolation measures, medical quarantine, forced evictions, and in rare cases running on health materials and equipment.
- Finally, the effective cooperation between public health sectors with police, security, and law enforcement agencies requires using the same definition of the terms, so it should set common guidance for the terms related to medical emergencies.

The greatest challenge for police, security, and law enforcement agencies may be during volunteering house quarantine cases (stay at your home or your area). People will need to go shopping for food or medical care. Consequently, we should care about educating and outreaching the public for the necessity of maintaining social distance for their health and safety. This could be done by choosing a proper means for isolation.

Another problem that may face police, security, and law enforcement agencies, concerning dealing with the prisoners. The problem elements are the mutual infectious cases between the two parties, which work in the police, security, and prisoners. As well as preventing disease prevailing between prisoners particularly in large, number prisons.

At last, in cases of transporting prisoners, the suggested solutions go on between the following:

- Using single cells for isolating the infectious prisoners or using isolation blocks in case of disease outbreak.
- Reducing physical communication between prisons personnel and the prisoners through using audiovisual aids and surveillance cameras.

The model law of the emergence of health authorities shows another form of the community cooperation form. Center Dominant Cooperation (CDC) with

Center for Law and Public's Health, in Georgetown and Johns Hopkins universities in the USA and representatives from various national organizations for developing Model State Emergency Health Powers Act (MSEHPA). This Model Law aims to assist US government in reviewing emergency public health authorities to make sure that it was enough for facing disease fears and modern biological terrorism. The model law helps in determining the emergency state and the measures that may be executed. There is no guidance for how to execute these measures, rule, and safety of the public health during applying these measures (The Model Act, USA 2020).[9]

On other hand, the problem of illegal foreigners who may not respond to the control measures of combating the voluntary diseases shall consider, if they believe that it will cause them to the risks of identification and deportation, a big problem on carrying out the quarantine or broad travel restriction.

Another problem is restricting the movement of people involved in criminal and gang activities. It was unknown how they would collaborate with the voluntary restriction and quarantine.

One of the best practices in this regard is "Smarter Crowdsourcing," a program based on organizing a series of online lectures gathering people who have experience and appropriate knowledge and then reach to innovative and practical remedies to combat the virus. Instead of meeting a group of fixed and stable expertise, you can use the online programs to facilitate on the expertise to participate by their time, knowledge and consult each other to find a practical solution that will be useful and helpful to the governments, enhancing the links between government, private sector, and citizens.

The forums have discussed issues like gathering information, data management, control wastes, stagnant water, and assessment of public awareness. Smarter Crowdsourcing initiatives included governmental local sources and non-profit institutions, with a view of understanding public health problems relevant to the epidemic, including methods of notifying citizens without making them panic, Welfare and evacuate populations who are most vulnerable to the risks and management of high demand on health services. More than sixty-five experts have participated in discussions continued for two months on the internet, the governmental officials keep informed by the results. Crowdsourcing program has developed a platform for informing citizens and others for maps and remote sensing, setting up a network of expertise to encourage medical staff, which will help police, security and law enforcement agencies to face epidemic challenges practically and realistically.

Conclusions and Recommendations

International practices and discussion of available options for facing security challenges relevant to threats of epidemic outbreaks have shown the main missions those officials of police, security, and law enforcement agencies should take into consideration. The first mission is to: Maintain the sustainability of the security operation of police and security forces. The second mission is to: Protect police and security forces and their families. The last mission is related to: Maintaining the community security and achieving safety for every person.

Achieving these missions requires various police, security, and law enforcement agencies must be able to pass the legal jurisdictional limitations to access the sources and necessary aids to face infection outbreaks. The importance of controlling the contaminated areas quickly and providing proper personal protective equipment for personnel of the police and security agencies. This requires wide community cooperation and approval on the compliance to the orders of the quarantine and isolation, the necessity of community awareness of public health threats, and following the necessary measures for preventing the passing of the infectious diseases.

We should benefit from the modern technological means and the artificial intelligence, internet sites, social media means to remotely accomplish the work, follow up on rumor spreading, early show up of the infectious cases whether in the security services or during surveillance, the outreach of the awareness in the security services, distributing the protective and personal hygiene equipment in the workplaces, setting a sustainable health strategy for the staff of the police and security services and their families for maintaining of the medical fitness.

The return of the security forces services should be systematical, allowing facing the epidemic in the security services or in the community, providing the forces that deal directly with the public with equipment and protective equipment. Consider in redistribution the forces stationed in the camps as if emergency forces or Special Forces, as well as we should put a plane for isolating the infected people inside these agencies. Providing the isolated cells for facing the potential of an outbreak the infection inside the prisons. At last, we should coordinate with the concerned agencies to dedicate the areas and equipment that allow for set up cantonment camps if necessary.

Notes

1 WHO. (2020, Jan 30). Statement on the second meeting of the International Health Regulations (2005) Emergency Committee regarding the outbreak of novel coronavirus (2019-nCoV). Retrieved on March 15, 2020. https://www.who.int/news-room/detail/30-01-2020-statement-on-the-second-meeting-of-the-international-health-regulations-%282005%29-emergency-committee-regarding-the-outbreak-of-novel-coronavirus-%282019-ncov%29
2 Saudi Ministry of Health. (2020, March 19) Command and Control Center, Statistics March 19, 2020. Retrieved on March 25, 2020. From the site. https://www.moh.gov.sa/CCC/Pages/default.aspx
3 The Guardian (2020, March 18). Murder inquiries could be hit if coronavirus reduces UK police numbers. Retrieved on 21. April 2020. https://www.theguardian.com/world/2020/mar/03/inquiries-to-be-halted-if-coronavirus-hits-police-numbers
4 Richards, E. P. (2006). The role of law enforcement in public health emergencies: Special considerations for an all-hazards approach. US Department of Justice, Office of Justice Programs, Bureau of Justice Assistance.
5 China's Ministry of Justice. (2020, March 7). Law Enforcement in the Time of the Coronavirus. Retrieved on 03/04/2020 from the website https://www.chinalawtranslate.com/en/law-in-the-time-of-the-coronavirus/.

6 WHO. (2019). Coronavirus disease (COVID-19) pandemic. https://www.who
   .int/emergencies/diseases/novel-coronavirus-2019 Retrieved on 20/05/2020
7 Toronto Police Service Board. (2019). Occupational Health and Safety Program,
   Toronto Police Service, Canada. Retrieved on 04/06/2020 from https://bit.ly
   /3jkGifm
8 Mamdouh Abdelmottlep. (2019). Introduction to Police Sciences, Dar alnahda
   alarabia, Cairo, Egypt, Page 380.
9 Centers for Law and the Public's Health at Georgetown and Johns Hopkins
   Universities. The Model State Emergency Health Powers Act. http://www.pub-
   lichealthlaw.net/ModelLaws/MSEHPA.php. Accessed March 17, 2020.

References

Abdelmottlep, M. 2019. *Introduction to police sciences.* Dar alnahda alarabia, Cairo,
   Egypt.
Centers for Law and the Public's Health at Georgetown and Johns Hopkins
   Universities. 2020. The model state emergency health powers act. Retrieved on
   March 17, 2020, from http://www.publichealthlaw.net/ModelLaws/MSEHPA
   .php.
China's Ministry of Justice. 2020, March 7. Law enforcement in the time of the
   coronavirus. Retrieved on April 3, 2020, from https://www.chinalawtranslate
   .com/en/law-in-the-time-of-the-coronavirus/.
Richards, E. P. 2006. *The role of law enforcement in public health emergencies: Special
   considerations for an all-hazards approach.* US Department of Justice, Office of
   Justice Programs, Bureau of Justice Assistance.
Saudi Ministry of Health. 2020, March 19. Command and control center, statistics
   March 19, 2020. Retrieved on March 25, 2020, from https://www.moh.gov.sa/
   CCC/Pages/default.aspx
The Guardian. 2020. Murder inquiries could be hit if coronavirus reduces UK police
   numbers. Retrieved on April 21, 2020, from https://www.theguardian.com/
   world/2020/mar/03/inquiries-to-be-halted-if-coronavirus-hits-police-numbers
Toronto Police Service Board. 2019. Occupational health and safety program,
   Toronto police service, Canada. Retrieved on June 4, 2020, from https://bit.ly
   /3jkGifm
WHO. 2019. Coronavirus disease (COVID-19) pandemic. Retrieved on May 20,
   2020, from https://www.who.int/emergencies/diseases/novel-coronavirus
   -2019
WHO. 2020, January 30. Statement on the second meeting of the international
   health regulations (2005) emergency committee regarding the outbreak of novel
   coronavirus (2019–nCoV). Retrieved on March 15, 2020, from https://www
   .who.int/news-room/detail/30-01-2020-statement-on-the-second-meeting
   -of-the-international-health-regulations-%282005%29-emergency-committee
   -regarding-the-outbreak-of-novel-coronavirus-%282019-ncov%29

15 Preventing the Next Pandemic
Promoting the Planetary Health

Rohan Gunaratna

Introduction

Natural resources have been used and abused in ways that have profoundly affected our environment. Our health and well-being are negatively impacted both short term and long term as a consequence of human activity. We can see that "pollution from landscape fires and the combustion of fossil and solid fuels results in respiratory diseases and millions of deaths, mostly among young children."[1] Household air pollution from burning

> solid fuels (wood, charcoal, crop residues, dung, and sometimes coal) for cooking and energy caused an estimated 2.6 million to 4.4 million deaths in 2010, mainly in women and children. Pollution caused by landscape fires, mainly related to deforestation and land clearing for industry and agriculture, is estimated to cause more than 300,000 premature deaths worldwide annually.[2]

Overfishing, warming, and acidification of water bodies harm coral reefs and fish supplies, resulting in food insecurity, disease, and poverty. Fish is an essential source of protein and vitamins such as iron, zinc, and omega-3 fatty acids; in fact, approximately 2.9 billion people receive 20% of their annual protein from fish. Around 90% of monitored fisheries are harvested at, or beyond, maximum sustainable yield limits. "Poor fish supply in Ghana, caused in part by overfishing, has led to food insecurity and an increase in bushmeat consumption, which increases the chances for transmission of zoonotic diseases like HIV and Ebola."[3]

> Extreme weather events related to global environmental change are a significant cause of illness and death. Monsoon rains across Pakistan in 2010 resulted in catastrophic flash floods, submerging a fifth of the country. The floods killed more than 1,900 people and displaced millions, leading to the consumption of unsafe drinking water and an increase in the incidence of waterborne disease.[4]

In response to the extreme drought in Sao Paulo in 2015, residents turned to water hoarding, creating ideal breeding grounds for dengue-carrying mosquitos.

DOI: 10.4324/9781003291909-16

This situation led to a 163% increase in dengue cases compared to the same period in 2014.

> Carbon dioxide emissions caused by human activity are altering the nutritional content of key crops, including wheat, rice, barley, and soy. This puts hundreds of millions of people, mostly in Africa and South Asia, at risk for vitamin deficiencies. Reductions in zinc content of food crops could put an additional 150 million people at risk for zinc deficiency, a key micronutrient for maternal and child health.[5]

Planetary health concerns itself with a need for serious governance, posing a threat to the sustainability of our human civilization, environment, and planet. Specifically, it seeks to confront three areas of challenges: "imagination challenges," such as failing to account for long-term human or environmental consequences of human progress; "research and information challenges," such as underfunding and lack of scope in research; and "governance challenges," such as delayed environmental action by governing bodies determined by unwillingness, uncertainty, or non-cooperation.

A primary ethical focus of planetary health research is human cooperation and non-cooperation in the form of conflict, nationalism, and competition. As one goal, the Lancet Commission on Health and Climate Change plans to use an accountability mechanism to track human cooperation and study the link between health, climate, and political action.[6]

> Likewise, nutrition and diet are important contributors to and indicators of planetary health. Scientists speculate that human population growth threatens the carrying capacity of the planet. Diets, agriculture, and technology must adjust to sustain population projections upwards of 9 billion while reducing harmful consequences on the environment through food waste and carbon-intensive diets. A focus of planetary health research will be nutritional solutions that are sustainable for the human species and the environment, and the generation of scientific research and political will to create and implement desired solutions. In January 2019, an international commission created the planetary health diet.[7]

Planetary health aims to seek further solutions to global human and environmental sustainability through collaboration and research across many sectors including the energy, agriculture, water, and health industries.

> Biodiversity loss, exposure to pollutants, climate change, and fuel consumption are all issues that threaten human and climate health. A number of researchers believe humanity's destruction of biodiversity and the invasion of wild landscapes created the conditions for malaria and new diseases such as COVID-19.[8]

Global Interest

Planetary health is an expanding scientific field and a social movement. The quality of human life has been extended. Life expectancy increased by more than

20 years in the past half century, jumping from 47 years in 1950–1955 to 69 years in 2005–2010.[9]

The term gained traction when the Rockefeller Foundation–Lancet Commission published on planetary health a report titled "Safeguarding human health in the Anthropocene epoch."[10] This paper defined planetary health as "the health of human civilisation and the state of the natural systems on which it depends." The approach emphasized on "the importance of a holistic view of human health, which is intrinsically linked to healthy ecosystems. The fast-paced field of planetary health matters for many reasons."[11]

The intention is to solve crises by addressing the root causes of global threats instead of wasting large amounts of resources addressing emergencies.

> Planetary Health is about leaving the state of emergency to ensure that no one is left behind, also in the long run. In this context, the root causes of this pandemic have a lot to do with the way we conceive our development and imagine success.[12]
>
> By recognising the urgency of Planetary Health, leaders are giving a change to durable development policies. A new report Preventing the Next Pandemic: Zoonotic diseases and how to break the chain of transmission, launched by the United Nations Environment Programme (UNEP) and the International Livestock Research Institute (ILRI) on 6 July 2020 identifies seven trends driving the increasing emergence of zoonotic diseases, those which jump between animal and human populations, including increased demand for animal protein; a rise in intense and unsustainable farming; the increased use and exploitation of wildlife; and the climate crisis. This suggests that human health, climate and biodiversity crises are not disconnected.[13]

The health of the planet necessitates solutions that are inclusive. Vaccination cannot be the sole answer to this pandemic's lingering problems. We can't have a meaningful recovery until we address inequalities, which is both desired and essential as stated by the UNEP Executive Director Inger Andersen.[14]

Pandemics are devastating our lives and our economies, and as we have seen over the past months, it is the poorest and the most vulnerable who suffer the most. For example, domestic energy consumption has risen substantially during the coronavirus lockdown. But it is not uncommon to address solutions from this pandemic through the lenses of developed countries. In the Global South, there has been a lack of access to clean energy services for decades. Almost 80–90% of households in developing countries, especially in Sub-Saharan Africa, lack access to clean cooking energy services, and must rely on polluting fuels (biomass and fossil fuels) and inefficient technologies such as open fires to prepare their food. The 2019 Sustainable Development Goals report estimates that 3 billion people are dependent on inefficient and highly polluting cooking technologies and fuels. This results in millions of premature deaths every year, in addition to other social, economic, and environmental risks and burdens.[15]

COVID-19 Transmission

COVID-19 has led to positive, but most likely, short-lived effects on a few aspects of environmental health. Reduced air pollution from vehicle traffic and industries has temporarily cleared the skies over major cities. Wildlife has emerged in parks and urban areas in the absence of human presence. Greenhouse gas emissions dropped early in the pandemic, displaying what we could achieve with significant change. COVID-19 was most likely transmitted from animals to humans; therefore much-needed attention is being placed on the human relationship to wildlife, with a renewed focus on wildlife trade, biodiversity, and habitat encroachment. Although these indicators are encouraging, it will be long before nature is healed. Much work remains to reverse the current trajectory of planetary health properly. Unfortunately, COVID-19 has also had some observable negative impacts on the environment. Plastic use is at an all-time high, and stay-at-home orders have disrupted waste management systems. Funding for frontline conservation efforts has dried up as ecotourism has halted and public and private funding has slowed, leading to increased poaching in some areas. Similarly, environmental research that supports wildlife and habitat conservation, climate change mitigation, improved food systems, and environmental health has faced funding reductions and travel restrictions.[16]

Because we are still in the midst of the COVID-19 crisis, it is too soon to definitively determine whether COVID-19 has or will impact Earth's systems and, therefore, global climate change or biodiversity and ecosystem loss. The research and human capacity needed to conduct these rigorous assessments require time and resources, and it could be years before we have a comprehensive understanding. Ongoing shutdowns and funding reductions will likely slow the pace of these assessments. In the meantime, it will be imperative to make strategic progress toward desired environmental outcomes and to reverse some of the harmful effects on our environment by adopting a new normal during and after COVID-19.

The ongoing COVID-19 pandemic has emphasized the importance of understanding the evolution of natural hosts in response to viral pathogens. In the past few decades, animal-origin viral diseases, especially bats-linked, have increased many folds in humans; this is known as cross-species transmissions. Although many of the illnesses are linked with bats, information on their ecological behavior and molecular aspects is limited, which could lead to more viral outbreaks.

COVID-19 is one of the worst zoonotic diseases, but it is not the first. Ebola, SARS, MERS, HIV, Lyme disease, Rift Valley fever and Lassa fever preceded it. In the last century we have seen at least six major outbreaks of novel coronaviruses. Sixty per cent of known infectious diseases and 75 per cent of emerging infectious diseases are zoonotic. Over the last two decades and before COVID-19, zoonotic diseases caused economic damage of USD 100 billion.[17]

The majority of sick animals do not infect humans, but if they do, "cross-species infections or viral host jumps have the potential to spread to humans," resulting in catastrophic epidemics.[18] Diseases such as measles and smallpox were likely caused by animal domestication as early as 5500 BCE. Zoonotic diseases have since played a role in the spread of HIV, Ebola, severe acute respiratory syndrome (SARS)/Middle East respiratory syndrome (MERS), and H1N1 swine flu, among others. COVID-19 is thought to be caused by a coronavirus that originated in animals according to scientists. The animal source of SARS-CoV-2, the virus triggering the COVID-19 pandemic, hasn't been established yet. It most likely originated from a bat species.

SARS-CoV-2 has first been reported from pneumonia patients in Wuhan city in the Hubei Province of China. These patients were trading at a wet animal market in the Hunan area. It is believed that SARS-CoV-2 is introduced from the animal kingdom to human populations during November or December 2019, as revealed from the phylogeny of the genomic sequences from the initially reported cases. The spillover of SARS-CoV-2 from animals to humans occurred at the beginning of December 2019, and the clinical cases appeared around the end of December. Genetic analysis showed that this novel virus is closely related to bat coronaviruses (CoVs) and is similar to but distinct from the SARS virus. Among the many questions unanswered for the COVID-19 pandemic are the origin of SARS-CoV-2 and the potential role of intermediate animal hosts in early animal-to-human transmission.[19] Bats are presumed reservoirs of diverse coronaviruses (CoVs), including progenitors of severe acute respiratory syndrome (SARS) and SARS-CoV-2, the causative agent of COVID-19. However, the evolution and diversification of these coronaviruses remain poorly understood. Although bats are considered the most likely natural host for SARS-CoV-2, the virus's origins remain unclear. The rapid spread of COVID-19 followed the initial animal-to-human spillover through human-to-human transmission. Genetic epidemiology had revealed that the spread from the beginning of December, when the first cases were retrospectively traced in Wuhan, was mainly by a human-to-human transmission and not due to continued spillover. These species cross jumping, spillover, and rapid transmission events are linked to viral characteristics, host diversity, and environmental feasibility. Exponential population growth, globalization, and environmental destruction will continue to accelerate the animal-to-human spillover effect.

Response

Emerging viruses are nearly impossible to control after they reach a specific threshold of infections and/or transmission rate, such as after spreading in humans in metropolitan areas, where quarantine and/or treatment are unfeasible. As a result, coordinated strategic planning is crucial for rapid responses required to protect against emerging viruses soon after their development. We don't know which virus will emerge or about its pathogenic or transmission properties, so planning must be all-encompassing. National and international planning is essential, as is utilizing scientific and diagnostic tools and developing systems for swiftly communicating outbreak information and prevention measures.

Preemptive strategies must include improved surveillance targeted to areas with a high risk of disease outbreak, pathogen monitoring in reservoirs or early in outbreaks, broad-based study to clarify the key steps that lead to emergence as well as modified versions of traditional quarantine or other control measures.

Human disease surveillance clearly must be associated with enhanced longitudinal veterinary and wild-animal infection surveillance. Vaccine strategies could be used in some control programs, but the current rate of development and approval of human vaccines is too low to allow control of most newly emerging virus diseases. Existing vaccines can be used to control the emergence of known viruses when sufficient lead time is available, as might veterinary vaccines which can be developed relatively quickly and used to combat outbreaks, along with the culling or quarantine measures that are now often used. New and improved vaccine technologies include molecularly cloned attenuated viruses that can be rapidly changed into the appropriate antigenic forms with sufficient efficacy and a low-risk level for use in the face of some outbreaks. Antiviral drugs may be used where available, although cost, logistic problems, and side effects may make them more difficult to use in a large-scale outbreak. They would likely work only in the context of other control measures.

Prevention

Although zoonotic disease prevention approaches vary per pathogen, several practices are proven as beneficial in reducing risk at the community and individual levels. Regulations for animal care in the agricultural sector reduce the risk of outbreaks of food-borne zoonotic diseases from goods such as meat, eggs, dairy, and certain vegetables. Requirements for safe drinking water and waste removal, as well as environmental regulations for protected surface water, are equally vital. When zoonotic diseases first appear in the community, education programs emphasizing hand washing after contact with animals and other behavioral changes can help to limit their spread.[20]

The emergence of new viral diseases by animal-to-human host switching has been, and will likely continue to be, a major source of new human infectious diseases. A better understanding of the many complex variables underlying such emergencies is of utmost importance to public health.[21]

Communication

Outbreaks like Nipah (1999), SARS (2003), H5N1 (2004), H1N1 (2009), MERS (2011), Ebola (2014), and Zika (2015) were all telltale signs that a new infectious illness might very well emerge and spread globally. However, there were no mechanisms in place to facilitate a global reaction to COVID-19.[22] Leaders have struggled to deal with COVID-19 as a community throughout the present pandemic. Pandemics do not adhere to national boundaries in a globalized world. Therefore, nations need to collaborate. While efforts are essential at the local, national, and regional levels to strengthen readiness, a set of actions are best coordinated globally.

> There is strong consensus in three recent reports – The Independent Panel for Pandemic Preparedness and Response (IPPPR), G20 High Level Independent Panel on Financing the Global Commons for Pandemic Preparedness and Response (HLIP), and the Pan-European Commission on Health and Sustainable Development (Pan-European Commission) – that new structures are needed to bring together political leaders to end this pandemic and prevent the next.[23]

"Therefore, a new Global Health Threats Council or Board should work with existing groups like the World Health Organization, the Global Fund, Gavi, CEPI, and not duplicate their work or activities." Governments of lower and middle-income nations must play an important role in any new structures to offer their experience and expertise in managing epidemics. The globe needs to move quickly, not be in a state of paralysis. Additionally, more funding is required to implement these adjustments.[24]

Funding

Since the COVID-19 pandemic started, a significantly increased investment in research, manufacturing, and distribution of COVID-19 tests, treatments, and vaccines has occurred. However, we have not seen the same increase in research and development (R&D) for diseases that may become the next pandemic.[25] Fighting the COVID-19 pandemic does not lower the chances of another health threat. The health and economic benefit of investing now and for future pandemic diseases has never been clearer. But major gaps in the world's capabilities continue, "such as in globally networked surveillance and research to prevent and detect emerging or escalating infectious diseases."[26]

> The mechanisms to mobilise global funding for these crucial tools are limited, leaving every country in our interconnected world vulnerable. We need governments to build collective financing mechanisms to transform the world's ability to prepare for and respond to pandemic threat.[27]

> Governments' contributions to new financing mechanisms, such as the US government established fund for Global Health Security and pandemic preparedness, must be in proportion to their ability to pay, this money must be in addition to overseas development assistance so it does not compete with other critical health and development priorities.[28]

Research and Development

At the start of the COVID-19 pandemic, little was known about the virus.[29] We struggled to diagnose, treat, and prevent the virus. Scientists therefore built on existing research on other coronaviruses, such as vaccines for MERS and new mRNA technology. Therefore, multiple vaccines were developed, approved, and manufactured faster than ever. We may not be so lucky next time.[30]

> Consider our response to Ebola, where failures to continue key research areas between outbreaks led to a delay in the development of usable diagnostics, treatments, and vaccines when the next outbreak hit. We must be prepared for all possible scenarios and that means more investment into R&D.[31]

We need a system that leads and supports collaborative R&D programs to deliver a full range of countermeasures, such as diagnostics, therapeutics, and vaccines, available to respond to a pandemic.[32] It will need to work with industries and global health organizations and have equitable access to its products. This can only be successful if leaders commit to transparency and openness in sharing the information they collect with foreign countries.[33]

Manufacturing

The world has witnessed what occurs when vaccinations and medications are developed in a limited number of countries during the COVID-19 pandemic. The worldwide supply is bought up by high-income nations, having left the virus to flourish everywhere else. The availability of these resources is a matter of both supply and delivery. The world necessitates a need to expand manufacturing capacity regionally. More individuals will have access to medicines and immunizations due to this. While attempts to expand production capacity may take many months to significantly affect COVID-19 vaccine supplies, developing regional manufacturing capacity will have long-term advantages for future pandemics throughout the world while also ensuring local demands are covered.

Surveillance

Globally, we did not have the right infrastructure to respond to COVID-19, so the initial spill led to an international outbreak. To prevent pandemics, we need to invest in three areas: surveillance, manufacturing, and coordinated research and development.

Finding new pathogens quickly is critical to containing them. There are too many global "dark spots" where new viruses cannot be identified – but building locally-owned, internationally-connected genomic surveillance networks will ensure we can spot potential dangers before they become a global problem. This network must work with local communities and be used between outbreaks to tackle other infectious diseases and urgent global threats. With sustainable, long-term investment, this network can inform powerful regional and international responses to all infectious diseases rapidly and efficiently.[34]

Planetary Consequences due to COVID-19

The science of planetary health contends that ecological systems impact human health, as seen by the vulnerabilities of impoverished communities, whose lack of power or control over their environment has put them in the greatest danger during this epidemic.

To slow the spread of the virus, schools were closed across the world. One year into the pandemic, almost half of the world's students were affected by school closures.

> Millions of girls in some countries might not be going back at all, putting them at risk of adolescent pregnancy, child marriage and violence. Businesses closed too, leading to the equivalent of 255 million full-time jobs lost, in terms of working hours, in 2020. Among the worst hit are workers in the informal economy, young people and women. Any economic recovery will likely be uneven, leading to greater inequality in the coming years.[35]

Millions of people have already fallen below the poverty line. In just a few months of COVID-19, extreme poverty went up for the first time in 20 years.[36]

Food

Large-scale and coordinated initiatives to fundamentally change the global food system have been hampered by the lack of globally defined scientific targets for healthy diets and sustainable food production. The EAT-Lancet Commission has set scientific targets proposing the increasing consumption of plant-based foods such as seeds, nuts, vegetables, fruits, and whole grains while restricting animal-source foods to make the necessary transition. These targets can be met by making healthy foods more affordable and available rather than unhealthy foods, enhancing the marketing of healthier foods, investing in sustainability education, employing healthcare services to provide dietary recommendations and treatments, and applying food-based dietary guidelines.

Transport

The importance of transportation in society and the economy cannot be overstated. For residents' quality of life and the earth's health, an efficient and accessible transportation infrastructure is critical. However, this industry continues to be one of the most significant environmental impacts we face. Decarbonizing the transportation sector by switching from gasoline to electric and hydrogen vehicles has the potential to significantly impact individuals' health. Research conducted by Mark Jacobson and colleagues at Stanford University showcases if all of the vehicles in the United States were powered by hydrogen fuel cells instead of fossil fuels, the drop in pollutants that cause asthma, respiratory problems, and other potentially life-threatening conditions would reduce deaths by up to 6,000 per year.[37] According to research published by the European Energy Agency, an electric automobile's electricity generation reduces carbon emissions by 17–30% compared to a petrol or diesel car. When low-carbon electricity is used, the emissions from electricity generation are greatly reduced.[38]

Energy

Improved air quality, better housing, healthier diets, and increased physical activity are all benefits of well-designed efforts to minimize emissions from fossil-fuel sources. Lowering fossil-fuel consumption to a level that keeps rising global temperatures to 1.5°C rather than 2°C may result in more than 100 million fewer premature deaths in the 21st century owing to improved air quality, with roughly 40% of the benefit coming in the next four decades. Depending on estimates, the expected benefits of these prevented deaths might cover a considerable percentage or all of the original mitigation expenses.

Awareness

Researchers can tackle, and funders can assist in creating interdisciplinary work further to develop evidence on the health effects of environmental change. Accessing the efficacy of national, global, and local policies reduces environmental damage and improves health, thus improving risk communication with governments and the public. Health professionals can assist in educating communities on the health effects of global environmental changes and advocate for policies that integrate health and environmental health at the primary level.

Multilaterals within the United Nations system can help define metrics to monitor planetary health, updating their use of integrated environmental and health assessment methodologies, and advocating for global and national reforms of tax, subsidy, and trade policies that support planetary health. Governments can best serve their constituents by enacting evidence-based policies throughout society that will promote human health and longevity whilst maintaining and preserving the environment allowing us to thrive. The business community can demonstrate leadership by improving and incorporating sustainability practices, and advocating for reforms throughout the global economy. "Civil society organisations can help by developing a broad public movement for social change, ultimately pressuring decision makers to implement needed policies and sustainable practices."[39]

Conclusion

With the increasing numbers and global spread of COVID-19, a need for global efforts relies greatly on the investigations executed at infection sites to trace different aspects of this virus outbreak. The one critical factor that must be researched is the origin of COVID-19 virus and the potential future of infectious diseases. Small sections of evidence revealed many cross-species jumping or spillovers from animals to humans may have caused these zoonotic coronaviruses. Detailed sero-logical investigation of all domestic and wild animals in proximity to humans is of utmost necessity to know and prevent the likely spillover of many other bat-related CoVs in the future. Rapid detection of spillovers above will only be possible by an effective and robust surveillance system for circulating viruses with high zoonotic potential in animals. The COVID-19 pandemic has provided a graphic demonstra-tion of the costs of a global health emergency. The research reinforced that climate change and its contributors, like fossil-fuel use and the global food system, have severe long-term complications on human health. As a result, some well-designed actions have been taken to mitigate and adapt to climate change, reducing mul-tiple adverse impacts on people's health. This can be done better if more people address inequities. "Science can assist policy-makers and individuals identify benefi-cial actions, trade-offs and priorities, from measures to improve air quality to more climate-friendly behaviours such as healthy and more sustainable dietary choices."[40]

Although a large-scale global disruption has occurred due to COVID-19, this has not only negatively affected the social, economic, and environmental domains of sustainable development. It has also created new opportunities for building a sustainable future, pertaining to growing concerns about climate change, biodiversity loss, and other challenges. All opportunities for trans-formative change must be urgently harnessed to improve human and planetary health.[41]

Such change requires going beyond building back better by nesting the economic domain of sustainable development within social and environmental domains, thereby challenging conventional economic thinking by viewing eco-nomic development not as an end goal, but as a means to improve the health and well-being of people and the planet. Recovery from the COVID-19 pandemic should focus on the ability to contain the disease. It is symbolic of the commit-ment and courage to challenge the status quo, envision what it means to thrive as people and planet, and go beyond building back better to deliver the future that humankind wants and needs.[42]

While the scale of the problems that global environmental changes pose to humans and our planet is immense, public health professionals are equipped with the skills, experience, and commitment to maintaining life support systems within planetary boundaries to allow humanity to thrive.

Systems thinking is critical for understanding how anthropogenic activities affect human and ecological environment health. When examining the effects of policies, using a systems-wide perspective encourages the evaluation of unin-tended repercussions at various geographical and temporal dimensions. It is criti-cal to organize information about the effects of human activities on health and natural systems, as well as to include various views, to ensure that policies are proposed in the proper situation.

Since the genesis of planetary health as a field, it has shaped two major pol-icy recommendations: adapting a food system that promotes plant-based diets, and reconstructing cities to reduce negative environmental consequences, whilst improving the health of surrounding people.

This will help mitigate humanity's impact on the planet while sustaining health gains made over the past century. We need to rely on more complex analytic approaches, informed by interdisciplinary collaboration between environmental, health, and behavioral scientists, that capture the dynamic relationships between human activities, human health, environmental change, and environmental degradation. Many more human and natural systems co-benefits remain to be identified. Public health professionals are well positioned to lead this effort and, must do so to preserve the health and longevity of the public and our planet.

The single biggest force on earth is nature. Despite advances in science and technology, human beings cannot effectively counter natural disasters and catastrophes such as hurricanes, tornadoes, epidemics, and pandemics. Just like human beings, the planet Earth is a living being. The planet Earth needs to be constantly nurtured and cared for to ensure its health and productivity. The constant and continuous abuse of our planet will result in far-reaching consequences and shocks like global warming and pandemics. When the threat reaches a threshold, like the outbreak of COVID-19, the scale, magnitude, and intensity of human activity depreciate, creating the opportunity for the planet Earth to recuperate and rejuvenate.

Governments worldwide should work together to protect the planet to ensure its health and well-being. During COVID-19, positive impacts on our planet were registered. Air quality improved as people mostly stayed indoors. Worldwide, biodiversity flourished and was protected from human interference. Rivers and lakes were restored. Air quality improved as people mostly stayed indoors. The world's most populous nation, China's "emissions of harmful gases and other pollutants dropped 25% at the start of the year 2020 and the quality of air improved up to 11.4% with respect to the start of the last year, in 337 cities across China."[43]

Far-reaching policies protecting and respecting the planet are vital for the future sustainability of the planet Earth.

The single most important lesson we can learn from the COVID-19 outbreak is to make the planet Earth's sustainability the norm.[44]

Notes

1 Panorama Perspectives: Conversations on Planetary Health, 2017. Planetary health 101: Information and resources report I. https://www.rockefellerfoun dation.org/wp-content/uploads/Planetary-Health-101-Information-and -Resources.pdf.
2 Ibid.
3 Ibid.
4 Ibid.
5 Ibid.
6 NCBI, 2020. ARS-CoV-2 jumping the species barrier: Zoonotic lessons from SARS, MERS and recent advances to combat this pandemic virus. https://www .ncbi.nlm.nih.gov/pmc/articles/PMC7396141/; Horton, Richard; Lo, Selina,

2015. Planetary health: A new science for exceptional action. *The Lancet* 386 (10007): 1921–1922. https://doi.org.10.1016/s0140-6736(15)61038-8.

7 Demaio, Alessandro R; Rockström, Johan, 2015. Human and planetary health: Towards a common language. *The Lancet* 386 (10007): e36–e37. https://doi .org/10.1016/s0140-6736(15)61044-3.

8 The Guardian, 2020. 'Tip of the iceberg': Is our destruction of nature responsible for COVID-19? *The Guardian*. https://www.theguardian.com/environment /2020/mar/18/tip-of-the-iceberg-is-our-destruction-of-nature-responsible-for -COVID-19-aoe.

9 Danzhen You et al., 2014. *Levels and trends in child mortality.* New York: United Nations, Inter-Agency Group for Child Mortality Estimation. HYPERLINK "https://childmortality.org/wp-content/uploads/2014/10/Levels-and -Trends-in-Child-Mortality-Report-2014.pdf" https://childmortality.org/wp -content/uploads/2014/10/Levels-and-Trends-in-Child-Mortality-Report -2014.pdf.

10 Sarah Whitmee et al., 2015. Safeguarding human health in the anthropocene epoch: Report of The Rockefeller Foundation–*Lancet* Commission on planetary health. *The Lancet* 386 (10007): 1973–2028.

11 Why Planetary Health can promote a more inclusive and durable pandemic recovery. https://www.csc-blog.org/en/why-planetary-health-can-promote-more -inclusive-and-durable-pandemic-recovery

12 Ibid.

13 Ibid.

14 Pedro Olinto et al., 2013. The state of the poor: Where are the poor, where is extreme poverty harder to end, and what is the current profile of the world's poor? *Economic Premise*, no. 125. https://reliefweb.int/report/world/state-poor-where-are-poor -where-extreme-poverty-harder-end-and-what-current-profile.

15 Ibid.

16 Milken Institute, 2020. Center for strategic philanthropy: A turning point for planetary health by Dr. Matthew Lurie (PhD). https://milkeninstitute.org/sites/default /files/reports-pdf/MI_Environment%20Report_R6%20%282%29_0.pdf.

17 Preventing the next pandemic: Zoonotic diseases and how to break the chain of transmission. UNEP. https://www.unep.org/news-and-stories/statements/pre -venting-next-pandemic-zoonotic-diseases-and-how-break-chain.

18 United Nations Secretariat, 2013. Department of economic and social affairs, population division. World population prospects: The 2012 revision, working paper no. ESA/P/WP.228. New York: United Nations. https://population.un .org/wpp/Publications/Files/ WPP2012_HIGHLIGHTS.pdf.

19 Evidence for SARS-CoV-2-related coronaviruses circulating in bats and pango-lins in Southeast Asia. *Nature*. https://www.nature.com/articles/s41467-021 -21240-1.

20 Zoonoses, 2020. Prevention and control. World Health Organization. https:// www.who.int/news-room/fact-sheets/detail/zoonoses.

21 WSV 2019: The First Committee Meeting of the World Society for Virology. SpringerLink. https://link.springer.com/article/10.1007/s12250-019-00189-y.

22 How to prevent another major pandemic. Wellcome. https://wellcome.org/ news/how-prevent-another-major-pandemic.

23 How to prevent another major pandemic | Wellcome. https://wellcome.org/ news/how-prevent-another-major-pandemic.

24 Ibid.

25 Opinion: Physician shortage underlines need for residency programs. https:// www.freep.com/story/opinion/contributors/2022/05/20/opinion-physician -shortage-residency-programs/9844427002/.

26 How to prevent another major pandemic | Wellcome. https://wellcome.org/news/how-prevent-another-major-pandemic.

27 Ibid.

28 Ibid.

29 Contactless payments and what they mean for healthcare. Rectangle Health. https://www.rectanglehealth.com/blog/contactless-payments-and-what-they-mean-for-healthcare/.

30 Opinion | Mark Meadows's PowerPoint plotters were crackpots. We may not be so lucky next time. https://www.washingtonpost.com/opinions/2021/12/13/mark-meadows-powerpoint-coup-plot-trump-crackpot/.

31 How to prevent another major pandemic. Wellcome. https://wellcome.org/news/how-prevent-another-major-pandemic.

32 How to prevent another major pandemic. Medical Xpress. https://medicalxpress.com/news/2021-12-major-pandemic.html.

33 How to prevent another major pandemic | Wellcome. https://wellcome.org/news/how-prevent-another-major-pandemic.

34 Ibid.

35 Examining the social and economic impacts of COVID-19. https://givingcompass.org/article/examining-the-social-and-economic-impacts-of-covid-19.

36 The Covid-19 effects on societies and economies. Wellcome. https://wellcome.org/news/equality-global-poverty-how-covid-19-affecting-societies-and-economies.

37 Hydrogen cars will save lives, 2005. Retrieved on May 2021 from https://www.nature.com/news/2005/050620/full/news050620-12.html.

38 EDF Energy, 2021. Benefits of electric cars on the environment. https://www.edfenergy.com/for-home/energywise/electric-cars-and-environment.

39 RSIS, 2020. Planetary health: A more resilient world post-COVID-19. rsis.edu.sg/rsis-publication/nts/planetary-health-a-more-resilient-world-post-COVID-19/?doing_wp_cron=1645411606.8603830337524414062500#.YhL9GJNBxJU.

40 The Royal Society, 2020. Retrieved on April 19, 2021, from https://royalsociety.org/-/media/policy/projects/climate-change-science-solutions/climate-science-solutions- health.pdf.

41 Beyond building back better: Imagining a future for human and planetary health. https://www.thelancet.com/action/showPdf? pii=S2542-5196%2821%2900262-X.

42 Ibid.

43 Khan, I.; Shah, D.; Shah, S.S., 2021. COVID-19 pandemic and its positive impacts on environment: An updated review. *International Journal of Environmental Science and Technology* 18 (2021): 521–530. https://doi.org/10.1007/s13762-020-03021-3.

44 For their research assistance, I wish to thank Inuri Hettithanthirige Tennakoon of the International Law College (Faculty of Laws), Panthéon-Sorbonne and Queen Mary School of Law, University of London and Kavindhya Wickramasinghe from the Faculty of Law, General Sir John Kotelawala Defence University, Sri Lanka.

Index

For Product Safety Concerns and Information please contact our EU
representative GPSR@taylorandfrancis.com
Taylor & Francis Verlag GmbH, Kaufingerstraße 24, 80331 München, Germany

* 9 7 8 1 0 3 2 2 7 2 2 4 5 *